Prentice Hall Health

review manual

for the EMT-Paramedic
Self-Assessment Exam Prep

Third Edition

Richard A. Cherry, MS, NREMT-P
Clinical Assistant Professor
Department of Emergency Medicine
SUNY Upstate Medical University
Syracuse, New York

Joseph J. Mistovich, M. Ed., NREMT-P
Chairperson and Professor
Department of Health Professions
Youngstown State University
Youngstown, Ohio

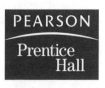

PEARSON

Prentice
Hall

Upper Saddle River, New Jersey 07458

Library of Congress Cataloging-in-Publication Data

Cherry, Richard A.
Prentice Hall Health review manual for the emt-paramedic self-assessment exam prep/
    Richard Cherry, Joseph Mistovich–3rd ed.
p. ; cm.
Rev. ed. of: Paramedic emergency care exam review/Richard A. Cherry.
2nd ed. c1997
Includes index.
ISBN 0-13-112869-8 (alk. paper)
1. Medical emergencies—Examinations, questions, etc. 2. Emergency
    medical personnel—Examinations, questions, etc.
[DNLM: 1. Emergency Medical Services—Examination Questions. 2. Emergency Medical
    Technicians–Examination Questions. WX 18.2 C522p 2004] I. Title: Review manual for the paramedic
    emergency care exam review. II. Cherry, Richard A. III. Mistovich, Joseph J. Paramedic emergency
    care exam review. IV. Title.
RC86.9C44 2004
616.02'5'076—dc22

2003015517

Publisher: Julie Levin Alexander
Publisher's Assistant: Regina Bruno
Executive Editor: Marlene McHugh Pratt
Assistant Editor: Monica Silva
Senior Managing Editor: Lois Berlowitz
Director of Production and Manufacturing: Bruce Johnson
Managing Production Editor: Patrick Walsh
Manufacturing Manager: Ilene Sanford
Manufacturing Buyer: Pat Brown
Production Liaison: Jeanne Molenaar
Production Editor: Emily Bush, Carlisle Communications, Ltd.
Design Director: Cheryl Asherman
Design Coordinator: Maria Guglielmo-Walsh
Cover and Interior Design: Janice Bielawa
Senior Marketing Manager: Katrin Beacom
Channels Marketing Manager: Rachele Strober
Composition: Carlisle Communications, Ltd.
Printing and Binding: Courier Westford
Cover Printer: Phoenix Color

Notice: The authors and the publisher of this book have taken care to make certain that the information given is correct and compatible with the standards generally accepted at the time of publication. Nevertheless, as new information becomes available, changes in treatment and in the use of equipment and procedures become necessary. The reader is advised to carefully consult the instruction and information material included in each piece of equipment or device before administration. Students are warned that the use of any techniques must be authorized by their medical adviser, where appropriate, in accord with local laws and regulations. The publisher disclaims any liability, loss, injury, or damage incurred as a consequence, directly or indirectly, of the use and application of any of the contents of this book.

Pearson Education LTD.
Pearson Education Singapore, Pte. Ltd
Pearson Education, Canada, Ltd
Pearson Education—Japan

Pearson Education Australia PTY, Limited
Pearson Education North Asia Ltd
Pearson Educación de Mexico, S.A. de C.V.
Pearson Education Malaysia, Pte. Ltd

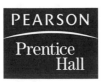

10 9 8 7 6 5 4 3 2
0-13-112869-8

Dedication

To my old guitar buddy, Mike Gambino,
who helped me change my life.

R.A.C.

In memory of my father, who provided me with the love and encouragement that allowed me to pursue my dreams. He will always be my inspiration to continue living life to its fullest, no matter what obstacles I encounter. To my beautiful wife Andrea, who continues to be my greatest supporter and my best friend. To my wonderful children, Katie, Kristyn, Chelsea, Morgan, and Kara for helping me get through another project. Your energy, hugs, kisses, and smiles make every day so much brighter! I love you all dearly.

J.J.M.

Contents

To the student. . .

This book is designed to help you prepare both for your certification exams and for the streets. I have provided for you a variety of questions covering every chapter of *Paramedic Care: Principles & Practice, Essentials of Paramedic Care,* and the USDOT Paramedic Curriculum. The questions test your knowledge, your understanding, and your ability to apply your knowledge in emergency medical scenarios. These scenarios are designed to help you develop the judgment necessary to solve real medical problems of real people. I have also provided the correct answer to each question, the rationale for the answer, and the page numbers from *Paramedic Care: Principles & Practice* (PCPP) and *Essentials of Paramedic Care* (EPC) where you will find more detailed explanation. The final ingredient is desire, which you must provide.

The great American poet Henry David Thoreau once wrote, "If one advances confidently in the direction of his dreams and endeavors to live the life which he has imagined, he will meet with a success unexpected in common hours." *Kaizen* is a Japanese word that means making a lifelong commitment to self-improvement. This Oriental philosophy encourages life satisfaction through continual personal and professional growth. It is a never-ending process of making small, incremental improvements in your life. If there were ever a group of people who should adopt the *kaizen* philosophy in their lives, it's EMS providers. Turning your professional life into an endless quest for perfection brings with it a measure of success. It is the journey—not the goal—that enriches our lives. It's like taking a cruise. The object is not to get to your destination as quickly as possible but to have fun getting there. Likewise, success is not a destination but a journey. When you make this commitment, you begin to reap the rewards immediately. The moment you set sail on this course, you and your future patients benefit from your increased commitment. Providing emergency medical care is a tremendous privilege. With this privilege comes responsibility to do your very best academic work. Think about how much patient care you will affect. Think about how many people's lives you will influence. Do so and you should begin to realize the tremendous responsibility you accept when you bear the title of paramedic.

The formula is simple. Turn your weaknesses into your strengths. The first step is to identify your weak areas. This step is difficult but critical. It's not easy because you must admit that you're not doing the job you could be doing. It's much easier to become complacent about your abilities. It's much easier to become comfortable with your present performance and accept your limitations as such. The consequences of this kind of attitude, however, are alarming. Patients suffer from your lack of knowledge and skill. Use this book of questions to identify your weak areas.

Once you have identified your weaknesses, make the personal commitment to improve in those areas. World-class athletes measure improvements by fractions of seconds and inches. They work tirelessly on making tiny improvements in the many aspects of their sport. They call it their personal best. You can achieve your personal best each year by making small, incremental improvements in the needed areas. By improving just one aspect of your craft each year, you make great strides. The short-term results are immediate—you enjoy EMS more because you are becoming better at it. We all enjoy doing the things that we do well. The long-term result is a rewarding career caring for those who are sick or injured.

Former Green Bay Packers football coach Vince Lombardi best described this attitude when he wrote, "Making the effort to be perfect is what life is all about. If you will not settle for anything less than the best, you will be amazed at what you can do with your lives. Winning isn't everything, but making the effort to win is. The difference between a successful person and an unsuccessful one is not a lack of knowledge, or a lack of strength, but a lack of will."

Remember, this is a lifetime journey. Don't try to do it all by Friday, but never give up your quest. You build a successful life one day at a time. Someone once asked former Miami Dolphins football coach Don Shula if it wasn't a waste of time trying to correct such a small flaw in his team's offense. Don's reply was "What's a small flaw?" That's striving for perfection. That's a commitment to excellence. That's *kaizen*. It's no wonder that his 1972 squad is still the only team ever to complete a perfect season. It's also no wonder that he still is the winningest coach in professional football history.

Why make learning a lifelong endeavor? American humorist Will Rogers once said, "Even if you are on the right track, you'll get run over if you just stand there." He was right. I don't believe in the status quo. Either you're getting better or you're getting worse. It's like walking up a down escalator. If you keep moving forward, you'll eventually end on top. You will at least stay in place. Once you slow down or stop, however, you begin to move downward until you eventually reach the bottom. A paramedic who fails to keep pace with the fast-moving world of emergency medicine soon becomes obsolete, even dangerous. This book is designed to help you maintain a high level of paramedic knowledge.

The road to excellence is not easy. It's easier to take the path of least resistance. It's easier to back away from excellence than it is to give everything you've got. While it's easier to let frustrations, distractions, and fatigue erode your performance, it's not satisfying in the long run. Making this commitment takes a tremendous amount of courage. If you fail, there are no excuses. You can look at yourself in the mirror and know that you gave it your very best. In that effort, you have not failed. When your paramedic career is over, you want to look back with no regrets.

Do you want to be great? Many talk the talk; few walk the walk. Many want to be great, but few are willing to pay the price. What is average? According to Notre Dame football coach Lou Holtz, "It's the best of the worst or the worst of the best. It's the top of the bottom or the bottom of the top. It's nowhere." Challenge yourself to make a commitment to excellence. If you believe in yourself, you can be as great as you want to be. You must have the courage, the determination, the dedication, and the competetive drive to do it. You must be willing to sacrifice the little things in life and pay the price for the things that are worthwhile. If you can do all these things, great things can happen.

Once you have made a commitment to a way of life, you put the greatest strength in the world behind you. We call it heart. Once you have made this commitment, nothing will stop you short of success. You have to want to. You have to have a raging desire to be the best you can be. It's not a part-time thing. Athletes call it competitive anger, and many use this motivational factor to spur them on to greatness. There have been few successful people who didn't have competitive anger driving their talents to the surface. Hall of Fame baseball player Ted Williams once said, "I wanted to be the greatest hitter who ever lived. A man has to have goals—for a day, for a lifetime—and that was mine, to have people say, 'There goes Ted Williams, the greatest hitter who ever lived.'" He was the greatest hitter because he made an unwavering commitment to excellence.

To succeed, you don't have to be the most experienced or the most talented, just the most tenacious. You must hold onto your goals and dreams. Your rewards for making a commitment to excellence cannot be measured financially. You will have the feeling of confidence and self-worth that comes from having accomplished something for yourself. This feeling will transfer into other areas of your life in more ways than you can ever imagine.

The essence of *kaizen* is adopting a positive attitude about everything you do. According to this philosophy, attitude is the most important thing you can develop in your life. While ability determines capability, attitude determines performance. You were born with certain abilities. Your attitude determines how close you come to realizing your full potential. Don't dwell on your shortcomings and limitations. Try to work around them. My father used to tell me that things turn out the best for those who make the best out of the way things turn out. Turn your weaknesses into strengths. Then measure yourself not by what you have done but by what you have done with your ability.

You don't have to be a sports fan to appreciate the tremendous difference a positive attitude makes. Victory doesn't always go to the strongest or fastest but to the one who wants it more. A positive attitude means believing in miracles. In sports, there are countless stories of people who overcame overwhelming odds to achieve their personal best. These people conceived the inconceivable, and then did it. When we hear of these triumphs, our usual response is "Unbelievable!"

With the proper attitude, you can do great things. Penn State football coach Joe Paterno describes this phenomenon: "The power of concentrating your brain, your whole body, your whole nervous system, your adrenaline, all your will on a single goal is an almost unbeatable concentration of force." David may have understood this before he went up against Goliath. After watching the 1980 United States hockey team win the Olympic gold medal in Lake Placid, I know I do. Anything is possible.

A positive attitude means making the best of your abilities. Pete Rose was not born with great strength, size, or speed. His natural talents were few. His most important talent was his attitude. No one got more out of himself on a baseball diamond than Pete Rose. As Pulitzer Prize–winning sports columnist Jim Murray wrote, "God made Babe Ruth and Mickey Mantle baseball players. Pete Rose made Pete Rose one."

A competitor finds a way to win. Competitors take bad breaks and use them to drive themselves just that much harder. Quitters take bad breaks and use them as reasons to give up. It's all a matter of pride. You'll never know what you can do unless you try. Life is short. Try as hard as you can. You owe it to your future patients and especially to yourself.

A positive attitude means adopting the work ethic. The only place success comes before work, hard work, is in the dictionary. Athletics teach the self-discipline of hard work and sacrifice necessary to reach a goal. Nowadays, too many people are looking for a shortcut. They want a free ride, a handout. For athletes, this shouldn't be true because they know what it takes. There are no shortcuts to success. Just the blood, sweat, and tears that produce results. Life resembles athletics. You must work hard to achieve anything. It's like the bank. Unless you make a deposit, you cannot make a withdrawal.

Some people say that good things happen to those who wait. I say that great things happen to those who work. American poet Robert Frost once wrote, "The world is full of willing people, some willing to work, others willing to let them." Boy, was he right. Don't spend your professional life on the sidelines watching others achieve greatness. Do it yourself. Make the effort to work *harder* to overcome your weaknesses.

A positive attitude means never becoming complacent and satisfied with the job you do. Always try to do it better. Develop an insatiable appetite for perfection. Like the author who writes a best-seller and wants to create another one. Like the painter who creates a masterpiece and wants to paint another one. Like the lawyer who wins the most prominent case in the nation and wants to win another one. It doesn't mean they have to do it. The great ones want to do it again. Great paramedics never end their search for better ways to treat their patients.

What are your weaknesses? Successful dieters say the best way to get started on a diet is to stand naked in front of a mirror (without holding in your stomach) for an honest evaluation. That's what this book is all about. Be self-critical, and make small improvements in those areas that need it most. Be patient. As any weekend golfer can tell you, improvement comes slowly. The difference between the possible and the impossible lies in your determination. You must have goals and dreams if you are ever going to do anything in this world. Set your goals in life, and go after them with all the drive, self-confidence, and determination that you possess. Good luck!

Richard A. Cherry

Introduction

SUCCESS ACROSS THE BOARDS: THE PRENTICE HALL HEALTH REVIEW SERIES

Prentice Hall Health is pleased to present *EMT-Paramedic Self-Assessment Exam Prep* as part of a review series on the various EMS education levels. The authoritative text gives you expert help in preparing for certifying examinations.

COMPONENTS OF THE SERIES

The series is made up of a book and CD combination.

ABOUT THE BOOK:

- **EMT-Paramedic Self-Assessment Exam Prep:** This manual has been designed to help students prepare for the written course and certification exams. It can also be used as a review for currently certified EMT-Paramedics. The multiple-choice items are similar to those found on teacher-made exams and certifying exams. Working through these items will help you assess your strengths and weaknesses in each section.

- **Answers and Rationales:** Correct answers and comprehensive rationales are provided and assist you in better understanding each item. Rationales for incorrect answers are typically presented so that you may also learn why that answer is incorrect. Additionally, page references from *Paramedic Care: Principles & Practice* (PCPP) and *Essentials of Paramedic Care* (EPC) are provided for a more detailed explanation of answers.

- **D.O.T. Objectives:** A complete presentation of the United States D.O.T. objectives can be found in the Appendix.

1 Introduction to Advanced Prehospital Care

DIRECTIONS Each of the questions or incomplete statements below is followed by suggested answers or completions. Select the **one answer** that is best in each case.

1. The paramedic of the twenty-first century is best described as
   A. a highly trained health care professional
   B. one who provides compassionate, efficient patient care
   C. a highly regarded member of society
   D. all of the above

2. Which of the following statements most accurately describes the paramedic?
   A. Paramedics function independently with their own license
   B. Paramedics may function only under the direction of an EMS system's medical director
   C. Paramedic credentialing or licensing is unnecessary in some states and provinces
   D. None of the above

3. The current paramedic curriculum was developed by which government agency?
   A. U.S. Department of Education
   B. U.S. Department of the Interior
   C. U.S. Department of Transportation
   D. U.S. Department of HHS

4. Which of the following statements is true regarding EMS research?
   A. There is much scientific data to support many prehospital practices
   B. Most prehospital practices are based on anecdotal data and tradition
   C. Paramedics are not expected to participate in EMS research
   D. Most questions and concerns regarding paramedic practice have been scientifically addressed

5. Which of the following are considered components of the expanded scope of paramedic practice?
   A. Critical care transport
   B. Primary care
   C. Industrial and sports medicine
   D. All of the above

answers & rationales

1.

D. Paramedics of the twenty-first century are highly trained health care professionals who provide compassionate, efficient, advanced prehospital emergency medical care. They are also more highly educated than their predecessors, which qualifies them to widen their scope of practice and accept a greater role in the future health care system. (PCPP 1–6   EPC 7)

2.

B. Paramedics receive credentialing or licensing from a state or provincial agency. While all paramedics must be certified or licensed, they may not practice independently. They may function only under the license and direction of an EMS system's medical director. (PCPP 1–6   EPC 6)

3.

C. As with all the previous paramedic curricula, the 1998 National Standard Paramedic Curriculum was developed by the U.S. Department of Trans-portation. Educators, physicians, providers, and representatives from all EMS-related organizations collaborated to design the curriculum. (PCPP 1–8   EPC 7)

4.

B. Believe it or not, most prehospital care is based on anecdotal data or tradition. EMS providers of the future must rely on scientific data to support the practice of prehospital emergency medical care. Without it, EMS, as we know it today, will surely not survive in the managed care environment. (PCPP 1–10   EPC 8)

5.

D. Increased education will allow paramedics to accept greater roles in the health care delivery system. These expanded roles include critical care transport, primary care, industrial medicine, and sports medicine. The new curriculum provides a greater educational foundation so paramedics can meet this challenge. (PCPP 1–10   EPC 8)

2

The Well-Being of the Paramedic

DIRECTIONS Each of the questions or incomplete statements below is followed by suggested answers or completions. Select the **one answer** that is best in each case.

1. Most paramedics are injured
   A. while lifting
   B. while working around motor vehicles
   C. by angry bystanders
   D. A and B

2. Which of the following elements of physical fitness is the most important to the paramedic?
   A. Cardiovascular endurance
   B. Muscular strength
   C. Flexibility
   D. All of the above

3. Your target heart rate is best described as
   A. your ideal resting heart rate
   B. your maximum heart rate during extreme exercise
   C. your ideal heart rate during a cardiovascular workout
   D. 50% of your resting heart rate

4. Isometric exercise is defined as exercise performed against
   A. stable resistance
   B. increasing resistance
   C. no resistance
   D. the range of motion

5. According to the author, you should hold a stretch for
   A. 30 seconds
   B. 1 minute
   C. 2 minutes
   D. 90 seconds

6. Which of the following is NOT an example of a daily recommended food?
   A. Whole wheat bread
   B. An orange
   C. A cup of caffeinated coffee
   D. A glass of 2% milk

7. Which of the following foods can acutally decrease the risk of cancer?
   A. Broccoli
   B. Charcoal-cooked lean meat
   C. High-fiber foods
   D. A and C

8. Which of the following exercises is no longer considered safe and effective?
   A. Sit-ups
   B. Abdominal crunches
   C. Bench presses
   D. Isometrics

9. _____ have the longest incubation periods.
   A. Whooping cough (pertussis) and German measles (rubella)
   B. Hepatitis and tuberculosis
   C. Influenza and pneumonia
   D. Chicken pox (varicella) and meningitis

10. You are about to assist a mother in delivering her baby at her home. Which of the following body substance isolation items is not considered necessary?
    A. Gown
    B. Gloves
    C. Eyewear
    D. HEPA mask

11. Which of the following is considered the most important infection control practice for the paramedic?
    A. Wearing latex gloves
    B. Wearing protective eyewear
    C. Washing your hands
    D. Disposing of needles appropriately

12. You have just finished a cardiac arrest call and have a dirty laryngoscope blade to clean. Which of the following procedures is **NOT** recommended?
    A. Sterilizing it with pressurized steam
    B. Using a germicidal chemical cleaning agent
    C. Soaking it in a bleach solution
    D. Sterilizing it by radiation

13. When using a bleach solution to disinfect a backboard, the recommended mix is 1 part bleach to _____ parts water.
    A. 1
    B. 10
    C. 100
    D. 1000

14. You just brought in a patient with tuberculosis, but you were unaware that the patient was infected. According to the Ryan White Act, the medical facility must notify your designated infection control officer within _____ hours.
    A. 24
    B. 48
    C. 8
    D. 72

15. Your patient has just been notified he has terminal, inoperable cancer. He refuses to believe the diagnosis and goes about his business in a normal fashion, avoiding all conversation on the subject. He is in which stage of the grieving process?
    A. Bargaining
    B. Depression
    C. Anger
    D. Denial

16. Another cancer patient yells at you for asking him questions and appears aggravated even to have to deal with you. During the call, you cannot do anything to please him. Which stage of grief does he appear to be in?
    A. Denial
    B. Anger
    C. Depression
    D. Acceptance

17. Another cancer patient appears sad and withdrawn and will not communicate with you or his family. Which stage of grief does this demonstrate?
    A. Denial
    B. Anger
    C. Depression
    D. Acceptance

18. If your cancer patient appears to have realized his fate and to have achieved a reasonable level of comfort with the anticipated outcome, he may be in what stage of grief?
    A. Denial
    B. Anger
    C. Depression
    D. Acceptance

19. When informing someone of the death of a loved one, you should use the term
    A. expired
    B. passed away
    C. dead
    D. none of the above

20. Which of the following physiological responses occurs during the alarm stage of stress?
    A. Heart rate and blood pressure fall
    B. Pupils constrict
    C. Adrenocorticotropic hormones are released
    D. Digestion increases

21. Which of the following best describes the resistance stage?
    A. The victim is beginning to cope
    B. Vital signs return to normal
    C. Resistance to the stressor becomes stronger
    D. All of the above

22. Which of the following may help in minimizing the stressful effects of the disruption in circadian rhythms seen in EMS shift work?
    A. Stick to your anchor sleeping time
    B. Eat a heavy meal just before bedtime
    C. Keep your bedroom light on and warm
    D. Sleep as much as possible on days off

23. When your coping mechanisms no longer buffer job stressors, which can compromise both your personal health and your well-being, you are said to suffer from
    A. post-traumatic stress disorder
    B. burnout
    C. anxiety
    D. demobilization

24. Which of the following is NOT a warning sign or physical symptom of stress?
    A. Heart palpitations
    B. GI distress
    C. Increased salivation
    D. Chest pain

25. A critical incident stress debriefing should occur _____ after the incident.
    A. <12 hours
    B. 12–24 hours
    C. immediately
    D. 24–72 hours

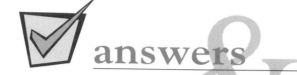

answers & rationales

1.

D. Most paramedics are injured while they are lifting, due to poor biomechanics and poor physical conditioning. Embarking on a lifelong program of reasonable physical fitness will increase your chances for a long EMS career. Paramedics also are injured at roadway scenes where ongoing traffic is not properly controlled and they are not mentally alert to the dangers. By making a commitment to physical fitness and proper lifting mechanics and by adhering to strict roadway safety procedures, paramedices can control both situations. (PCPP 1–17   EPC 33)

2.

D. Cardiovascular endurance (aerobic capacity), muscular strength, and flexibility are equally important elements in any program of physical fitness for paramedics. Some type of aerobic training, such as jogging, swimming, biking, or even walking briskly, is essential to build up enough endurance to work long shifts in the streets. Strength conditioning, such as weight lifting, is important to be able to carry patients and the multitude of equipment up and down flights of stairs. Flexibility exercises, such as stretching, are important in avoiding pulled muscles and ensure a full range of motion of your joints in the variety of movements you will perform during a shift. (PCPP 1–17   EPC 33)

3.

C. Your target heart rate is the rate at which you receive the maximum aerobic benefit while exercising. You can approximate yours by subtracting your age from 220. Then subtract your resting heart rate from this number. Finally multiply this number by 0.7 and add it to your resting heart rate to calculate your target heart rate. Try to maintain this rate while running, walking, biking, or swimming for at least 20–30 minutes a few times per week. (PCPP 1–18   EPC 33)

4.

A. Isometric exercise is active exercise performed against a stable, or immobile, resistance. You simply contract your muscle against an immovable resistance. (PCPP 1–18   EPC 33)

5.

B. Flexibility means that you can work your joints through their full range of motion. You can accomplish this by stretching your muscles before and after workouts. Hold the stretch for at least 60 seconds and avoid bouncing. An excellent comprehensive stretching program is yoga. (PCPP 1–18 EPC 33)

6.

C. The major food groups include breads and grains, vegetables, fruits, dairy products, and meat/fish. You should minimize your intake of fat, salt, sugar, cholesterol, and caffeine. Instead of a piece of apple pie, try an apple. (PCPP 1–19   EPC 34)

7.

D. Some foods can decrease the risk of some cancers. Broccoli and foods high in fiber can decrease the risk. Anything cooked on charcoal can actually increase it. (PCPP 1–21   EPC 35)

8.

A. The old-fashioned sit-up is no longer considered a beneficial exercise because of the abnormal stress it puts on your lumbar spine. To get that "six-pack" look, do abdominal crunches, which target only the rectus abdominus muscles. A variation on the basic crunch is to twist gently to either side during the crunch to target the oblique muscles. A strong abdominal section helps stabilize the spine, especially during lifting. (PCPP 1–21   EPC 35)

9.

B. The incubation period is the time between contact with a disease organism and the appearance of the first symptoms. Tuberculosis (2 to 6 weeks), hepatitis B and C (weeks or months), and AIDS (months or years) have long incubation periods, so you may not experience symptoms of such diseases for a long time following your exposure. Paramedics are at high risk for disease transmission. Consider the blood and body fluids of all patients as potentially dangerous, and take the necessary body substance isolation precautions. (PCPP 1–24 EPC 38)

10.

D. Common sense is the key to answering this question. You are trying to avoid body fluids that you should suspect are infectious. Splashing during childbirth is common. Gloves, protective eyewear, masks, and gowns are all reasonable protective measures to take. A HEPA (high-efficiency particulate air) mask is unnecessary unless your patient also has confirmed or suspected tuberculosis. (PCPP 1–26   EPC 39)

11.

C. While gloves, protective eyewear, and proper needle disposal are all essential components of a reasonable infection control policy, simply washing your hands is considered the most important. Not everyone knows how to do it properly. First, lather well with soap and water. Then scrub for at least 15 seconds, making sure to get underneath your fingernails (ideally with a brush). Then point your hands down while you rinse so that the soap and water run away from your body. Finally dry your hands on a clean towel. It sounds simple, but sometimes the simplest things are the most effective. (PCPP 1–27   EPC 40)

12.

C. Soaking in a bleach solution is appropriate for disinfecting objects that have come in direct contact with a patient's intact skin. For items such as a laryngoscope, which is inserted into your patient's mouth and is covered with oral secretions, this is ineffective and inappropriate. Sterilization by heat, steam, or radiation is recommended for killing all microorganisms on an object. However, since these methods are all impractical in the field, there are EPA-approved solutions for sterilization you can use. (PCPP 1–29   EPC 41)

13.

C. The recommended bleach solution mix is 1 part bleach to 100 parts water. (PCPP 1–29   EPC 41)

14.

B. According to the Ryan White Act, the medical facility must notify your infection control officer that your patient had tuberculosis within 48 hours. Your officer should notify you that you have been exposed, and your employer must arrange for you to be evaluated and followed up by a physician or other appropriate health care professional. This also pertains to occupational exposure to AIDS, hepatitis, diphtheria, meningitis, plague, hemorrhagic fever, and rabies. (PCPP 1–30   EPC 42)

15.

D. The patient in denial exhibits the inability or refusal to believe the reality of the event. It is a defense mechanism that can last for hours, days, weeks, or even months. During this stage, the person puts off dealing with the inevitable event. (PCPP 1–31   EPC 41)

16.

B. Often patients or their families will aim their anger at you. This rage is just a frustration related to their inability to control the situation. Just remember to remain calm; do not take it personally, and allow them to vent their feelings. Quite often this is all they need, it is inexpensive, and you are providing the best care possible—comfort, understanding, and compassion. (PCPP 1–31   EPC 41)

17.

C. People who despair at their fate and misfortune may enter the depression stage. During this stage, they withdraw into their private world and may choose not to communicate with you or even their closest and most intimate friends and loved ones. During this stage, provide reassurance and gentle guidance. (PCPP 1–31   EPC 42)

18.

D. In the end, grieving people generally come to accept their situation as inevitable. They realize, even while others may still be angry or depressed, that their fate has been cast. They appear to have achieved a reasonable level of comfort with the anticipated outcome. In these cases, the family may need your support more than the patient. (PCPP 1–31   EPC 42)

19.

C. When informing someone of the death of a loved one, help him work through the denial stage by using the word "dead." Avoid euphemisms such as expired, passed away, or moved on. Recognize that the family will cope with death in much the same manner as they deal with everyday stressors. (PCPP 1–33   EPC 45)

20.

C. During the alarm stage, the body prepares to defend itself against a perceived stressor by initiating the "fight or flight" response. This dates back to prehistoric times, when man needed all his abilities to fight or run away from the saber-toothed tiger. As the body responds to stress, the endocrine system releases epinephrine and norepinephrine. These hormones cause increases in pulse and blood pressure (to deliver more oxygenated blood to vital organs), dilated pupils (to improve vision), excessive perspiration (to decrease body temperature), increased muscle tension (to anticipate increased muscle use), and increased blood glucose levels (to supply fuel to vital tissues). (PCPP 1–35 EPC 46)

21.

D. The resistance stage begins as the victim adapts to the stressor. It is brought on by the use of various coping mechanisms. Vital signs return to normal. As adaptation develops, resistance to the particular stressor increases. (PCPP 1–35   EPC 46)

22.

A. Disrupting the normal circadian rhythm can add to paramedic job stress. Some tips to reduce the effects of this disruption include sleeping in a cool, dark room; not eating a heavy meal before bedtime; turning off your telephone; lowering the volume on your answering machine; and sticking to your "anchor" time for sleeping on your day off. Your anchor time is the time when you can rest without interruption, even on your days off. It is the time when you get your best rest. (PCPP 1–36   EPC 47)

23.

B. Many a paramedic career has been prematurely ended because of burnout. When the coping mechanisms no longer keep you afloat, burnout is inevitable. Paramedics need to develop interests outside of EMS and cultivate strong relationships and support to help them withstand the many and varied stressors of paramedic life. (PCPP 1–36 EPC 47)

24.

C. Many of the physiological reactions to stress are mediated by the sympathetic nervous system. Stress triggers an increase in sympathetic tone by releasing norepinephrine and epinephrine. Examples of signs and symptoms are heart palpitations, GI distress, and chest pain. Sympathetic stimulation causes decreased secretion from the salivary glands, resulting in dry mouth. (PCPP 1–37   EPC 48)

25.

D. Following a critical incident, you and your crew may require a critical incident stress debriefing. This is a process designed to help rescuers work through their responses to a critical incident within 24 to 72 hours. (PCPP 1–39   EPC 49)

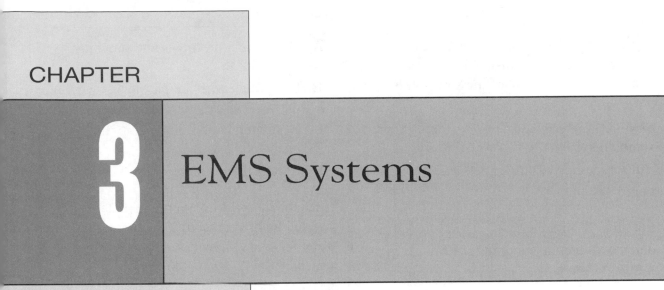

CHAPTER

3

EMS Systems

DIRECTIONS Each of the questions or incomplete statements below is followed by suggested answers or completions. Select the **one answer** that is best in each case.

1. The type of EMS system in which various levels of responders are dispatched to calls depending on the severity of the situation is known as a
   A. multilevel system
   B. standard system
   C. call screening system
   D. tiered system

2. In 1966, the "White Paper"
   A. deleted all federal funding for EMS
   B. outlined deficiencies in emergency care
   C. established the "15 components" of an EMS system
   D. appropriated over $200 million for EMS

3. Which of the following was **NOT** a requirement to receive federal dollars from the EMS Systems Act of 1973?
   A. Training
   B. Mutual aid
   C. Consumer participation
   D. Medical direction

4. State EMS agencies are usually responsible for all of the following **EXCEPT**
   A. contracting local medical directors
   B. enacting EMS legislation
   C. licensing and certifying field personnel
   D. enforcing statewide EMS regulations

5. Who has the ultimate authority in all patient care-related issues in a local EMS system?
   A. State EMS director
   B. System medical director
   C. Chief paramedic on duty
   D. Local EMS coordinator

6. Which of the following is an example of direct medical control?

A. Developing protocols and standing orders
B. Consulting with the physician by radio during an emergency call
C. Designing continuing quality improvement activities
D. Conducting chart reviews

7. Paramedic field interventions that are completed before contacting the medical control physician are known as
   A. indirect medical control orders
   B. the 4 "Ts"
   C. intervener physician protocols
   D. standing orders

8. Which of the following is an important area in which to educate the public?
   A. How to easily access the EMS system
   B. How to initiate basic life support procedures
   C. How to recognize a medical emergency
   D. All of the above

9. Which of the following is a component of a modern E-911 system?
   A. Instant call-back capabilities
   B. Automatic caller location
   C. Instant routing of the call
   D. All of the above

10. A system of emergency medical dispatching introduced by the Salt Lake City Fire Department, which standardizes every aspect of dispatching emergency vehicles, is known as
    A. priority dispatching
    B. pre-arrival dispatching
    C. triage dispatching
    D. call screening

11. System status management determines ambulance placement based on
    A. projected call volumes and locations
    B. signed contracts
    C. political sectors
    D. geographical boundaries

12. Which of the following is a nationally recognized level of EMT?
    A. EMT–Critical Care
    B. EMT–Ambulance
    C. EMT–Intermediate
    D. EMT–Cardiac Technician

13. The National Standard Paramedic Curriculum is divided into three specific learning domains. Which of the following is NOT a domain?
    A. Delineative
    B. Affective
    C. Psychomotor
    D. Cognitive

14. The process by which an agency or association grants recognition to an individual who has met its qualifications is known as
    A. licensure
    B. certification
    C. reciprocity
    D. censure

15. The process by which a government agency grants permission to engage in a given occupation to an individual who has attained the degree of competency required to ensure the public's protection is known as
    A. licensure
    B. certification
    C. reciprocity
    D. censure

16. The process by which an agency grants credentials to an individual who has comparable credentials from another agency is known as

    A. licensure
    B. certification
    C. reciprocity
    D. consensus

17. Which of the following is NOT a responsibility of the National Registry of EMTs?
    A. Administering testing materials
    B. Establishing national standards
    C. Assisting in evaluating training programs
    D. Licensing and certifying EMTs in each state

18. NASAR, NAEMSP, and NAEMT are examples of
    A. professional organizations
    B. EMS journals
    C. licensing agencies
    D. national testing agencies

19. In 1970, the MAST program was established to
    A. raise the blood pressure in shock victims
    B. bring military air medical transport capabilities to civilian accident scenes
    C. lower the evacuation times for wounded soldiers in Vietnam
    D. raise funds to establish regional EMS systems

20. Which two organizations have developed equipment lists for EMS services?
    A. NAEMT and National Registry of EMTs
    B. NAEMSP and U.S. Department of Transportation
    C. ACS and ACEP
    D. SAEM and JEMS Magazine

21. The KKK standards deal with
    A. ambulance safety and design
    B. minimum standard medical protocols
    C. training and education of field personnel
    D. air evacuation of trauma victims

22. Hospital categorization is important because
    A. not every patient can afford every hospital
    B. receiving facilities have varying capabilities
    C. not all patients can be transported to the appropriate facility
    D. it is impossible to match patient needs with hospital resources

23. Quality assurance differs from quality improvement in that
    A. quality assurance deals with patient perceptions of quality
    B. quality improvement is an objective look at clinical care
    C. quality assurance is often viewed as punitive and negative
    D. quality improvement does not elicit customer satisfaction information

24. Research in EMS is important in order to
    A. justify future funding allocations
    B. scientifically evaluate paramedical care
    C. weigh the benefits versus the risks of certain prehospital treatments
    D. all of the above

25. The public utility model and the fail-safe franchise are examples of
    A. CQI programs
    B. KKK standards
    C. system financing
    D. dispatching protocols

answers & rationales

1.

D. A "tiered" system is one in which basic life support first responders are dispatched unless advanced life support is needed. In that case, both are simultaneously dispatched to the emergency, and the first responders initiate care until the higher level arrives. (PCPP 1–47   EPC 9)

2.

B. In 1966, the National Academy of Sciences–National Research Council published a paper titled "Accidental Death and Disability, the Neglected Disease of Modern Society." The "White Paper," as it is better known, focused national attention on the problem of inadequate emergency medical care. It suggested guidelines for developing regional EMS systems, training prehospital care providers, and upgrading ambulances and their equipment. This landmark publication set off a series of federal and private funding initiatives. (PCPP 1–51   EPC 11)

3.

D. Of the 15 necessary components, the 2 that are missing are the most interesting. The authors of this legislation never foresaw the need to ensure medical direction and physician involvement in EMS system design. Neither did they see the need to ensure the financial stability of these programs in the event that the "soft" federal dollars became scarce. Both of these oversights led EMS in the wrong direction. (PCPP 1–51   EPC 11)

4.

A. State EMS agencies are typically responsible for allocating funding to local systems, enacting legislation concerning the prehospital practice of medicine, licensing and certifying field providers, enforcing all state EMS regulations, and appointing regional advisory councils. Hiring a local system medical director is the responsibility of the local EMS administrative agency. (PCPP 1–53   EPC 13)

5.

B. The local EMS system medical director is the ultimate authority in all patient care-related issues in the local EMS system. All prehospital patient care activities are extensions of this physician's license. Only a physician is licensed to practice medicine. This doctrine is known as "delegation of authority." (PCPP 1–53   EPC 13)

6.

B. Direct medical control exists when prehospital providers communicate directly with the physician at a medical control or resource hospital. The physician's direction is usually based on established protocols for managing specific problems. This physician assumes responsibility and gives treatment orders for patients. Direct medical control physicians should be experienced in emergency medicine. (PCPP 1–54   EPC 13)

7.

D. Paramedic field interventions that are completed before contacting the medical control physician are known as standing orders. Standing orders are established by indirect medical control prior to the emergency call. They allow paramedics to perform certain procedures without a direct order from the base station physician. (PCPP 1–55   EPC 14)

8.

D. The public is an essential but often overlooked component of an EMS system. An EMS system should have a plan for educating the public about recognizing an emergency situation, accessing the EMS system, and initiating basic life support procedures. (PCPP 1–55   EPC 14)

9.

D. The basic emergency telephone service is a toll-free service that enables the caller to dial three digits, 911, to reach a single public safety answering point. Enhanced 911 (E-911) provides automatic location of the caller, instant routing of the call to the appropriate emergency service agency, and instant call-back capabilitities if the caller hangs up too soon. (PCPP 1–56   EPC 15)

10.

A. A system of emergency medical dispatching introduced by the Salt Lake City Fire Department, which standardizes every aspect of dispatching emergency vehicles, is known as priority dispatching. In this system, medical dispatchers are trained to medically interrogate the distressed caller, prioritize symptoms, select the appropriate response, and give lifesaving pre-arrival instructions. These protocols are designed and approved by the system medical director. (PCPP 1–58   EPC 16)

11.

A. System status management is an emergency medical dispatching tool used to place ambulances and crews strategically around an EMS coverage area. The system status manager relies on projected call volumes and locations rather than geographical or political traditions. It is used to reduce response times. (PCPP 1–58   EPC 16)

12.

C. The National Registry of EMTs recognizes and the U.S. Department of Transportation develops training curricula for three levels of field providers: EMT–Basic, EMT–Intermediate, and EMT–Paramedic. There exist, however, approximately 30 various levels of field providers nationwide. (PCPP 1–60 EPC 17)

13.

A. The U.S. Department of Transportation's National Standard Curricula all have three specific domains: cognitive (knowledge), psychomotor (skills), and affective (attitudes and values). The well-rounded paramedic excels in all three areas. He is knowledgeable, skillful, and a professional provider of compassionate emergency medical care. (PCPP 1–59   EPC 17)

14.

B. Certification is the process by which an agency or association grants recognition to an individual who has met its qualifications. It is not a license to practice but rather a statement that a person has fulfilled predetermined requirements. Each paramedic must maintain current certification by following the guidelines established by the certifying agency. (PCPP 1–59   EPC 17)

15.

A. A license is permission to engage in a given occupation. A government agency grants licensure to individuals who have attained the degree of competency required to ensure the public's protection. A state grants licenses to teachers, physicians, nurses, and barbers. Some states also license their paramedics. (PCPP 1–59   EPC 17)

16.

C. Reciprocity is the process by which an agency grants automatic certification or licensure to an individual who has comparable credentials from another agency. Some states grant automatic paramedic certification to persons who hold a paramedic card from another state. Others grant certification to individuals who are nationally registered. (PCPP 1–60   EPC 17)

17.

D. The National Registry is an agency that prepares and administers standardized testing materials, assists in developing and evaluating training programs, establishes the qualifications for registration, and plays a major role in enabling reciprocity by establishing the national minimum standards for competency. (PCPP 1–62   EPC 18)

18.

A. Belonging to a national EMS organization is an excellent way to communicate with members from other parts of the country. Some national organizations include the National Association for Search and Rescue (NASAR), the National Association of EMS Physicians (NAEMSP), and the National Association of EMTs (NAEMT). (PCPP 1–63 EPC 18)

19.

B. In 1970, the Military Assistance to Safety and Traffic (MAST) program was established. This demonstration project set up 35 programs nationwide to test the feasibility of using military helicopters and paramedical personnel in civilian medical emergencies. (PCPP 1–64)

20.

C. In 1983, the American College of Surgeons (ACS) Committee on Trauma recommended a standard set of equipment to be carried by providers of basic life support services. In 1988, the American College of Emergency Physicians (ACEP) published a recommended list of advanced life support (ALS) supplies and equipment to be carried by ALS units. Both sets of recommendations serve as excellent guidelines for any prehospital EMS system. (PCPP 1–64   EPC 19)

21.

A. In 1974, responding to a request from the U.S. Department of Transportation, the General Services Administration developed the KKK standards, which established federal specifications for ambulances. The original guidelines and the subsequent revisions are aimed at improving ambulance design and safety features. (PCPP 1–64   EPC 19)

22.

B. Since all hospitals are not equal in terms of emergency and support service capabilities, hospital categorization is an important component of an EMS system. It identifies the readiness and capability of a hospital and its staff to receive and effectively treat emergency patients. Categorization resulted from the realization that patients have varying degrees of illness and injury and that receiving facilities have varying capabilities to provide initial or definitive care. (PCPP 1–66   EPC 20)

23.

C. Quality assurance programs are primarily designed to maintain continuous monitoring and measurement of the quality of clinical care delivered. They emphasize evaluation of response times, adherence to protocols, patient survival, and other indicators. They are often viewed as punitive and negative. (PCPP 1–68   EPC 21)

24.

D. In order to provide a scientific basis for prehospital EMS, a formal, ongoing research program is an essential component of the system. Research is necessary to justify future funding allocations, to scientifically evaluate paramedical care, and to weigh the benefits versus the risks of certain prehospital treatments. (PCPP 1–69   EPC 23)

25.

C. The public utility model and the fail-safe franchise are examples of system financing. In these systems, municipalities establish the design and standards for the contract bid and periodically, usually every three or four years, hold wholesale competition for the market. (PCPP 1–70   EPC 24)

4 Roles and Responsibilities of the Paramedic

DIRECTIONS Each of the questions or incomplete statements below is followed by suggested answers or completions. Select the **one answer** that is best in each case.

1. Your number one priority during an emergency response is
   A. patient care
   B. personal gratification
   C. insurance information
   D. safety

2. You respond to a major automobile collision involving multiple patients. Which of the following patients would receive priority-1 transport?
   A. 45-year-old with no vital signs
   B. 6-year-old with lower leg fracture and normal vital signs
   C. 25-year-old with abdominal bruising and signs of shock
   D. 68-year-old with mild respiratory distress and seat belt burns

3. When confronted with a serious unfamiliar medical situation that is not clearly outlined in your local protocols, you should
   A. improvise ALS procedures
   B. contact medical direction for guidance
   C. transport the patient BLS
   D. none of the above

4. To receive optimum care, your critical trauma patient should be transported to which of the following facilities?
   A. Level I trauma center
   B. Level II trauma center
   C. Level III trauma center
   D. The closest hospital, regardless of the designation

5. You have a critical burn patient. The nearest rural hospital is 10 minutes away. The burn center is 45 minutes away. Your patient's HMO, per the family, directs you to take him to another facility that is 30 minutes away but that does not have burn treatment capabilities. On what should you base your transport decision?
   A. The needs of this patient
   B. Knowledge of the capabilities of the hospitals in question
   C. Advice from your medical direction physician
   D. All of the above

6. The rules that govern the conduct of members of a particular group or profession are called
   A. ethics
   B. morals
   C. standards
   D. principles

7. Professionalism is exhibited by all of the following EXCEPT
   A. setting high standards
   B. seeking self-improvement
   C. earning the respect of your peers
   D. aiming for the minimum standard

8. Upon learning that he has made a mistake, the professional will
   A. blame someone else
   B. accept the responsibility
   C. blame the equipment
   D. request a new partner

9. Placing yourself in the shoes of the patient is practicing
   A. sympathy
   B. integrity
   C. empathy
   D. diplomacy

10. You have not placed a traction splint on a patient since your last refresher class two years ago. On your next call, your patient has an isolated midshaft femur fracture and requires traction. You fumble with the splint but manage to apply it with some discomfort to your patient. How could this have been avoided?

A. Practice with the splint during down time
B. Have your partner apply it
C. Transport the patient with a fixation splint
D. Use blankets and straps to stabilize the leg

answers & rationales

1.

D. Always remember that the number one priority during any emergency response is your personal safety. You can do your patient no good if you become a victim yourself. Never let your guard down because the most placid and safe scene can instantly become deadly. (PCPP 1–77   EPC 25)

2.

C. Priority-1, or immediate, transport is for patients who require definitive care that you cannot provide on the scene. The patient with signs of shock and abdominal bruising probably has an intra-abdominal hemorrhage. He needs surgery and whole blood replacement, neither of which you can provide. In his case, perform a rapid trauma assessment while you prepare for immediate transport. Perform all other assessments and treatments en route to the hospital. (PCPP 1–79)

3.

B. You will eventually encounter an unfamiliar situation that confuses you. It happens to everyone. In these cases, your best friend is the medical direction physician, who is there to help you sort out the problem and guide your care. All you have to do is call. (PCPP 1–80)

4.

A. Receiving facilities are designated by the level of care they can provide. The American College of Surgeons categorizes trauma centers by levels. A Level I trauma center provides the highest level of care. (PCPP 1–81)

5.

D. As a paramedic, you will be confronted with situations that call for quick decision making under pressure. Your patient's very life may depend on

your decision. You can base that decision on knowledge, experience, your patient's best interest, and guidance from your medical direction physician. (PCPP 1–81)

6.

A. Ethics are the rules of conduct that govern members of a particular group or profession. Examples of ethical codes for EMS include the EMT Code of Ethics and the EMT Oath. They are not laws or morals but rather guidelines for the behavior expected from professionals. (PCPP 1–85 EPC 60)

7.

D. Professionalism describes the conduct or qualities that characterize a practitioner in a particular field or occupation. Professionals take pride in their work and earn the respect of their peers by the way they conduct daily business. They are the role models who set high standards for themselves and their colleagues. The professional paramedic promotes only excellent patient care. (PCPP 1–85 EPC 28)

8.

B. When a professional makes a mistake, he does only three things: He admits it, he learns from it, and he tries never to repeat it. Professionals accept the responsibility for their actions and do their best to place their patients' best interest first, not their egos. Professionals don't complain, blame others, or make excuses for poor performance. (PCPP 1–87   EPC 29)

9.

C. By identifying with your patient's situation and trying to understand his feelings, you are practicing empathy. You can show empathy by being supportive and reassuring; having a calm, compassionate demeanor; and demonstrating respect for others. All customers want only two things: They want their problem solved, and they want to feel good. Treat your customers well, and you will be a king in their eyes. (PCPP 1–88   EPC 30)

10.

A. Professional paramedics spend the vast majority of their time preparing for the next emergency call.

Being a paramedic means accepting the responsibility of being the leader in the prehospital phase of emergency medical care. Leaders understand that performance requires preparation. The end of the training program marks only the beginning of the paramedic's education. Any skill erodes when not used. The key to confidence on the scene is competence. The key to competence is practice. (PCPP 1–89   EPC 29)

5 | Illness and Injury Prevention

DIRECTIONS Each of the questions or incomplete statements below is followed by suggested answers or completions. Select the **one answer** that is best in each case.

1. The study of the factors that influence the frequency, distribution, and causes of injury, disease, and other health-related events in a population is called
   A. holography
   B. epidemiology
   C. pathophysiology
   D. demographics

2. In a lawsuit based on the wrongful death of a 50-year-old man, a jury might assess damages based on that man's loss of _____ years as a wage earner.
   A. 40
   B. 20
   C. 15
   D. 10

3. Components of an injury-surveillance program might include
   A. injury risk
   B. teachable moments
   C. primary prevention
   D. all of the above

True or False—Identify whether the following statements are true or false:

4. ____ Low birth weight is a key indicator of poor health at time of birth.

5. ____ 33% of deaths among children result from an injury.

6. ____ The front seat of a car is the best seat for children 12 years old or younger.

7. ____ Car-pedestrian incidents are the most frequent cause of injury to children under 6 years of age.

8. ____ Fire and burn injuries occur in the highest numbers in the very young.

9. ____ The majority of firearm-related deaths are unintentional.

10. ____ Alcohol is a factor in about half of motor vehicle crashes.

11. ____ The elderly are at higher risk for falls.

12. ____ Back injuries account for almost one-quarter of all disabling injuries.

13. ____ Alzheimer's disease is a contributing factor in elderly trauma.

14. ____ About 500 children die each year from falls.

15. ____ HMOs often mandate shorter hospital stays and premature discharges from the hospital.

1.

B. The study of the factors that influence the frequency, distribution, and causes of injury, disease, and other health-related events in a population is known as epidemiology. Many injuries result from interaction with potential hazards and can be predicted. Studying these factors is the first step in prevention. (PCPP 1–97   EPC 52)

2.

C. The "years of productive life" calculation is made by subtracting the deceased's age from 65. In this case, 65 − 50 = 15. (PCPP 1–97   EPC 53)

3.

D. As medical professionals, paramedics should take part in an injury-surveillance program. This involves identifying potential injury risks, maintaining related injury statistics, teaching prevention to patients and others immediately following an incident, and developing prevention programs to keep injuries from occurring. (PCPP 1–97 EPC 53)

4.

T. Low birth weight is a key indicator of poor health at time of birth. (PCPP 1–102   EPC 56)

5.

T. 33% of deaths among children result from an injury. (PCPP 1–102   EPC 56)

6.

F. The front seat of a car is the best seat for children 12 years old or younger. (PCPP 1–102   EPC 56)

7.

F. Car-pedestrian incidents are the most frequent cause of injury to children under 6 years of age. (PCPP 1–103   EPC 56)

8.

T. Fire and burn injuries occur in the highest numbers in the very young. (PCPP 1–103   EPC 56)

9.

F. The majority of firearm-related deaths are unintentional. (PCPP 1–103   EPC 57)

10.

T. Alcohol is a factor in about half of motor vehicle crashes. (PCPP 1–103   EPC 57)

11.

T. The elderly are at higher risk for falls. (PCPP 1–103   EPC 57)

12.

T. Back injuries account for almost one-quarter of all disabling injuries. (PCPP 1–103   EPC 57)

13.

T. Alzheimer's disease is a contributing factor in elderly trauma. (PCPP 1–103   EPC 57)

14.

F. About 500 children die each year from falls. (PCPP 1–103   EPC 56)

15.

T. HMOs often mandate shorter hospital stays and premature discharges from the hospital. (PCPP 1–104   EPC 57)

6 Medical/Legal Aspects of Advanced Prehospital Care

DIRECTIONS
Each of the questions or incomplete statements below is followed by suggested answers or completions. Select the **one answer** that is best in each case.

1. The Fourth Amendment is an example of _____ law.
   A. legislative
   B. administrative
   C. regulatory
   D. constitutional

2. The *Miranda* ruling is an example of _____ law.
   A. common
   B. regulatory
   C. legislative
   D. criminal

3. Statutory law is another name for _____ law.
   A. administrative
   B. constitutional
   C. civil
   D. legislative

4. The OSHA regulations are an example of _____ laws.
   A. legislative
   B. administrative
   C. common
   D. civil

5. Homicide and rape are examples of wrongs against society and are tried in
   A. criminal court
   B. tort court
   C. civil court
   D. none of the above

6. Which of the following is an example of a tort case?
   A. Divorce
   B. Suicide
   C. Contract dispute
   D. Malpractice

7. A "Medical Practice Act"
   A. defines the scope of practice for allied health care professionals
   B. is a national standard for allied health care professionals
   C. outlines ethical behavior guidelines for medical paraprofessionals
   D. is unnecessary in states that license their paramedics

8. Which of the following statements is true?
   A. Paramedics may practice independently
   B. Paramedics may practice only under the license of a physician
   C. Paramedics cannot be found criminally liable for practicing without a license
   D. Paramedics do not require a "Medical Practice Act"

9. If, after you question an order from medical direction that you feel is inappropriate, the physician still wants you to carry it out, you should
   A. carry the order out as directed
   B. refuse the order and document the incident
   C. transport the patient BLS
   D. call another hospital

10. Which of the following circumstances are you mandated to report to the proper authority?
    A. Circumstances listed in your state's laws
    B. Child and spousal abuse
    C. Animal bites
    D. B and C

11. Laws that protect health care workers from liability in the event they stop and render roadside care are known as
    A. Good Samaritan laws
    B. res ipsa loquitor laws
    C. Ryan White laws
    D. negligence laws

12. Negligence is defined as
    A. bringing a lawsuit involving no physical harm
    B. deviating from the standard of care
    C. failing to prove proximate cause
    D. all of the above

13. Which of the following is **NOT** a necessary component of a successful negligence suit?
    A. Duty to act
    B. Breach of duty
    C. Proximate cause
    D. Unlawful consent

14. Which of the following would be considered a breach of duty?
    A. Malfeasance
    B. Misfeasance
    C. Nonfeasance
    D. All of the above

15. In a res ipsa loquitor claim, the burden of proof rests with the
    A. plaintiff
    B. defendant
    C. medical advisory council
    D. district attorney

16. You are on the scene of an automobile crash and are taking a quick report of the crash from a police officer when you suddenly notice that your EMT partner just pulled a driver out of the window without any regard for immobilization. In this case, you could be held liable under which doctrine?

    A. Delegation of authority
    B. Proximate liability
    C. Borrowed servant
    D. You are not responsible for the actions of this EMT

17. All medical records are confidential. Under which of the following circumstances can a patient's medical record be released?
    A. A court order or subpoena
    B. Third-party billing requirements
    C. Patient consent
    D. All of the above

18. Stating on the air that "We've got Joe Jones again, and he's drunk and obnoxious as usual" could place the paramedic in danger of being liable for
    A. assault
    B. battery
    C. libel
    D. slander

19. Writing on the run sheet that a certain patient "probably has AIDS from deviant homosexual activity" could place the paramedic in danger of being sued for
    A. assault
    B. defamation of character
    C. libel
    D. slander

20. Informed consent means
    A. the adult patient is mentally competent
    B. the patient understands the treatment and the risks
    C. the patient agrees to the treatment
    D. all of the above

21. Which of the following would **NOT** fall under the concept of implied consent?
    A. An unconscious diabetic in insulin shock
    B. A 5-year-old in anaphylactic shock with no parent present

C. A mentally retarded person with bilateral fractured femurs

D. A diabetic who awakens following 50% dextrose therapy and refuses transport

22. Who is required to give informed consent for an emancipated minor?
    A. Parent
    B. Legal guardian
    C. No one
    D. Police officer

23. If your diabetic patient awakens following dextrose therapy and now absolutely refuses transport to the hospital, even after speaking with your medical direction physician on the phone, what should you do?
    A. Have the patient sign a release form and document the incident thoroughly
    B. Transport the patient against his wishes
    C. Have the patient placed in custody by the police and transport
    D. Leave and return with a court order to transport

24. Failure to formally transfer the patient to medical staff in the emergency department could place the paramedic in danger of being held liable for
    A. false imprisonment
    B. unlawful consent
    C. abandonment
    D. patient endangerment

25. Threatening to defibrillate a patient if he does not quiet down could place a paramedic in danger of being held liable for
    A. assault
    B. battery
    C. libel
    D. slander

26. Starting an IV on a competent patient who absolutely refuses one could place the paramedic in danger of being held liable for
    A. assault
    B. battery
    C. libel
    D. slander

27. Transporting a patient to the hospital against his will could place the paramedic in danger of being held liable for
    A. false imprisonment
    B. kidnapping
    C. unlawful consent
    D. assault and battery

28. If a question arises concerning the validity of advanced directives, such as "Do Not Resuscitate" orders or "Living Wills," the paramedic should
    A. contact your medical direction physican
    B. ignore all such orders and run the code
    C. accept and honor all such orders
    D. run a "slow code" in these cases

29. Which of the following statements is true concerning prehospital documentation?
    A. If you do not write it down, you did not do it
    B. A well-documented run sheet can be your best defense in court
    C. Intentional alterations of the run sheet are considered admissions of guilt
    D. All of the above

30. A paramedic's best defense against potential legal liability is
    A. purchasing medical malpractice insurance
    B. documenting as little as possible on the run sheet
    C. relying on Good Samaritan immunity
    D. practicing excellent prehospital care

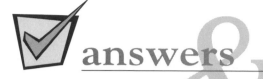

1.

D. Constitutional law is based on the U.S. Constitution, which sets forth our basic government structures and personal protections. The Fourth Amendment protects people from unreasonable searches and seizures by the government. (PCPP 1–112 EPC 74)

2.

A. Common law is based on precedents. It is also called case law and judge-made law and is derived from society's acceptance of customs and norms. In the *Miranda* case, the U.S. Supreme Court ruled that if a suspect has not been read his rights, involuntary statements made by the suspect will not be admissible in court. (PCPP 1–112 EPC 74)

3.

D. Legislative law is also called statutory law and is created by lawmaking bodies such as Congress and state assemblies. It takes precedence over common law. (PCPP 1–112 EPC 74)

4.

B. Administrative law, such as the Occupational Safety and Health Administration (OSHA) standards, is enacted by government agencies at either the state or the federal level. The agency is authorized to make regulations based on a standard and enforce those regulations. If a paramedic ambulance company violates an OSHA standard, it can suffer penalties and fines. (PCPP 1–112 EPC 74)

5.

A. Criminal law deals with crimes against society and their punishments. Criminal litigations are legal actions taken by the state against the offending individual. Homicide and rape are examples of criminal wrongs. To convict requires proof beyond a reasonable doubt. (PCPP 1–113 EPC 75)

6.

D. Tort law, a branch of civil law, deals with civil wrongs committed by one individual against another. A medical malpractice suit is an example of a tort action against a paramedic. Unlike in a criminal case, only a preponderance of evidence (50% + 1) is needed to win the case. (PCPP 1–113 EPC 75)

7.

A. A "Medical Practice Act" is specific state legislation that defines the scope and role of the paramedic and other allied health care professionals. It establishes the requirements for those who will be allowed to practice and identifies certification and licensing procedures. Medical practice acts differ from state to state. (PCPP 1–114 EPC 76)

8.

B. Paramedics are not licensed to practice independently. They may function only under the supervision of a licensed physician through delegation of authority. This supervision may be direct (in person, on radio) or indirect (through protocols, standing orders). Failure to adhere to this requirement could make the paramedic criminally liable for practicing medicine without a license. In some states, this constitutes a felony, punishable by fines or imprisonment. (PCPP 1–114 EPC 76)

9.

B. As a paramedic, you practice under the license of the physician giving you orders. However, you are still held responsible for your own actions. In this case, if you are sure the order is contraindicated and potentially harmful to your patient, you must refuse the order and document the incident thoroughly. (PCPP 1–114   EPC 76)

10.

A. Each state enacts its own laws concerning mandatory reporting. Some states require paramedics to report a long list of circumstances, while others do not. You must become familiar with the circumstances under which you are required to make a report, or you may be criminally and civilly liable for your inaction. (PCPP 1–115   EPC 77)

11.

A. Laws that protect off-duty health care workers from liability in the event they stop and render roadside care are known as Good Samaritan laws. A person is immune from liability for assisting at the scene of a medical emergency if he acts in good faith, is not grossly negligent, and does not accept payment for services. Unfortunately, grossly negligent is a subjective term, and the plaintiff's attorney will portray the paramedic as such. A jury of nonmedical civilians will listen to testimony and decide the outcome. In many cases, the Good Samaritan defense has not held up in court. (PCPP 1–116   EPC 78)

12.

B. Negligence is defined as deviating from accepted standards of care. In medicine, negligence is synonymous with malpractice. Paramedics can be negligent by not performing to the standard of care (failure to immobilize the c-spine), by performing beyond their training and certification (any skill not approved by the local medical director), or by performing at a substandard level (unrecognized esophageal intubation of a breathing patient). (PCPP 1–116   EPC 78)

13.

D. To win a negligence case, the plaintiff's attorney must prove that a paramedic's breach of duty caused harm to the patient. Once again, in a tort case, only a preponderance of evidence is needed to win. (PCPP 1–117   EPC 79)

14.

D. Breach of duty also means deviating from the standard of care. It can take the form of malfeasance (performing a wrongful act, such as assaulting your patient), misfeasance (performing improperly, such as failing to recognize an esophageal intubation), or nonfeasance (failing to perform an indicated procedure, such as immobilizing the spine). (PCPP 1–117   EPC 79)

15.

B. When the doctrine of res ipsa loquitor is invoked, the burden of proof shifts from the plaintiff to the defendant. Res ipsa loquitor is Latin for "the thing speaks for itself," meaning that the damages could not have occurred in the absence of the paramedic's negligence. For example, only the paramedic could have inserted the endotracheal tube into the patient's esophagus. (PCPP 1–118   EPC 80)

16.

C. As a paramedic, one of your responsibilities is supervising the actions of other EMS providers—in this case, your EMT partner. You may be liable for any negligent act he commits under the borrowed servant doctrine. (PCPP 1–120   EPC 82)

17.

D. It is true that all medical records are confidential. But there are special circumstances in which the release of medical information is not only practical, but also essential. These include patient consent, when other medical providers need to know, a subpoena, and third-party billing requirements. (PCPP 1–121   EPC 83)

18.

D. Slander is the act of injuring a person's character, name, or reputation by false or malicious spoken words. Information transmitted over the radio should be limited to essential matters of patient care. Such a medical report should never contain the patient's name or the paramedic's subjective opinions. (PCPP 1–122   EPC 84)

19.

C. Libel is the act of injuring a person's character, name, or reputation by false or malicious writings. Allegations of libel can be avoided by respecting the patient's confidentiality. The medical record should be accurate and confidential; slang and labels should be avoided. Never write anything on the run report that could be construed as libel. (PCPP 1–122   EPC 84)

20.

D. Informed consent must be obtained from every conscious, mentally competent adult before treatment can be started. To give informed consent, the adult patient must be mentally competent, understand the treatment and the risks, and agree to be treated. (PCPP 1–122   EPC 85)

21.

D. Unconscious patients cannot express consent. When treating the unconscious patient, the consent is considered to be implied. With implied consent, it is assumed that the patient would want lifesaving treatment if he were able to provide expressed consent. (PCPP 1–123   EPC 85)

22.

C. An emancipated minor is considered an adult and can give informed consent. This is a person under 18 years old who is married, pregnant, a parent, a member of the armed forces, or financially independent and living away from home. (PCPP 1–124   EPC 86)

23.

A. Competent patients have the right to be left alone. This patient, now awake and competent, has every legal right to refuse your help. Respect his wishes, but document that you informed him of the dangers of refusing help, and make sure he understands the risks involved in refusing. You can only document everything and hope for the best. (PCPP 1–124   EPC 86)

24.

C. Abandonment is the termination of the paramedic-patient relationship without assuring continuation of the care. Paramedics should not initiate care and then arbitrarily discontinue it. Physically leaving a patient unattended on an emergency department stretcher may be grounds for abandonment if the patient's condition deteriorates. (PCPP 1–127   EPC 88)

25.

A. Assault is defined as unlawfully placing a person in apprehension of immediate bodily harm without his consent. Threatening to defibrillate a patient if he does not quiet down could place a paramedic in danger of being sued for assault. Assault can be either a criminal or a civil offense. (PCPP 1–127 EPC 88)

26.

B. Battery is the unlawful touching of another individual without his consent. Starting an IV on a competent patient who absolutely refuses one could place the paramedic in danger of being sued for battery. Battery also could be a criminal or a civil offense. (PCPP 1–127   EPC 88)

27.

A. Everyone has the right to be left alone. False imprisonment is defined as unlawful and unjustifiable detention. Transporting a patient to the hospital against his will could constitute false imprisonment. In these cases, paramedics should ensure that the transportation is medically justified. (PCPP 1–128   EPC 89)

28.

A. When questions concerning the validity of "Do Not Resuscitate" orders or "Living Wills" arise in the field, paramedics should contact medical direction physician. Paramedics do not have the legal authority and are not in the position to evaluate the validity of such documents. (PCPP 1–130   EPC 91)

29.

D. A complete, well-written run report is a paramedic's best protection in a malpractice proceeding. To the court, observations and treatments not documented on the run report were not performed. The medical record should never be altered because this may amount to an admission of guilt by the paramedic. (PCPP 1–134   EPC 93)

30.

D. A paramedic's best defense against potential legal liability is practicing the highest quality of patient care, which includes good documentation. (PCPP 1–135   EPC 93)

7

Ethics in Advanced Prehospital Care

DIRECTIONS Each of the questions or incomplete statements below is followed by suggested answers or completions. Select the **one answer** that is best in each case.

1. The rules or standards that govern the behavior of members of a particular group or profession are known as
   A. morals
   B. laws
   C. ethics
   D. consequences

2. Social, religious, or personal standards of right and wrong are known as
   A. morals
   B. laws
   C. ethics
   D. consequences

3. Your EMS agency functions under the philosophy that whatever you decide in the field is the correct course of action and is all right. This is an example of
   A. autonomy
   B. consequentialism
   C. ethical relativism
   D. beneficence

4. John, a paramedic, treats every patient with the same skill, compassion, and effort. This is an example of
   A. autonomy
   B. justice
   C. consequentialism
   D. beneficence

5. Your patient is a 56-year-old competent female who refuses all treatment and transport after falling on the sidewalk and twisting her ankle. You abide by her wishes and allow her to refuse your care. This is an example of
   A. nonmaleficence
   B. autonomy
   C. ethical relativism
   D. justice

6. After an emergency run, you wonder whether you should have initiated advanced life support procedures. As you review the circumstances, you wonder, if asked, how you will defend your actions to your medical director. This is known as the _____ test.
   A. relevance
   B. universalizability
   C. interpersonal justifiability
   D. impartiality

7. Which of the following statements is true regarding advanced directives?
   A. Always follow the family's wishes
   B. Accept verbal DNR orders from other health care providers
   C. When in doubt, resuscitate
   D. Never accept a prehospital advanced directive

8. You are on the scene with a competent patient who refuses care. To exercise this right, the patient must have
   A. the mental faculties to evaluate the risk/benefit ratio
   B. an attorney in attendance to validate the documents
   C. a physician consultation with the patient
   D. an advanced directive on letterhead

9. Which of the following would normally receive the highest-priority care in a multiple-patient incident?
   A. A visiting president
   B. A critically injured soldier in war
   C. The least injured person in a motor vehicle collision
   D. A visiting movie star

10. How does emergency medicine differ from the other medical disciplines?

    A. HMOs can dictate that an emergency care facility is off limits

    B. Good Samaritan statutes generally do not protect off-duty emergency providers who stop and offer roadside care

    C. Emergency departments agree to provide care to anyone who asks for it

    D. None of the above

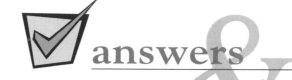

answers & rationales

1.

C. The rules or standards that govern the behavior of members of a particular group or profession are known as ethics. Every profession has a set of ethics developed by that profession. General ethical guidelines for EMS providers include the EMT Oath and the EMT Code of Ethics. (PCPP 1–141   EPC 60)

2.

A. Social, religious, or personal standards of right and wrong are known as morals. Just as ethical standards guide your actions as a paramedic, so will your own personal morals. (PCPP 1–141   EPC 60)

3.

C. Ethical relativism means that each person gets to decide how to behave and whatever decision that person makes is all right. The obvious lack of direction and guidelines often results in gross errors in judgment. For example, Charles Manson made some decisions that most people would agree were reprehensible. (PCPP 1–142   EPC 60)

4.

B. Justice is the obligation to treat all patients fairly, regardless of age, race, religion, ability to pay, or cultural background. Every patient encountered by the EMS system deserves justice. (PCPP 1–144 EPC 61)

5.

B. A competent adult has the right to be left alone. Respecting the patient's right allows the patient to practice autonomy. Just remember to follow your medical director's guidelines for refusal of care and document the incident thoroughly. (PCPP 1–144   EPC 61)

6.

C. Asking whether you can defend or justify your actions to others is using the interpersonal justifiabil-ity test. Soliciting other opinions helps a paramedic navigate through the sometimes murky waters of emergency medicine. (PCPP 1–147   EPC 63)

7.

C. Whenever you doubt the validity of an advanced directive, resuscitate the patient. During a crisis, a paramedic is not trained to judge the validity of a legal document. (PCPP 1–149   EPC 65)

8.

A. In order for an adult to refuse care, he must be competent. This means he must have the mental ability to understand the situation and what is recommended by the care providers and must be able to weigh the risks and the benefits. If your patient is refusing care against your advice, make sure to identify the risks clearly, with particular emphasis on the worst case scenario. (PCPP 1–152   EPC 67)

9.

A. Triage is a French word meaning "to sort." Triaging medical care is a necessity fraught with different rules for different situations. For example, in civilian life the most injured and salvageable patient gets the highest priority. In war, the least injured soldier gets the highest priority in order to return him to the fighting. A visiting dignitary, such as the president or vice president, immediately receives special treatment because of his importance. (PCPP 1–152   EPC 68)

10.

C. While most other health care professionals can pick and choose their patients, those who provide emergency medicine have a special obligation to care for anyone who presents in the emergency department, regardless of his ability to pay. This is one reason why emergency medicine is a unique specialty. (PCPP 1–153   EPC 68)

8

General Principles of Pathophysiology

DIRECTIONS Each of the questions or incomplete statements below is followed by suggested answers or completions. Select the **one answer** that is best in each case.

1. The basic unit of life is the
   A. nucleus
   B. tissue
   C. organ
   D. cell

2. The three main components of a cell are the
   A. cell membrane, cytokine, and nucleus
   B. cell membrane, nucleus, and organelles
   C. cytoplasm, organelles, and nucleus
   D. organelles, cytoplasm, and cell membrane

Match the following cellular terms with their respective definitions:

3. _____ Nucleus
4. _____ Cytosol
5. _____ Golgi
6. _____ Mitochondrion
7. _____ Lysosome
8. _____ Peroxisome
9. _____ Phagocyte

A. Scavenger cell
B. Packages enzymes and mucus
C. Clear liquid portion of cytoplasm
D. Neutralizes alcohol and toxins
E. Energy factory
F. Contains DNA
G. Contains digestive enzymes

10. The structure that surrounds the cell and protects it from the outer environment is the
    A. membrane
    B. wall
    C. mitochondrion
    D. cytoplasm

11. The skin, mucous membranes, and intestinal tract lining are examples of
    A. muscle tissue
    B. connective tissue
    C. nerve tissue
    D. epithelial tissue

12. The only muscle tissue that can contract without external stimulation is
    A. cardiac muscle
    B. smooth muscle
    C. skeletal muscle
    D. connective muscle

13. Bones, cartilage, and fat are examples of
    A. epithelium
    B. organelles
    C. connective tissue
    D. organ systems

14. The type of muscle found in the inner lining of hollow organs is
    A. skeletal muscle
    B. epithelial muscle
    C. smooth muscle
    D. connective muscle

15. The natural tendency of the body to maintain a constant, stable internal environment is called
    A. osmosis
    B. organism stability
    C. hemostasis
    D. homeostasis

16. Ductless glands that secrete their hormones directly into the bloodstream are called _____ glands.
    A. lipophilic
    B. endocrine
    C. exocrine
    D. paracrine

17. _____ respond to changes in arterial PCO_2 levels.
    A. Baroreceptors
    B. Neuroreceptors
    C. Chemoreceptors
    D. Alpha receptors

18. _____ respond to changes in blood pressure.
    A. Baroreceptors
    B. Neuroreceptors
    C. Chemoreceptors
    D. Alpha receptors

19. As your blood pressure falls, your body initiates a series of mechanisms to increase it. These mechanisms then begin to subside as your blood pressure returns to normal. This process is known as a/an
    A. positive feedback loop
    B. enhanced compensatory mechanism
    C. pathological homeopathic episode
    D. negative feedback loop

20. Your fractured tibia is placed in a cast for 6 weeks. When the cast is removed, you notice that your calf muscle is smaller. This is an example of cell
    A. atrophy
    B. hypertrophy
    C. hyperplasia
    D. dysplasia

21. Your father has a long history of heart disease and now is diagnosed with congestive heart failure. You notice on the X-ray that his heart is enlarged and at the physical exam that his point of maximal impulse is nearly at the anterior axillary line. This is an example of
    A. atrophy
    B. hypertrophy
    C. hyperplasia
    D. metaplasia

22. You have smoked for years. From the years of inhaled irritants, your ciliated columnar epithelial cells have been replaced by stratified squamous epithelial cells. This is an example of
    A. metaplasia
    B. hypertrophy
    C. hyperplasia
    D. dysplasia

23. After years of sitting in the tripod position, your emphysema patient has developed calloused elbows. This is an example of
    A. atrophy
    B. hypertrophy
    C. hyperplasia
    D. dysplasia

24. The most common cause of cellular injury is
    A. hypoglycemia
    B. hypoxia
    C. hypersensitivity
    D. anabolism

25. Which of the following statements is true regarding anaerobic metabolism?
    A. The cells cease to metabolize
    B. There is a marked increase in ATP production
    C. The sodium-potassium pumps increase their rates
    D. The cells metabolize without oxygen

26. Which of the following is a common result of a chemical injury?
    A. Altered coagulation
    B. Enzymatic reactions
    C. Cell death
    D. All of the above

27. A pathogen's virulence is its
    A. ability to cause damage
    B. number of microorganisms
    C. ability to ward off the immune system
    D. none of the above

28. Which of the following statements is true regarding immunologic and inflammatory injuries?
    A. They pose no threat to life
    B. They rarely injure healthy body cells
    C. They often alter the cell membrane
    D. Injured body cells rarely repair themselves

29. Most diseases are caused by
    A. environmental factors
    B. genetic factors
    C. a combination of environmental and genetic factors
    D. all of the above

30. Which of the following best illustrates the process of anabolism?
    A. Using calcium to build bone
    B. Breaking down bone to release calcium
    C. Storing glucose in the form of glycogen
    D. Phagocyte migration

31. The most common result from cellular injury is
    A. fatty change
    B. apoptosis
    C. necrosis
    D. cellular swelling

32. Which of the following statements is true regarding the process of apoptosis?
    A. It is always pathological
    B. It is a normal form of homeostasis
    C. The cells multiply and invade healthy cells
    D. Gas gangrene is a common result

33. Which of the following is NOT a type of gangrene?
    A. Gas
    B. Wet
    C. Dry
    D. Caseous

34. Water makes up approximately _____ of total body weight.
    A. 30%
    B. 60%
    C. 80%
    D. None of the above

35. Where is most of this water is found?
    A. Between the cells
    B. In the blood vessels
    C. In the cells
    D. None of the above

36. As we age, our total body water
    A. increases
    B. decreases
    C. stays the same
    D. varies with the individual

37. All of the following happen when your fluid levels drop EXCEPT
    A. ADH is secreted
    B. the kidneys reabsorb sodium
    C. more urine is excreted
    D. water shifts into the intravascular compartment

38. All of the following are signs of dehydration EXCEPT
    A. poor skin turgor
    B. sacral edema
    C. sunken fontanels
    D. tachycardia

39. Dehydrated patients should receive
    A. an isotonic solution
    B. lactated Ringer's
    C. normal saline
    D. all of the above

40. A positively charged ion is called a/an
    A. cation
    B. anion

C. colloid

D. crystalloid

41. The chief extracellular cation that regulates fluid distribution is
    A. bicarbonate
    B. sodium
    C. potassium
    D. magnesium

42. The chief intracellular cation that aids in electrical impulse transmission is
    A. magnesium
    B. sodium
    C. potassium
    D. calcium

43. The cation that plays a major role in muscle contraction is
    A. bicarbonate
    B. sodium
    C. potassium
    D. calcium

44. The principal buffer of the acid-base system is
    A. bicarbonate
    B. sodium
    C. potassium
    D. magnesium

45. Electrolytes are measured in
    A. mg/kg
    B. mEq/L
    C. mEq/dl
    D. mcg/L

46. The movement of water through a semipermeable membrane from an area of low solute concentration toward an area of high solute concentration is called
    A. diffusion
    B. facilitated diffusion
    C. active transport
    D. osmosis

47. Infusing a hypotonic solution into the bloodstream causes water to move
    A. into the cells
    B. into the blood vessel
    C. out of the cells
    D. none of the above

48. The movement of solute particles through a semipermeable membrane from an area of high solute concentration toward an area of low solute concentration is called
    A. diffusion
    B. facilitated diffusion
    C. active transport
    D. osmosis

49. Infusing a hypertonic solution into a blood vessel will cause all of the following to happen EXCEPT
    A. an osmotic gradient toward the vein
    B. a fluid shift into the blood vessel
    C. an increase in blood pressure
    D. a decrease in intravascular blood volume

50. A solution with the same osmolarity as blood plasma is said to be
    A. hypotonic
    B. hypertonic
    C. isotonic
    D. none of the above

51. In a freshwater drowning, what happens as water enters the pulmonary capillaries?
    A. It remains in the capillaries
    B. It quickly diffuses into the cells
    C. It draws additional fluid into the blood vessel
    D. None of the above

52. Sodium is transported out of the cell against the gradient in a process called
    A. facilitated diffusion
    B. facilitated transport
    C. passive diffusion
    D. active transport

53. The insulin/glucose relationship is an example of
    A. facilitated diffusion
    B. facilitated transport
    C. passive diffusion
    D. active transport

54. Oncotic force is created by _____ in the intravascular space.
    A. cations
    B. sodium ions
    C. plasma proteins
    D. potassium ions

55. Filtration is caused by
    A. oncotic force
    B. sodium and potassium ions
    C. plasma proteins
    D. hydrostatic pressure

56. Which of the following can cause tissue edema?
    A. Increased oncotic force
    B. Decreased hydrostatic pressure
    C. Decreased capillary permeability
    D. Lymphatic channel obstruction

57. Osmoreceptors are located in the _____ _____.
    A. medulla
    B. aortic arch
    C. hypothalamus
    D. pituitary

58. The majority of blood volume consists of
    A. red blood cells
    B. plasma
    C. platelets
    D. white blood cells

59. The percentage of red blood cells in the blood is called
    A. homeostasis

B. hematocrit
    C. hemoglobin
    D. hematoma

60. Red blood cells make up what percentage of total blood volume in the healthy adult?
    A. 20
    B. 45
    C. 55
    D. 60

61. A patient with blood infusing suddenly develops fever, chills, nausea, hives, tachycardia, and hypotension. You suspect a transfusion reaction. Which of the following should you do?
    A. Stop the IV
    B. Infuse normal saline
    C. Monitor the patient closely
    D. All of the above

62. Hespan, dextran, and albumin are examples of
    A. colloids
    B. crystalloids
    C. isotonic solutions
    D. hypotonic solutions

63. After infusing a colloid solution, you should expect
    A. a decrease in blood pressure
    B. a fluid shift into the bloodstream
    C. rapid diffusion of its solute particles into the tissues
    D. an osmotic gradient toward the intracellular compartment

64. The normal pH for the human body is
    A. 7.0–8.0
    B. 7.35–7.45
    C. 7.3
    D. 7.5

65. The fastest mechanism for correcting the body's acid-base abnormalities is the
    A. respiratory system

B. renal system

C. buffer system

D. none of the above

66. A patient with a pH of 7.2 and a $PaCO_2$ of 52 torr is in a state of

A. respiratory acidosis

B. respiratory alkalosis

C. metabolic acidosis

D. metabolic alkalosis

67. A probable cause of this patient's condition is

A. near-drowning

B. amphetamine drug overdose

C. antacid ingestion

D. excessive vomiting

68. The reasons behind the pH and $PaCO_2$ abnormalities include

A. an increase in carbon dioxide elimination

B. an increase in bicarbonate concentration

C. a decrease in carbon dioxide retention

D. none of the above

69. Immediate management of a patient with this condition includes

A. coaching the patient to breathe slower

B. administering sodium bicarbonate

C. ventilating with positive pressure

D. none of the above

70. Which of the following is true regarding a patient in alkalosis?

A. The pH is abnormally low

B. The hydrogen ion concentration is abnormally high

C. There are no bicarbonate ions present

D. None of the above

71. Management of a patient in respiratory alkalosis includes

A. hyperventilating

B. coaching and reassuring

C. breathing into a paper bag

D. administering sodium bicarbonate

Match the following acid-base derangements with their possible causes:

72. ____ Respiratory acidosis

73. ____ Respiratory alkalosis

74. ____ Metabolic acidosis

75. ____ Metabolic alkalosis

A. Unchecked diabetes

B. Strangulation

C. Diuretic overuse

D. Anxiety

76. Which of the following diseases is considered purely genetic in origin?

A. Asthma

B. Diabetes

C. Heart disease

D. Sickle cell disease

77. For which of the following diseases is positive family history NOT considered a risk factor?

A. Breast cancer

B. Colon cancer

C. Lung cancer

D. Rectal cancer

78. Which statement best describes the difference between Type I and Type II diabetes?

A. Type I is more prevalent

B. Type II is more severe

C. In Type II, the pancreas produces no insulin

D. None of the above

79. A bleeding disorder caused by a genetic clotting factor deficiency is known as

A. hemophilia

B. hemochromatosis

C. hemoglobinuria

D. hemolytic anemia

80. Which of the following cardiac diseases is NOT caused by a genetic factor?
    A. Coronary artery disease
    B. Hypertension
    C. Cardiomyopathy
    D. Mitral valve prolapse

81. The primary cause of renal failure is
    A. an infectious process
    B. hypertension
    C. a sodium deficiency
    D. hyperkalemia

82. Which of the following factors is related to gout?
    A. Uremia
    B. Crystal deposits in the joints
    C. Hereditary metabolic disorder
    D. All of the above

83. Which of the following gastrointestinal disorders is believed to be caused by the *H. pylori* bacteria?
    A. Crohn's disease
    B. Peptic ulcer disease
    C. Cholecystitis
    D. Lactose intolerance

84. Which of the following neuromuscular disorders is caused by the destruction of the myelin sheath by the autoimmune system?
    A. Huntington's disease
    B. Parkinson's disease
    C. Multiple sclerosis
    D. Alzheimer's disease

85. Which of the following factors does NOT affect the heart's stroke volume?
    A. Heart rate
    B. Preload
    C. Afterload
    D. Contractile force

86. Stroke volume could be increased by all of the following EXCEPT
    A. increasing venous return
    B. increasing contractile force
    C. decreasing afterload
    D. promoting venodilation

87. The amount of blood pumped from the heart in one contraction is called
    A. preload
    B. afterload
    C. stroke volume
    D. tidal volume

88. Which of the following statements best illustrates the Frank-Starling mechanism?
    A. The greater the afterload, the greater the stroke volume
    B. The less the stroke volume, the less the afterload
    C. The greater the preload, the greater the stroke volume
    D. The less the preload, the greater the afterload

89. In order to decrease the workload on the heart in a patient with CHF, you should
    A. place the victim in Trendelenberg
    B. administer a drug that dilates the veins
    C. administer a fluid challenge
    D. hyperventilate the patient

90. The amount of blood pumped by the heart in 1 minute is called
    A. minute volume
    B. stroke volume
    C. cardiac output
    D. contractile volume

91. The amount of resistance against which the heart must pump in order to eject blood is called
    A. stroke volume

B. end-diastolic volume

C. afterload

D. pulse pressure

92. Baroreceptors constantly monitor for changes in
    A. oxygen levels
    B. carbon dioxide levels
    C. heart rate
    D. blood pressure

93. Stimulation of the baroreceptors causes all of the following EXCEPT
    A. peripheral vasodilation
    B. increased cardiac output
    C. increased heart rate
    D. bronchodilation

94. Peripheral vascular resistance is dependent on
    A. vessel diameter
    B. fluid viscosity
    C. vessel length
    D. all of the above

95. The greatest change in peripheral resistance occurs in the
    A. aorta
    B. arteries
    C. arterioles
    D. capillaries

96. Which of the following is a component of the "Fick principle"?
    A. Adequate FiO_2
    B. Adequate hematocrit
    C. Adequate diffusion of gases
    D. All of the above

97. Anaerobic metabolism results in which of the following?
    A. Inefficient energy
    B. Increased pyruvic acid formation
    C. Glycolysis
    D. All of the above

98. The first stage of glucose breakdown is known as
    A. the Krebs cycle
    B. the citric acid cycle
    C. glycolysis
    D. aerobic metabolism

99. The second stage of glucose breakdown is known as
    A. the Krebs cycle
    B. progressive metabolism
    C. glycolysis
    D. anaerobic metabolism

100. Which of the following happens during the shock state?
    A. The Krebs cycle produces increased energy
    B. Glycolysis creates pyruvic acid
    C. Pyruvic acid degrades into lactic acid
    D. B and C

101. In the absence of an adequate supply of glucose for the cells, the body will do all of the following EXCEPT
    A. gluconeogenesis
    B. glycogenolysis
    C. lipolysis
    D. glycolysis

102. Which of the following is the hallmark of decompensated shock?
    A. Hypotension
    B. Unconsciousness
    C. Tachycardia
    D. Dysuria

103. Which of the following would distinguish cardiogenic shock from other forms of shock?
    A. Warm skin
    B. Tachycardia
    C. Pulmonary edema
    D. Hypotension

104. Which of the following drugs would you administer to increase contractile force without affecting heart rate?
   A. Dopamine
   B. Dobutamine
   C. Atropine
   D. Epinephrine

105. Which of the following is **NOT** considered supportive treatment for prehospital hypovolemic shock?
   A. Colloid administration
   B. Crystalloid administration
   C. Hemorrhage control
   D. Pneumatic antishock garment

106. Which of the following would distinguish neurogenic shock from other forms of shock?
   A. Warm skin
   B. Tachycardia
   C. Altered mental status
   D. Hypotension

107. Prehospital management of neurogenic shock includes all of the following **EXCEPT**
   A. vasopressors
   B. IV crystalloids
   C. maintenance body temperature
   D. atropine

108. Prehospital management of anaphylactic shock includes all of the following **EXCEPT**
   A. vasopressors
   B. IV crystalloids
   C. inhaled beta antagonists
   D. antihistamines

109. Which of the following would distinguish septic shock from other forms of shock?
   A. High fever
   B. Tachycardia
   C. Altered mental status
   D. Hypotension

110. The mortality rate for a patient with MODS is
   A. 100%
   B. 60–90%
   C. 30–60%
   D. 80–95%

111. Which of the following is a result of MODS?
   A. Decreased capillary permeability
   B. Massive vasoconstriction
   C. Increased aerobic metabolism
   D. Clotting abnormalities

112. How long does MODS typically take to result in death?
   A. 24 hours
   B. 3 days
   C. 1 week
   D. 3 weeks

113. Which of the following statements is true regarding bacteria?
   A. They are multicell organisms
   B. They cannot reproduce independently
   C. They bind to host cells for support
   D. They contain an organized nucleus

114. Most antibiotics are designed to kill or inhibit bacteria by
   A. consuming the host cell
   B. weakening the cell membrane
   C. introducing bradykinins into the area
   D. surrounding the host cell and cutting off nourishment

115. *Clostridium botulinum* and *Clostridium tetani* are caused by
   A. endotoxins
   B. extracellular antibodies
   C. exotoxins
   D. intracellular antigens

116. When endotoxins are released into the bloodstream, they can cause
   A. widespread clotting
   B. capillary damage
   C. fever
   D. all of the above

117. Fever is caused by
   A. pathogens
   B. pryogens
   C. bacteria
   D. exotoxins

118. Most infections are caused by
   A. bacteria
   B. viruses
   C. fungi
   D. mycoses

119. Which of the following is an example of a dormant virus?
   A. HIV
   B. Botulinum tetani
   C. Varicella zoster
   D. All of the above

120. Which of the following statements explains why viruses are difficult to treat?
   A. The host cell must also be destroyed
   B. No effective drugs have been developed
   C. Viruses mutate frequently
   D. All of the above

121. Which of the following is NOT one of the body's three chief lines of self-defense against infection and injury?
   A. Anatomical barriers
   B. Endocrine system
   C. Inflammatory response
   D. Immune response

122. Which of the following statements is true regarding the inflammatory response?

   A. It is specific
   B. It is slow acting
   C. It is transient and has no memory
   D. It involves one plasma protein system and one blood cell type

123. Which of the following statements is true regarding active acquired immunity?
   A. It is part of your genetic makeup
   B. It is temporary
   C. It can be from an injected serum
   D. It is generated by exposure to an antigen

124. Which of the following immunoglobulins has memory and remembers certain antigens?
   A. IgM
   B. IgG
   C. IgA
   D. IgE

125. The thoracic duct is a receptacle for
   A. venous blood
   B. lymph
   C. immunoglobulins
   D. arterial blood

126. Which of the following substances is likely to produce an immune response?
   A. Amino acid
   B. Protein
   C. Monosaccharide
   D. Fatty acid

127. Which of the following statements best describes the function of the thoracic duct?
   A. It collects venous blood prior to the vena cava
   B. It receives lymph from the body
   C. It manufactures and secretes lymph
   D. It connects the spleen with the subclavian vein

128. Not all antigens elicit an immune response. Ones that do not probably are not
    A. large enough
    B. complex enough
    C. foreign enough
    D. all of the above

129. The universal recipient is blood type
    A. A
    B. B
    C. AB
    D. O

130. The universal donor is blood type
    A. A
    B. B
    C. AB
    D. O

131. Lymphocytes are generated from stem cells in the bone marrow that eventually mature into
    A. B lymphocytes
    B. T lymphocytes
    C. thrombocytes
    D. all of the above

132. B lymphocytes mature following travel through the
    A. thymus gland
    B. thalamus
    C. spleen
    D. thoracic duct

133. B lymphocytes then develop
    A. antibodies to specific antigens
    B. cells that memorize antigens
    C. a swift response to destroy the antigen
    D. all of the above

Match the following immunoglobulins with their respective functions:

134. ____ IgA
135. ____ IgD
136. ____ IgE
137. ____ IgG
138. ____ IgM
    A. Recognizes repeat antigen invasions
    B. Contributes to allergic and anaphylaxis reactions
    C. Present in body secretions
    D. Produced first in primary immune response
    E. Little known, little understood

139. Antibodies produced in the laboratory that are specific to a single antigen are called
    A. isotypic
    B. allotypic
    C. monoclonal
    D. idiotypic

140. The first line of defense against pathogens is the _____ immune system.
    A. secretory
    B. cell-mediated
    C. humoral
    D. pathogenic

141. Which of the following statements is true regarding T lymphocytes?
    A. The cell-mediated immunity they create is long lasting
    B. They attack pathogens directly
    C. They produce antibodies that attack the pathogens
    D. All of the above

142. Proteins produced by white blood cells that regulate immune responses by binding with and affecting the function of the cells that produced them or of other nearby cells are called
    A. cytokines
    B. monoclonal antibodies
    C. interleukins
    D. Th cells

143. Which of the following is **NOT** a function of the inflammatory response?
    A. Walling off the inflamed area
    B. Developing a memory for foreign substances
    C. Promoting healing
    D. Stimulating the immune response

144. The inflammatory response includes
    A. increased capillary permeability
    B. selected vasoconstriction and vasodilation
    C. mobilization of leukocytes and plasma proteins
    D. all of the above

145. The chief activator(s) of the inflammatory response is/are the
    A. spleen
    B. thymus gland
    C. mast cells
    D. leukocytes

146. Which of the following can trigger mast cell degranulation?
    A. Trauma
    B. Snake venom
    C. Bee sting
    D. All of the above

147. Which of the following is released as a result of mast cell degranulation?
    A. Histamine
    B. Serotonin
    C. Chemotactic factors
    D. All of the above

148. Which of the following causes the same effects as histamine but is longer lasting?
    A. Leukotrienes
    B. Prostaglandins

    C. Lysosomes
    D. Bradykinin

149. The plasma protein system that consists of 11 proteins that work in a cascade manner to destroy invading organisms is the _____ system.
    A. kinin
    B. complement
    C. coagulation
    D. prostaglandin

150. The plasma protein system that forms a network at the site of inflammation and whose end is to produce fibrin is the _____ system.
    A. kinin
    B. complement
    C. coagulation
    D. prostaglandin

151. The plasma protein system that causes vasodilation, extravascular smooth muscle contraction, increased permeability, and chemotaxis is the _____ system.
    A. kinin
    B. complement
    C. coagulation
    D. prostaglandin

152. The inflammatory process includes all of the following **EXCEPT**
    A. red blood cell exudate
    B. vascular response
    C. increased permeability
    D. margination

153. Neutrophils, eosinophils, and basophils are also known as
    A. lymphokines
    B. granulocytes
    C. interleukins
    D. cytokines

154. Cells that work like the Pac-Man® video game by eating up the enemy cells are called
A. interleukins
B. lymphocytes
C. phagocytes
D. monocytes

Match the following cellular products with their respective definitions:

155. ____ Interleukin
156. ____ Lymphokine
157. ____ Interferon
158. ____ Cytokine
159. ____ MIF
160. ____ MAF

A. Stimulates monocytes to become macrophages
B. Acts as a messenger between cells
C. Prevents virus migration
D. Inhibits macrophage migration from the site
E. Stimulates the lymphocyte response
F. Enhances macrophage activity

161. Which of the following is NOT a chief manifestation of acute inflammation?
A. Increased body temperature
B. Increased heart rate and blood pressure
C. Increased leukocytes
D. Increased plasma proteins

162. Fibroblasts are cells that
A. produce pus
B. secrete collagen
C. wall off the offending pathogens
D. secrete macrophages

163. Pus is comprised of all of the following EXCEPT
A. dead cells
B. bits of dead tissue
C. tissue fluid
D. fibroblasts

164. Sometimes people with tuberculosis have hard-walled structures caused by microbacteria that resist destruction by macrophages. These are called
A. leukophages
B. diapedesis
C. granulomas
D. mast cells

165. As you inspect a patient's exudate, you observe that it contains thick, purulent pus. You suspect the infection is
A. viral
B. bacterial
C. parasitic
D. almost healed

166. A scab is comprised of all of the following EXCEPT
A. epithelial cells
B. fibrin
C. erythrocytes
D. leukocytes

167. The filling of a wound by the inward growth of healthy tissues from the wound edge is known as
A. epithelialization
B. contraction
C. granulation
D. maturation

168. The scab is eventually separated from the wound surface during a process called
A. epithelialization
B. contraction
C. granulation
D. maturation

169. The inward movement of wound edges during healing that eventually brings the wound edges together is called
A. epithelialization
B. contraction

C. granulation

D. maturation

170. Which of the following can cause dysfunctional healing during inflammation?

A. Hypovolemia

B. Excess fibrin in the wound

C. Bleeding

D. All of the above

171. The use of steroid drugs can cause dysfunctional healing during reconstruction by

A. suppressing epithelialization

B. inhibiting collagen synthesis

C. stimulating collagen synthesis

D. all of the above

172. You have an allergic reaction to pollen every spring. This is an example of a(n)

A. autoimmunity

B. alloimmunity

C. hypersensitivity

D. isoimmunity

173. Hyperthyroidism is an example of

A. autoimmunity

B. alloimmunity

C. allergy

D. isoimmunity

174. All of the following are clinical indications of an IgE-mediated hypersensitivity response EXCEPT

A. urticaria

B. peripheral vasoconstriction

C. laryngeal edema

D. abdominal cramping

175. Which of the following statements is true regarding stress?

A. It is a state of physical arousal

B. It is a state of psychological arousal

C. It exists to some degree in everyone

D. All of the above

176. Any agent or situation that causes stress is called a/an

A. antagonist

B. stressor

C. alarmist

D. none of the above

177. Which of the following is NOT part of the body's response to stress?

A. Epinephrine and norepinephrine are released

B. The pulse rate and blood pressure decrease

C. The pupils dilate

D. Blood glucose levels increase

178. Which of the following best describes the alarm stage?

A. It occurs at the first exposure to the stressor

B. It results in a sympathetic nervous system activation

C. If resistance is low, the response can be overwhelming

D. All of the above

179. Which of the following statements best describes the resistance stage?

A. The victim is beginning to cope

B. Vital signs return to normal

C. Resistance to the stressor becomes stronger

D. All of the above

180. Which of the following statements best describes the exhaustion stage?

A. The victim no longer can adapt to the stressor

B. Alarm stage signs reappear

C. Alarm stage signs are more difficult to reverse

D. All of the above

181. Another term for dynamic steady state is
    A. hemostasis
    B. turnover
    C. burnout
    D. homeostasis

182. Which of the following is NOT a catecholamine?
    A. Norepinephrine
    B. Adrenalin
    C. Cortisol
    D. Epinephrine

Match the following physiological effects with their respective adrenergic receptors:

183. ____ Peripheral vasoconstriction
184. ____ Increased heart rate
185. ____ Bronchoconstriction
186. ____ Bronchodilation
187. ____ Increased cardiac contractions
188. ____ Vasodilation

    A. Alpha 1
    B. Alpha 2
    C. Beta 1
    D. Beta 2

189. Which of the following statements best describes the role of cortisol in the stress response?
    A. It is both helpful and harmful
    B. It promotes and hastens the healing process
    C. It increases the immune response
    D. It decreases blood glucose levels

190. All of the following hormones show an increase during the stress response EXCEPT
    A. growth hormone
    B. testosterone
    C. prolactin
    D. adrenocorticotropic hormone

answers & rationales

1.

D. The basic unit of life is the cell. It contains all the necessary components to turn essential nutrients into energy and to carry on essential life functions. (PCPP 1–161   EPC 96)

2.

D. The three main components of a cell are the cell membrane (semipermeable outer covering), the cytoplasm (thick, viscous fluid), and the organelles (inner structures). (PCPP 1–161   EPC 97)

Matching (PCPP 1–163   EPC 98)

3. **F**	Nucleus	**A.**	Scavenger cell
4. **C**	Cytosol	**B.**	Packages enzymes and mucus
5. **B**	Golgi		
6. **E**	Mitochondrion	**C.**	Clear liquid portion of cytoplasm
7. **G**	Lysosome		
8. **D**	Peroxisome	**D.**	Neutralizes alcohol and toxins
9. **A**	Phagocyte		
		E.	Energy factory
		F.	Contains DNA
		G.	Contains digestive enzymes

10.

A. The cell membrane is a semipermeable structure that surrounds the cell and protects it from the outer environment. (PCPP 1–164   EPC 99)

11.

D. Epithelial tissue lines body surfaces and protects the body. Certain types of epithelial tissue perform specialized functions, such as secretion, absorption, diffusion, and filtration. (PCPP 1–165   EPC 100)

12.

A. Cardiac muscle tissue is found only within the heart. It has the unique capability of spontaneous contraction without external stimulation. This property is called automaticity. (PCPP 1–165 EPC 100)

13.

C. Connective tissue is the most abundant tissue in the body. It provides support, connection, and insulation. (PCPP 1–165   EPC 100)

14.

C. The type of muscle found in the inner lining of hollow organs, such as the intestines, airways, and blood vessels, is called smooth muscle. It is generally under the control of the involuntary or autonomic component of the central nervous system. (PCPP 1–165   EPC 100)

15.

D. The natural tendency of the body to maintain a constant, stable internal environment is called homeostasis. The paramedic should understand this process in order to recognize how the body attempts to correct underlying problems. (PCPP 1–167   EPC 102)

16.

B. Endocrine glands are ductless and secrete their hormones directly into the circulatory system. Examples include the pancreas, pituitary gland, thyroid, parathyroid, adrenal gland, and gonads. Glands that release their secretion into the epithelial surfaces of the body are called exocrine glands. Examples of these secretions are mucus, sweat, and saliva. (PCPP 1–167   EPC 102)

17.

C. As the name suggests, chemoreceptors respond to changes in chemistry. Our chemoreceptors, located in the medulla, the carotid arteries, and the aortic arch, sense changes in pH, PO_2, and PCO_2. (PCPP 1–168   EPC 102)

18.

A. As the name suggests, baroreceptors respond to changes in pressure in our circulatory system. They are located in the carotid sinus and the aortic arch. They are stretch receptors that stretch with increased pressure in the blood vessel. (PCPP 1–168 EPC 102)

19.

D. A negative feedback loop occurs when the body attempts to reverse, or compensate for, a pathophysiological process. In this example, the body tries to increase blood pressure through a series of compensatory mechanisms until the pressure returns to normal, similar to a thermostat that triggers the furnace to turn on when the temperature drops below your setting. (PCPP 1–169   EPC 103)

20.

A. Atrophy is a decrease in cell size resulting from a decreased workload. If you don't use it, you lose it. Muscle atrophy is common after a prolonged immobilization. (PCPP 1–170   EPC 265)

21.

B. Hypertrophy is an increase in cell size resulting from an increased workload. Body builders increase muscle bulk and strength by increasing the stress on the muscle groups. The heart and kidneys can also hypertrophy through an increased workload. (PCPP 1–171   EPC 265)

22.

A. Metaplasia is the replacement of one type of cell by another type of cell that is not normal for that tissue. One reason COPD patients cannot clear their lungs of mucus efficiently is that the normal ciliated columnar epithelial cells have been replaced by nonciliated stratified squamous epithelial cells—no cilia, no clearance. (PCPP 1–171 EPC 266)

23.

C. Hyperplasia is an increase in the number of cells, resulting from an increased workload. Calloused elbows are simply an increase in epidermal cells in response to the stress of leaning on the elbows (tripod position) in an effort to breathe easier. (PCPP 1–171   EPC 266)

24.

B. Hypoxia, decreased oxygen to the tissues, is the most common cause of cellular injury. Hypoxia can be the result of ventilation (airway, breathing, oxygen concentration) or perfusion (circulation). Left untreated, the cells and tissues die (infarct). (PCPP 1–172   EPC 267)

25.

D. During anaerobic metabolism, the cells continue to do their jobs but without an adequate oxygen supply. The result is a marked decrease in ATP production and an increase of harmful acids. If oxygen is applied in time, the condition is reversible. If not, it is irreversible, and cell death is imminent. (PCPP 1–172   EPC 267)

26.

D. Cellular injury due to chemical products is common, especially among children. Chemical injuries can cause disruption of the cell membrane, resulting in enzymatic reactions, altered coagulation, and cell death. (PCPP 1–173   EPC 267)

27.

A. A pathogen's virulence refers to its ability to cause damage. This is dependent on its ability to invade and destroy cells, produce toxins, and produce hypersensitivity reactions. (PCPP 1–173   EPC 267)

28.

C. The inflammatory and immunologic processes are essential to the destruction of foreign substances and aid in healing. Unfortunately cell membranes are often destroyed, and healthy cells are often damaged. Fortunately, once the foreign cells are destroyed, the damaged cells repair themselves. (PCPP 1–173   EPC 268)

29.

D. Some diseases are caused by environmental factors (bacterial invasion), some by genetic defect, and others by the combined effects of both. (PCPP 1–174   EPC 268)

30.

A. Anabolism is the constructive phase of metabolism, in which cells convert nonliving substances (such as calcium) into living cytoplasm (such as bone). The body uses the calcium in the blood and uses it to build bone. As blood calcium levels drop, the body catabolizes the bone to release the needed calcium. (PCPP 1–174   EPC 269)

31.

D. The most common result from cellular injury is swelling. This occurs due to damage to the cell membrane leading to increased permeability. Without a stable cell membrane, proper intra- and extra-cellular fluid and electrolyte levels will not be maintained. (PCPP 1–175   EPC 270)

32.

B. The process of apoptosis is a normal form of bodily housekeeping. The body rids itself of damaged and dead cells by having the injured cell release a digestive enzyme that destroys the cell. Then phagocytes come along and clear the digested cells away. (PCPP 1–176   EPC 270)

33.

D. Gangrene comes in three varieties: gas (a bacterial infection releasing gas bubbles), dry (a coagulative process affecting the skin of the lower extremities), and wet (liquefactive necrosis of the internal organs). (PCPP 1–176   EPC 270)

34.

B. Water is the most abundant substance in the human body. In fact, it accounts for approximately 60% of total body weight. (PCPP 1–176   EPC 104)

35.

C. Approximately 75% of total body water (TBW) is found within the intracellular compartment. This compartment is found inside the body's cells. Refer to the following chart: (PCPP 1–177   EPC 105)

Compartment	Percentage of TBW	Volume in 70 kg Adult
Intracellular fluid	75.0	31.50 L
Extracellular fluid	25.0	10.50 L
Interstitial fluid	17.5	7.35 L
Intravascular fluid	7.5	3.15 L

36.

B. As we age, our TBW decreases. Refer to the following chart: (PCPP 1–177   EPC 105)

Age	TBW
Infant	75–80%
1 year	70–75%
Late childhood	65–70%
Early adulthood	65–70% males
	60–65% females
Late adulthood	45–55%

37.

C. When your fluid levels drop, the pituitary gland at the base of the brain secrets ADH, or antidiuretic hormone. ADH causes the kidneys to reabsorb more water back into the bloodstream and excrete less urine. (PCPP 1–178   EPC 106)

38.

B. Clinically the dehydrated patient exhibits dry mucous membranes and poor skin turgor. As the dehydration becomes more severe, the pulse will quicken, and the blood pressure will drop. In infants, the anterior fontanel may be sunken. (PCPP 1–179   EPC 107)

39.

D. Treatment for dehydration is fluid replacement. Since you cannot determine electrolyte deficits in the field, you should use isotonic solutions, such as normal saline or lactated Ringer's. For mild to moderate dehydration, run the infusion at 100–200 ml per hour. (PCPP 1–179   EPC 107)

40.

A. Electrolytes are substances that dissociate into charged particles when placed in water. Ions with a positive charge are called cations. (PCPP 1–181 EPC 109)

41.

B. Sodium is the most prevalent cation in the extracellular fluid. It plays a major role in regulating the distribution of water. (PCPP 1–182 EPC 109)

42.

C. Potassium is the most prevalent cation in the intracellular fluid. It plays an important role in the transmission of electrical impulses. (PCPP 1–182 EPC 109)

43.

D. Calcium has many physiological functions. It plays a major role in muscular contraction as well as nerve impulse transmission. (PCPP 1–182 EPC 109)

44.

A. Bicarbonate is the principal buffer of the body. It neutralizes the highly acidic hydrogen ion and other organic acids. (PCPP 1–182 EPC 109)

45.

B. Electrolytes are usually measured in milliequivalents per liter (mEq/L). (PCPP 1–182 EPC 110)

46.

D. Osmosis is the movement of water across a semipermeable membrane from an area of lesser solute concentration to an area of greater solute concentration. This movement occurs until the solute concentrations on both sides are equal. (PCPP 1–183 EPC 110)

47.

A. Infusing a hypotonic solution into the bloodstream causes water to move from the bloodstream into the cells. This occurs because water tends to move from areas of low solute concentration, which in this case will be the bloodstream, toward areas of higher solute concentration, which in this case will be the interstitial spaces and cells. (PCPP 1–183 EPC 110)

48.

A. Diffusion is the movement of solutes from an area of greater concentration to an area of lesser concentration. This movement occurs until the solute concentrations on both sides are equal. (PCPP 1–183 EPC 110)

49.

D. Infusing a hypertonic solution into a blood vessel will cause an osmotic gradient, which shifts water into the blood vessel. This will cause an increase in blood pressure. (PCPP 1–183 EPC 110)

50.

C. A solution with the same osmolarity as blood plasma is isotonic. Isotonicity is a state in which solutions on opposite sides of a semipermeable membrane have equal concentrations. (PCPP 1–183 EPC 110)

51.

B. In a freshwater drowning, water enters the pulmonary capillaries and quickly diffuses into the cells. This occurs because freshwater is hypotonic. (PCPP 1–183 EPC 110)

52.

D. Sodium is transported out of the cell by a process called active transport. Active transport is a biochemical process in which substances use energy to move across the cell membrane against the normal gradient. Active transport is faster than diffusion, but it requires the expenditure of energy. (PCPP 1–184 EPC 111)

53.

A. The insulin/glucose relationship is an example of facilitated diffusion. Facilitated diffusion is a biochemical process in which a substance is selectively transported across a membrane using helper proteins and requires energy. (PCPP 1–184 EPC 112)

54.

C. Oncotic force or pressure is caused by the presence of plasma proteins in the blood, which make the blood hypertonic and draw water into the bloodstream. This is the principal force that returns water to the blood from the capillary beds following cellular respiration. (PCPP 1–185 EPC 112)

55.

D. While oncotic force pulls water into the intravascular space, hydrostatic pressure forces water out. This process, known as filtration, is caused by the pressure increase in the arteries during systole. Normally these opposing processes equal out. When they do not, the result is tissue edema or poor turgor. (PCPP 1–185 EPC 112)

56.

D. Tissue edema is caused by an increase in hydrostatic pressure, a decrease in oncotic force, increased capillary permeability, or a blocked lymph channel. In these cases, water remains in the interstitial spaces and cannot be absorbed into circulation. (PCPP 1–186   EPC 113)

57.

C. Osmoreceptors, located in the hypothalamus, monitor for changes in the osmolarity of the blood. When the blood has less fluid, the osmoreceptors stimulate the release of antidiuretic hormone (ADH), which stimulates water reabsorption in the kidneys. (PCPP 1–187)

58.

B. Plasma makes up approximately 55% of the total blood volume. It consists of 92% water, 6–7% proteins, and a small portion containing electrolytes, lipids, enzymes, clotting factors, glucose, and other dissolved substances. (PCPP 1–187   EPC 120)

59.

B. The percentage of blood occupied by red blood cells is referred to as the hematocrit. Normal hematocrit in the healthy person is approximately 45%. (PCPP 1–187   EPC 121)

60.

B. Red blood cells account for approximately 45% of the total blood volume. This percentage is known as the patient's hematocrit. (PCPP 1–187 EPC 121)

61.

D. Signs and symptoms of a transfusion reaction include fever, chills, hives, hypotension, palpitations, tachycardia, flushing of the skin, headache, loss of consciousness, nausea and vomiting, and shortness of breath. If you suspect a transfusion reaction, stop the IV, infuse normal saline, and monitor the patient closely. (PCPP 1–189   EPC 1499)

62.

A. Hespan, dextran, and albumin are examples of colloids. Colloids are solutions that contain proteins or other high molecular weight molecules that tend to remain in the intravascular space for an extended period of time. (PCPP 1–189   EPC 450)

63.

B. Colloids create a colloid osmotic pressure and tend to attract water into the intravascular space. Colloids

draw water from the interstitial spaces and the intracellular compartment in order to increase the intravascular blood volume. (PCPP 1–189   EPC 450)

64.

B. The normal pH for the human body is 7.35–7.45. (PCPP 1–191   EPC 113)

65.

C. There are three major mechanisms to remove acids from the body. The fastest mechanism is often referred to as the buffer system, or the bicarbonate buffer system. This system works in seconds. (PCPP 1–192   EPC 113)

66.

A. A patient with a pH of 7.2 and a $PaCO_2$ of 52 torr is in a state of respiratory acidosis. (PCPP 1–195 EPC 276)

67.

A. A probable cause of this patient's condition could be a near-drowning. Respiratory acidosis is caused by the retention of carbon dioxide. This can result from impaired ventilation due to problems occurring in either the lungs or the respiratory center of the brain. (PCPP 1–195   EPC 276)

68.

D. The reasons behind this patient's pH and $PaCO_2$ levels include a decrease in carbon dioxide elimination and an increase in carbon dioxide retention. (PCPP 1–195   EPC 276)

69.

C. Immediate management of the patient in respiratory acidosis is aimed at improving ventilation and oxygenation. Vigorously ventilate this patient with positive pressure and 100% oxygen. (PCPP 1–195 EPC 276)

70.

D. Alkalosis is a state in which the patient's hydrogen ion concentration is abnormally low and the pH is high. (PCPP 1–195   EPC 276)

71.

B. Management of a patient in respiratory alkalosis is aimed at helping the patient retain carbon dioxide.

Respiratory alkalosis results from the excessive elimination of carbon dioxide. This can occur with anxiety or after climbing to a high altitude. It can also occur as a compensatory mechanism in shock and a variety of other serious hypoxic conditions. For this reason, withholding oxygen from this patient could prove to be a fatal mistake. Simply place your patient on a rebreather mask with 10–15 liters/minute oxygen flow, and coach him to breathe slowly. (PCPP 1–195   EPC 276)

Matching   (PCPP 1–195   EPC 276)

72. **B**   Respiratory acidosis   **A.** Unchecked diabetes
73. **D**   Respiratory alkalosis   **B.** Strangulation
74. **A**   Metabolic acidosis   **C.** Diuretic overuse
75. **C**   Metabolic alkalosis   **D.** Anxiety

76.
D. Diseases such as sickle cell and cystic fibrosis are considered purely genetic because they are caused by a defect in a single gene. The others have genetic and environmental components. (PCPP 1–198 EPC 278)

77.
C. Risk factors for diseases include environmental (lifestyle) and genetic factors. Of these, only lung cancer is considered strictly environmental. It usually is caused by inhaling smoke, asbestos, arsenic, or nickel. (PCPP 1–199   EPC 279)

78.
D. Diabetes is the most common endocrine disease. Type I (juvenile onset) is characterized by a pancreas that produces little or no insulin. Type II (adult onset) is more common but less severe because the pancreas does produce some, but not enough, insulin. (PCPP 1–200   EPC 280)

79.
A. Hemophilia is a bleeding disorder caused by a genetic clotting factor deficiency inherited usually by males from the mother. (PCPP 1–201   EPC 281)

80.
C. Most cardiovascular diseases are genetic in origin with environmental factors contributing. Cardiomyopathy, an exception, is thought to be primarily due to infectious disease, toxic exposure,

connective tissue disease, or nutritional deficiency. (PCPP 1–201   EPC 281)

81.
B. The primary cause of chronic renal failure is hypertension. Acute renal failure is caused by prerenal factors (shock, dehydration, vasopressor drugs), renal factors (trauma, nephrotoxic drugs, infection), and postrenal factors (enlarged prostate, ureter or bladder cancer). (PCPP 1–201 EPC 282)

82.
D. Gout is a condition with hereditary and environmental factors. It is characterized by crystal deposits in the joints (especially the big toe), causing a great deal of pain. Crystals form because of high levels of uric acid in the blood (uremia) caused by a genetic abnormality. (PCPP 1–202   EPC 282)

83.
B. The causes of peptic ulcer disease (PUD) include the *Helicobacter pylori* bacteria, diet, stress, and alcohol consumption. (PCPP 1–202   EPC 282)

84.
C. Although the exact cause is unknown, multiple sclerosis seems to be the result of a destruction of the myelin sheath by an autoimmune response. It affects the nerves of the eyes, the brain, and spinal cord. (PCPP 1–203   EPC 283)

85.
A. The amount of blood ejected by the heart at one contraction is referred to as the stroke volume. Stroke volume is determined by preload, afterload, and contractile force. (PCPP 1–204   EPC 222)

86.
D. Stroke Volume could be increased by increasing the venous return, by increasing the contractile force of the heart, and by decreasing the afterload. (PCPP 1–204   EPC 222)

87.
C. The amount of blood pumped from the heart in one contraction is called stroke volume. It is measured

in ml. Normal stroke volume in the healthy adult at rest is 60–100 ml. (PCPP 1–204 EPC 222)

88.

C. The greater the volume of the preload is, the more the ventricles are stretched. The greater the stretch, up to a certain point, the greater the subsequent cardiac contraction. This is referred to as the Frank-Starling mechanism. (PCPP 1–204 EPC 223)

89.

B. For a patient in severe congestive heart failure (CHF), you want to decrease the workload on the heart by decreasing preload. You could accomplish this by administering drugs such as nitroglycerin, furosemide, and morphine, which dilate the veins. Dilating the veins causes pooling of blood on the venous side and decreases preload. (PCPP 1–204 EPC 223)

90.

C. The amount of blood pumped by the heart in 1 minute is called cardiac output. Cardiac output is calculated by stroke volume times heart rate. (PCPP 1–204 EPC 223)

91.

C. The amount of resistance against which the heart must pump is called afterload. The heart must overcome this resistance in order to eject blood. Afterload is determined by the degree of peripheral vascular resistance. Peripheral resistance is determined by the degree of vasoconstriction present on the arterial side. (PCPP 1–204 EPC 223)

92.

D. Baroreceptors are located in the carotid bodies and the arch of the aorta. These stretch receptors closely monitor blood pressure by the amount of stretch. (PCPP 1–205 EPC 223)

93.

A. Baroreceptors are stretch receptors that stretch with increased pressure. When they detect reduced flow and pressure, they send messages to the brain to stimulate the sympathetic nervous system. This results in increased heart rate and cardiac output to increase circulation and bronchodilation. (PCPP 1–205 EPC 223)

94.

D. Blood flow through a blood vessel is determined by peripheral resistance and pressure within the system. Peripheral resistance is defined as resistance to blood flow and is dependent on three factors: the length of the vessel, the diameter of the vessel, and blood viscosity. (PCPP 1–205 EPC 223)

95.

C. There is very little resistance to blood flow through the aorta and arteries. A significant change in peripheral resistance occurs at the arteriole level. This is because the inside diameter of the arteriole is much smaller as compared to the aorta and arteries. Additionally the arteriole has a pronounced ability to change its diameter as much as fivefold in response to local tissue needs and autonomic nervous system signals. (PCPP 1 206 EPC 224)

96.

D. The movement and utilization of oxygen in the body depend on the following conditions: an adequate concentration of inspired oxygen, appropriate movement of oxygen across the alveolar-capillary membrane into the bloodstream, an adequate number of red blood cells to carry the oxygen, proper tissue perfusion, and efficient off-loading of oxygen at the tissue level. These conditions are collectively known as the Fick principle. (PCPP 1–207 EPC 225)

97.

D. During periods of inadequate tissue perfusion, cell metabolism switches from an aerobic to an anaerobic mode. Results of this process are inefficient energy, an increase in pyruvic acid formation, and glycolysis. (PCPP 1–209 EPC 285)

98.

C. The first stage of glucose breakdown is known as glycolysis, which does not require oxygen and creates pyruvic acid. This stage is anaerobic. (PCPP 1–209 EPC 285)

99.

A. The second stage of glucose metabolism is the Krebs cycle. During this stage, oxygen degrades the pyruvic acid into carbon dioxide and water and releases energy in the form of ATP (adenosine triphosphate). (PCPP 1–209 EPC 285)

100.

D. During the shock state, the absence of oxygen for cellular metabolism results in glycolysis, which creates pyruvic acid. The pyruvic acid degrades into lactic acid, reducing oxygen transport by red blood cells and furthering cell hypoxia. (PCPP 1–209   EPC 285)

101.

D. In the absence of an adequate glucose supply, the body will derive energy from fats (lipolysis), convert glycogen into glucose (glycogenolysis), and create glucose from protein (gluconeogenesis). (PCPP 1–210   EPC 286)

102.

A. Decompensated shock means that your compensatory mechanisms no longer can maintain adequate perfusion. During this stage, the peripheral vasculature reopens, enlarging the circulatory tank and dropping the blood pressure. (PCPP 1–212   EPC 287)

103.

C. A major difference between cardiogenic shock and other forms of shock is the presence of pulmonary edema, usually caused by left ventricular failure. (PCPP 1–213   EPC 289)

104.

B. If you wish to increase blood pressure by increasing the force of contractions but do not wish to increase myocardial oxygen demands and consumption, administer dobutamine (a positive inotrope with no chronotropic properties). (PCPP 1–213   EPC 290)

105.

A. Prehospital supportive treatment for hypovolemic shock includes hemorrhage control, administration of crystalloids, and, in some cases, the pneumatic antishock garment. (PCPP 1–214   EPC 290)

106.

A. Neurogenic shock causes massive vasodilation because of the lack of sympathetic innervation, which causes the vessels to constrict. This causes the skin, normally pale and cool from vasoconstriction, to be pink and warm. (PCPP 1–214 EPC 290)

107.

D. Prehospital management of neurogenic shock includes IV fluids (to fill the enlarged tank), vasopressors (to reduce tank size), and maintenance of body temperature. (PCPP 1–214   EPC 291)

108.

C. Prehospital management of anaphylactic shock includes IV crystalloids (to refill the tank), vasopressors (to vasocontrict and relieve swollen airway tissue), corticosteroids (to reduce inflammation), antihistamines (to block histamine receptors), and inhaled beta agonists (to dilate the airways). (PCPP 1–216   EPC 292)

109.

A. Septic shock is caused by an infection that enters the bloodstream and is carried throughout the body. The pyrogens cause massive vasodilation. High fever is a common finding except in the elderly or very young. (PCPP 1–216   EPC 292)

110.

B. MODS stands for multiple organ dysfunction syndrome, a massive inflammatory response that follows a variety of serious diseases. It is the major cause of death following sepsis, trauma, and burn injuries. (PCPP 1–217   EPC 293)

111.

D. As a result of MODS, a cascade of responses produces massive vasodilation, increased permeability of the capillaries, cardiac dysrhythmias, endothelial damage, and clotting abnormalities. (PCPP 1–217   EPC 293)

112.

D. MODS usually takes about 3 weeks to cause death. The most important time is the first 24 hours. If you can recognize the signs of early MODS (low-grade fever, tachycardia, dyspnea, altered mental status, and a general hypermetabolic-hyperdynamic state) and provide supportive measures, that is your patient's only chance for survival. (PCPP 1–218   EPC 295)

113.

C. Bacteria are single-cell organisms that lack an organized nucleus and can reproduce independently. They require a host cell to supply food and other support. They are classified according to their appearance underneath a microscope following the application of gram stains. (PCPP 1–220   EPC 296)

114.

B. Most broad-spectrum antibiotics are designed to kill bacteria or inhibit their growth by destroying the bacterial cell membrane, allowing phagocytes to ingest and destroy the pathogen. (PCPP 1–220   EPC 296)

115.

C. Exotoxins are poisonous proteins secreted by bacterial cells during their growth that cause problems elsewhere in the body. Examples include *Clostridium botulinum*, which causes a cholinergic blockade, resulting in paralysis, and *Clostridium tetani*, which causes spastic muscle rigidity. (PCPP 1–220   EPC 296)

116.

D. Endotoxins are complex molecules contained in the cell walls of certain gram-negative bacteria that can be released when the bacterial cell is attacked by an antibiotic. When released, the endotoxin can cause widespread clotting, capillary damage, hypotension, respiratory distress, and fever. This condition is known as septicemia, or sepsis. (PCPP 1–221   EPC 297)

117.

B. As macrophages attempt to destroy bacteria, they release substances known as pyrogens, which cause an increase in temperature and thus aid in the destruction of the pathogens. (PCPP 1–221   EPC 297)

118.

B. Most infections are caused by viruses, the intracellular parasites that invade the cells of the organism they infect. They cannot grow without the assistance of another organism. (PCPP 1–221   EPC 297)

119.

C. In some cases, a virus can become dormant in a host cell for years. A common example is the varicella zoster virus, which causes chicken pox in childhood and reappears as shingles in adulthood, sometimes decades later. (PCPP 1–221   EPC 297)

120.

D. Viruses are difficult to treat because once they infect a cell, they can be killed only by killing the cell; no drug has been developed that will leave the host cells unharmed. In addition, viruses mutate frequently. (PCPP 1–222   EPC 298)

121.

B. There are three chief lines of self-defense against infection and injury: anatomical barriers (skin and epithelium), the inflammatory response, and the immune response. (PCPP 1–222   EPC 298)

122.

C. The inflammatory response is characterized by the following: it is fast, nonspecific, and transient (having no memory); it involves multiple plasma protein systems and multiple blood cell types. The immune response is just the opposite. (PCPP 1–223   EPC 299)

123.

D. Active acquired immunity is generated by an exposure to an antigen and is long lasting. Just the opposite, passive acquired immunity is transferred to a person from an outside source and is temporary. (PCPP 1–224   EPC 300)

124.

B. Immunoglobulin G (IgG) has memory and remembers particular antigens that have entered the body. This is part of the humoral immunity system. (PCPP 1–224)

125.

B. The thoracic duct lies in the left thorax and is the larger of two main ducts that receive lymph from the body. The contents of this duct drain into the left subclavian vein and reenter the bloodstream. (PCPP 1–226)

126.

B. Large molecules, such as proteins, polysaccharides, and nucleic acids, are the most likely to produce an immune response. Smaller molecules such as fatty acids, monosaccharides, and amino acids, are less likely to produce such a response. (PCPP 1–226)

127.

B. The thoracic duct is the main receptacle of lymph from the body. It is located on the left side of the body and empties into the left subclavian vein, returning its contents to general circulation. (PCPP 1–226)

128.

D. Not all antigens cause a reaction. To elicit an immune response, they must be large enough, foreign enough, and complex enough, and they must be found in sufficient numbers in addition to having the proper chemical structure. (PCPP 1–226)

129.

C. Persons with type AB blood are referred to as universal recipients. These people do not have antibodies to either A or B, since they carry both antigens. In an emergency, they can receive blood of any type. (PCPP 1–228   EPC 301)

130.

D. Type O blood does not contain either the A or the B antigen. In an emergency, it can be administered to a patient of any blood type. Because of this, persons with type O blood are referred to as universal donors. (PCPP 1–228   EPC 301)

131.

D. Lymphocytes are generated from stem cells in the bone marrow. From there, they mature into thrombocytes, erythrocytes, and various forms of leukocytes (including B lymphocytes and T lymphocytes). (PCPP 1–229   EPC 300)

132.

C. B lymphocytes mature as they travel through a set of lymphoid tissues, including the spleen and lymph nodes. They then become involved in humoral immunity. (PCPP 1–229   EPC 300)

133.

D. Mature B lymphocytes begin to develop antibodies to specific antigens, memory cells to recognize foreign antigens, and an immune response to the antigen. This is known as humoral immunity. (PCPP 1–229   EPC 300)

Matching (PCPP 1–233   EPC 1396)

134. C	IgA	A.	Recognizes repeat antigen
135. E	IgD		invasions
136. B	IgE	B.	Contributes to allergic and ana-
137. A	IgG		phylaxis reactions
138. D	IgM	C.	Present in body secretions
		D.	Produced first in primary im-
			mune response
		E.	Little known, little understood

139.

C. Monoclonal antibodies are produced in the laboratory to react to a single antigen. These pure antibodies are experimental and are used to identify infectious organisms, type blood and tissue, and treat autoimmune diseases and cancer. (PCPP 1–234)

140.

A. The secretory immune system is the body's first line of defense against invading pathogens. Its antibodies (IgA, IgM, IgG) are contained in tears, sweat, saliva, mucus, and breast milk. Its main defense is against ingested or inhaled pathogens. (PCPP 1–235)

141.

B. T lymphocytes, as opposed to B lymphocytes, attack pathogens directly and are short lived. They do not produce antibodies, and the cell-mediated immunity they create is temporary. (PCPP 1–235)

142.

A. Proteins produced by white blood cells that regulate immune responses by binding with and affecting the function of the cells that produced them or of other nearby cells are called cytokines. Cytokines are the messengers of the immune system that help to regulate cell function during both inflammatory and immune responses. (PCPP 1–236)

143.

B. During each phase of the inflammatory response, the components of inflammation work together to destroy and remove unwanted substances, wall off the infected or inflamed area, promote healing, and stimulate the immune response. (PCPP 1–241   EPC 303)

144.

D. The inflammatory response includes increased capillary permeability (to increase circulation at the injured site), selected vasoconstriction and vasodilation (to direct blood where needed), and the mobilization of leukocytes and plasma proteins (to destroy and remove the invader). (PCPP 1–242   EPC 304)

145.

C. The chief activators of the inflammatory response are the mast cells. The mast cell resembles a bag of granules, which, when activated, empties its contents into the extracellular environment. (PCPP 1–242   EPC 304)

146.

D. Degranulation is the process by which mast cells empty their granules into the extracellular environment. This occurs when the mast cells are stimulated by physical injury (trauma), chemical agents (venom, toxins), or hypersensitivities (bee sting, shellfish). (PCPP 1–242   EPC 304)

147.

D. During degranulation, histamine, serotonin, and chemotactic factors are released. Histamine and serotonin alter blood flow, while the chemotactic factors attract leukocytes to the injured site. (PCPP 1–243   EPC 304)

148.

A. Leukotrienes, also known as slow-reacting substances of anaphylaxis (SRS–A), have actions similar to histamine and chemotactic factors but promote slower and longer lasting effects. Leukotriene blockers, a new class of drug, are designed to decrease the inflammatory process of asthma. (PCPP 1–243   EPC 305)

149.

B. The complement system is comprised of 11 proteins that, when stimulated, work in a cascade manner to destroy invading organisms. There are two pathways involved: a slower classic pathway that is activated by an antigen-antibody complex and a faster alternate pathway that acts as the first line of inflammatory defense. (PCPP 1–244)

150.

C. The coagulation system, also called the clotting system, forms a network at the site of inflammation and also works in a cascade manner. The coagulation cascade is activated either extrinsically (injury to vessel wall) or intrinsically (exposure to collagen). The end product of the clotting cascade is fibrin. (PCPP 1–246   EPC 881)

151.

A. The kinin system, with bradykinin as its chief product, causes increased permeability, vasodilation, extravascular smooth muscle contraction, and chemotaxis. (PCPP 1–246   EPC 305)

152.

A. The inflammation sequence includes vascular response (selective constriction and dilation), increased permeability, margination (adherence of leukocytes to vessel walls), and exudation of white blood cells. (PCPP 1–247   EPC 922)

153.

B. Neutrophils (the first scavengers), eosinophils (parasite eaters), and basophils (similar to histamine) are types of granulocytes. They mobilize to destroy and remove invading organisms. (PCPP 1–248   EPC 922)

154.

C. Phagocytes are cells that destroy the enemy cells by swallowing them up. The most important phagocytes are macrophages and neutrophils. (PCPP 1–248   EPC 922)

Matching   (PCPP 1–249)

155. E	Interleukin	**A.**	Stimulates monocytes to become macrophages
156. A	Lymphokine		
157. C	Interferon	**B.**	Acts as a messenger between cells
158. B	Cytokine		
159. D	MIF	**C.**	Prevents virus migration
160. F	MAF	**D.**	Inhibits macrophage migration from the site
		E.	Stimulates the lymphocyte response
		F.	Enhances macrophage activity

161.

B. The three chief manifestations of acute inflammation include fever (to create a hostile environment for the invading pathogen), increased leukocytes in the blood (to destroy and remove the pathogen), and increased plasma proteins (to inhibit and control the inflammatory response). (PCPP 1–250   EPC 306)

162.

B. Fibroblasts are cells that secrete collagen, a critical factor in wound healing. (PCPP 1–250   EPC 306)

163.

D. Pus is a liquid mixture of dead cells (neutrophils, lymphocytes, macrophages), bits of dead tissue, and tissue fluid. It usually collects in a cavity formed by dead leukocytes. (PCPP 1–250   EPC 306)

164.

C. Granulomas are hard-walled structures caused by microbacteria that resist destruction by macrophages. Patients with tuberculosis and leprosy often have them for life. (PCPP 1–250   EPC 306)

165.

B. In persistent bacterial infections, the exudate may contain thick, purulent pus, as with a cyst or abscess. (PCPP 1–251   EPC 307)

166.

A. A scab is a protective layer comprised of a mesh of fibrin, red blood cells, and white blood cells. This is the first step of the healing process. (PCPP 1–252   EPC 307)

167.

C. Granulation is the first step in repair, in which the wound is filled in by healthy tissue from the wound edge. This tissue is filled with capillaries and lymph channels. (PCPP 1–252   EPC 922)

168.

A. During epithelialization, the scab (original clot) dissolves, while epithelial cells move in under the scab and separate it from the wound surface to provide a protective covering for the healing wound. (PCPP 1–252   EPC 922)

169.

B. Myofibroblasts in the granulation tissues contract and begin to move inward. This process, known as contraction, occurs 6–12 days after the injury. (PCPP 1–252   EPC 923)

170.

D. Dysfunctional healing during inflammation can be caused by bleeding (takes up space and is a breeding ground for infection), hypovolemia (no circulation = no healing), or an excess of fibrin in the wound (causes adhesions). (PCPP 1–253   EPC 925)

171.

A. Taking steroids suppresses the epithelialization process and causes dysfunctional healing. (PCPP 1–253   EPC 926)

172.

C. An allergy is an exaggerated response to an environmental antigen. Many people have this type of hypersensitivity from seasonal allergies. (PCPP 1–254   EPC 308)

173.

A. Conditions such as rheumatic fever and hyperthyroidism are classified as autoimmunity disorders and are a type of hypersensitivity. (PCPP 1–254 EPC 308)

174.

B. Clinical indicators of an IgE-mediated hypersensitivity response include urticaria and hives, vasodilation and hypotension, laryngeal edema and bronchospasm, abdominal cramping and nausea, and headache and dizziness. (PCPP 1–255   EPC 309)

175.

D. Stress is defined as a state of physical or psychological arousal that exists to some degree in everyone. (PCPP 1–262   EPC 312)

176.

B. Any agent or situation that causes stress is called a stressor. A stressor can be physical (illness, injury, temperature extremes), psychological (taking a test), or emotional (love, hate, anger). (PCPP 1–262   EPC 312)

177.

B. As the body responds to stress, the neurological system and endocrine system release epinephrine and norepinephrine. These hormones cause increases in pulse and blood pressure (to deliver more oxygenated blood to vital organs), dilated pupils (to improve vision), excessive perspiration (to decrease body temperature), increased muscle tension (to anticipate increased muscle use), and increased blood glucose levels (to supply fuel to vital tissues). (PCPP 1–262   EPC 312)

178.

D. An alarm stage reaction occurs at the first exposure to the stressor. The signs include the normal responses of the sympathetic nervous stimulation (see answer 177). If the victim's resistance is lowered, the stress response may be overwhelming. (PCPP 1–262   EPC 312)

179.

D. The resistance stage begins as the victim adapts to the stressor. It is brought on by the use of various coping mechanisms. Vital signs return to normal. As adaptation develops, resistance to the particular stressor increases. (PCPP 1–262   EPC 312)

180.

D. Prolonged exposure to the same stressors may lead to exhaustion of the victim's adaptation capabilities. The alarm stage signs reappear, but they are now much more difficult to reverse. (PCPP 1–263 EPC 313)

181.

D. Another term for dynamic steady state is homeostasis. This describes the body's attempt to maintain a constant, stable internal environment while its components are always changing. (PCPP 1–263 EPC 313)

182.

C. The hormones epinephrine (adrenalin) and norepinephrine (noradrenalin) are known as catecholamines. Catecholamines stimulate the alpha and beta receptors of the sympathetic nervous system. (PCPP 1–264   EPC 314)

Matching   (PCPP 1–265   EPC 315)

183.	**A**	Peripheral vasoconstriction	**A.** Alpha 1
			B. Alpha 2
184.	**C**	Increased heart rate	**C.** Beta 1
185.	**A**	Bronchoconstriction	**D.** Beta 2
186.	**D**	Bronchodilation	
187.	**C**	Increased cardiac contractions	
188.	**D**	Vasodilation	

189.

A. During the stress response, the anterior pituitary gland secretes adrenocorticotropic hormone (ACTH), which, in turn, stimulates the adrenal cortex to secrete cortisol. Cortisol appears to have both beneficial and harmful effects on a body in stress. But it is believed that the overall net effect of cortisol secretion aids in the homeostatic process. (PCPP 1–266   EPC 316)

190.

B. During the stress response, growth hormone, prolactin, and ACTH are released. Testosterone levels are decreased during stress. (PCPP 1–267)

9 General Principles of Pharmacology

DIRECTIONS Each of the questions or incomplete statements below is followed by suggested answers or completions. Select the **one answer** that is best in each case.

1. Furosemide, diazepam, and meperidine are examples of
   A. chemical names
   B. trade names
   C. brand names
   D. generic names

2. Lasix®, Valium®, and Demerol® are examples of
   A. trade names
   B. chemical names
   C. official names
   D. generic namcs

3. Atropine and digitalis are examples of drugs derived from
   A. plants
   B. minerals
   C. animals
   D. synthetics

4. Insulin is an example of a drug derived from
   Λ. plants
   B. minerals
   C. animals
   D. synthetics

5. Calcium chloride and magnesium sulfate are examples of drugs derived from
   A. plants
   B. minerals
   C. animals
   D. synthetics

6. The first drug legislation in the United States was the
   A. Narcotics Act
   B. Pure Food and Drug Act
   C. Federal Food, Drug, and Cosmetic Act
   D. Durham-Humphrey Amendment

7. The Federal Food, Drug, and Cosmetic Act of 1938 requires that
   A. all ingredients be placed on the label
   B. all opium by-products be classified according to schedules
   C. all prescriptions be filled within 72 hours
   D. all of the above

8. The Harrison Narcotic Act of 1915 regulates the sale of
   A. cocaine
   B. morphine
   C. all drugs
   D. barbiturates and amphetamines

9. The Controlled Substances Act of 1970 establishes
   A. schedules for abusive drugs
   B. time limits for filling prescriptions
   C. prohibitions on refills for classified drugs
   D. all of the above

10. Examples of Schedule I drugs, which have a high abuse potential and no medically acceptable medical indications, are
    A. diazepam and methadone
    B. heroin and LSD
    C. Vicodin and phenobarbital
    D. cocaine and opium

11. Examples of Schedule II drugs, which have a high abuse potential but accepted medical indications, are
    A. mescaline and lorazepam
    B. heroin and codeine
    C. cocaine and morphine
    D. diazepam and phenobarbital

12. Examples of Schedule III drugs, which have a lower abuse potential than Schedule I and II drugs and have accepted medical indications, are
    A. Vicodin and Tylenol with codeine
    B. heroin and morphine
    C. diazepam and lorazepam
    D. none of the above

13. Examples of Schedule IV drugs, which have a low abuse potential and accepted medical indications, are
    A. morphine and codeine
    B. phenobarbital and lorazepam
    C. Vicodin and Tylenol with codeine
    D. heroin and LSD

14. Which of the following statements is true regarding over-the-counter drugs?
    A. They are usually a higher dose than their prescribed counterparts
    B. They still require a physician's order to administer in the field
    C. They present a higher risk to patients taking them
    D. All of the above

15. Adenosine is administered into the bloodstream, is distributed to all body regions, and is rapidly metabolized by red blood cells. This information is known as its
    A. bioequivalence
    B. bioassay
    C. pharmacokinetics
    D. pharmacodynamics

16. Arrange the following phases of the FDA drug approval process from first to last:
    A. Perform postmarketing analysis
    B. Determine pharmacokinetics by testing on healthy adults

    C. Conduct double-blind studies to determine side effects
    D. Test diseased adults to determine therapeutic dose

17. With the rigid FDA standards for drug approval, why did thalidomide cause so many birth defects?
    A. There was no FDA program then
    B. Thalidomide was an aberration
    C. Women and children are excluded during the first three testing phases
    D. None of the above

18. Which of the following statements is FALSE regarding the administration of drugs to a pregnant woman?
    A. Her altered anatomy and physiology may alter the drug's pharmacokinetics
    B. The drug may pass through the placenta and reach the fetus
    C. Therapeutic levels for the mother may be toxic levels for the fetus
    D. All drugs are considered contraindicated for the pregnant woman

19. Why do infants and young children pose special considerations when dosing drugs?
    A. They have a higher free drug availability than adults
    B. They have a much greater proportion of extracellular fluid
    C. They have overdeveloped blood-brain barriers
    D. The newborn's metabolic rate is much higher than an adult's

20. Which of the following statements is true regarding drug administration to geriatric patients?
    A. Depressed liver function may alter biotransformation
    B. Their gastric motility increases with age

C. Compromised renal function may increase elimination

D. All of the above

21. You administer epinephrine 1:1000 subcutaneously to a patient in severe anaphylactic shock. Which of the following statements is true?
    A. The drug probably will be readily absorbed into the bloodstream
    B. Subcutaneous blood flow during the shock state is increased
    C. Capillary bed shutdown may impede drug absorption
    D. None of the above

22. Which of the following affects a drug's rate of absorption?
    A. Its concentration
    B. Its pH
    C. Its solubility
    D. All of the above

23. You administer via IV a lidocaine bolus of 1mg/kg followed by a 2mg/min IV drip. The initial bolus is called the _____ dose, and the drip is called the _____ dose.
    A. initial, follow-up
    B. loading, maintenance
    C. preceding, following
    D. large, small

24. Sodium bicarbonate is administered to patients who overdose on tricyclic antidepressants because it
    A. lowers the pH and facilitates protein binding
    B. lowers the pH and encourages diffusion into the cells
    C. raises the pH and encourages protein binding

D. raises the pH and increases the free drug availability

25. Your chest pain patient takes warfarin daily. Why would it be dangerous to administer aspirin to him?
    A. Aspirin reacts unpredictably with warfarin
    B. There is a high incidence of anaphylactic shock
    C. Neither is a protein-bound drug
    D. Aspirin causes an increase in free warfarin availability

26. In order to cross the blood-brain barrier or the placenta barrier, a drug should be
    A. ionized
    B. lipid soluble
    C. protein bound
    D. all of the above

27. Which organ(s) is/are responsible for the majority of the biotransformation process?
    A. Liver
    B. Kidneys
    C. Intestines
    D. Lungs

28. Renal excretion of drugs can be affected by
    A. glomerular filtration
    B. blood pressure
    C. change in the urine pH
    D. all of the above

29. Which of the following is a NOT an enteral route?
    A. Rectal
    B. Buccal
    C. Umbilical
    D. Sublingual

Match the following liquid drug forms with their respective definitions:

30. ____ Tincture
31. ____ Suspension
32. ____ Emulsion
33. ____ Spirit
34. ____ Elixer

A. Alcohol and water solvent with flavorings
B. Volatile drug in alcohol
C. Extracted with alcohol
D. Oily solvent
E. Preparation that precipitates when left alone

35. The force of attraction between a drug and a receptor is known as
   A. agonism
   B. antagonism
   C. affinity
   D. efficacy

36. A drug's ability to produce the expected response is known as
   A. agonism
   B. antagonism
   C. affinity
   D. efficacy

37. Which of the following statements is true regarding the drug/receptor response?
   A. Drugs can inhibit a cell's normal function
   B. Drugs can stimulate a cell's normal function
   C. Drugs can impart a new function to a cell
   D. A and B

38. Drugs that bind to a receptor and produce a response are known as
   A. antagonists
   B. agonists
   C. biotransformers
   D. lytics

39. Drugs that bind to a receptor and block a response are known as
   A. antagonists
   B. agonists
   C. inhibitors
   D. mimetics

40. Morphine and naloxone are two drugs that, when both are present at a target cell, exhibit _____ antagonism.
   A. noncompetitive
   B. irreversible
   C. competitive
   D. partial

41. Repeating boluses of lidocaine until the desired effect is reached is an example of
   A. synergism
   B. potentiation
   C. cumulative action
   D. agonism

42. The enhancing effect of taking promethazine with morphine is an example of
   A. antagonism
   B. potentiation
   C. synergism
   D. cumulative action

43. A patient who once took 5 mg of diazepam each day now requires 10 mg. This is an example of
   A. potentiation
   B. tolerance
   C. becoming refractory
   D. untoward effect

44. An individual reaction to a drug that is unusually different from that normally seen is called a/an
   A. hypersensitivity
   B. idiosyncrasy

C. adverse reaction

D. untoward effect

45. Drugs with a low therapeutic index
    A. are difficult to titrate
    B. have a narrow therapeutic range
    C. are easy to overdose
    D. all of the above

True or False—Identify whether the following statements are true or false:

46. _____ Infants and elderly patients are susceptible to having an altered response to drugs.

47. _____ A given amount of drug will have a lower concentration in a person with lower body mass.

48. _____ Fat distribution alters drug concentration.

49. _____ A patient's environment may alter the physiological or psychological response to drugs.

50. _____ An empty stomach can aid in drug absorption.

51. _____ Renal failure may increase drug elimination.

52. _____ Liver failure may decrease drug metabolism.

53. _____ Derangements in acid-base may alter absorption and elimination of drugs.

54. _____ A patient's mental state has no effect on the drug response.

55. _____ A patient's genetics may alter drug absorption and biotransformation.

56. Drugs that relieve the sensation of pain are known as
    A. anesthetics
    B. analgesics
    C. neuroleptics
    D. anxiolytics

57. Morphine is an example of a/an
    A. narcotic analgesic
    B. opioid antagonist
    C. opioid agonist/antagonist
    D. nonopioid analgesic

58. Besides pain relief, which of the following is an indication for using morphine?
    A. Hypotension
    B. Respiratory failure
    C. Pulmonary edema
    D. COPD

59. Ibuprofen is an example of a/an
    A. NSAID
    B. nonopioid analgesic
    C. antipyretic
    D. all of the above

60. Which of the following drugs would you use to treat a heroin overdose?
    A. Morphine
    B. Diazepam
    C. Naloxone
    D. Nalbuphine

61. Sometimes diazepam, lorazepam, or promethazine is given concurrently with an analgesic in order to
    A. prolong or intensify the effects
    B. reduce the side effects
    C. aid in biotransformation
    D. compete for the receptor site

62. Which of the following is an example of an agonist/antagonist?
    A. Pentazocine
    B. Nalbuphine
    C. Butorphanol
    D. All of the above

63. Drugs that induce a loss of the sensation of touch or pain are known as
    A. anesthetics
    B. analgesics
    C. neuroleptics
    D. anxiolytics

64. Lidocaine is an anesthetic injected into the skin surrounding a wound site prior to suturing. Often epinephrine is added to the lidocaine. Why?
    A. Epinephrine potentiates lidocaine
    B. They work synergistically to decrease pain
    C. Epinephrine reduces the side effects of lidocaine
    D. Epinephrine decreases the systemic absorption of lidocaine

65. Which of the following drugs has been used since the nineteenth century as an ophthalmic anesthetic?
    A. Lidocaine
    B. Cocaine
    C. Halothane
    D. Nitrous oxide

66. Which of the following classes is an example of a sedative-hypnotic drug?
    A. Benzodiazepines
    B. Barbiturates
    C. Neuroleptics
    D. A and B

67. Both benzodiazepines and barbiturates work by
    A. decreasing blood flow to an innervated area
    B. causing a neuromuscular blockade
    C. increasing GABA receptor effects
    D. decreasing endorphin release

68. Which of the following is a benzodiazepine antagonist?

A. Xylocaine
B. Flumazenil
C. Naloxone
D. Lorazepam

Match the following antiseizure medications with their respective mechanisms of action:

69. ____ Carbamazepine (Tegretol)
70. ____ Phenytoin (Dilantin)
71. ____ Valproic acid (Depakote)
72. ____ Diazepam (Valium)
73. ____ Phenobarbital (Luminal)

A. Inhibits calcium channel influx
B. Increases GABA response
C. Inhibits sodium channel influx

74. Amphetamines, methylphenidates, and methylxanthines work by
    A. decreasing the effects of excitatory neurotransmitters
    B. increasing the effects of inhibitory neurotransmitters
    C. increasing the effects of excitatory neurotransmitters
    D. none of the above

75. Which of the following drugs is used as an appetite suppressant to treat obesity?
    A. Dexedrine
    B. Adenosine
    C. Ritalin
    D. Theophylline

76. Which of the following drugs is used to treat the hyperactive disorder known as ADHD?
    A. Methylphenidate (Ritalin)
    B. Theophylline
    C. Dexedrine
    D. Amphetamine sulfate

77. Which of the following is an example of a methylxanthine?

A. Caffeine
B. Aminophylline
C. Theophylline
D. All of the above

78. Psychotherapeutic medications work by
    A. regulating excitatory and inhibitory neurotransmitters
    B. causing total autonomic blockade
    C. stabilizing GABA receptors
    D. releasing endorphins

79. Common side effects of antipsychotic medications include
    A. neuroleptic convulsions
    B. extrapyramidal symptoms
    C. cholinergic cascades
    D. preganglionic stimulation

80. Treatment for the above condition includes
    A. 50% dextrose IV
    B. dopamine IV
    C. diphenhydramine IV
    D. haloperidol IM

81. Which of the following drug classes is used to treat depression?
    A. Selective serotonin reuptake inhibitors
    B. Monoamine oxidase inhibitors
    C. Tricyclic antidepressants
    D. All of the above

82. TCAs work by
    A. increasing norepinephrine influx
    B. inhibiting norepinephrine reuptake
    C. increasing the reuptake of serotonin
    D. B and C

83. SSRIs work by blocking the reuptake of
    A. serotonin
    B. norepinephrine
    C. dopamine
    D. all of the above

84. MAO inhibitors work by
    A. promoting the release of norepinephrine
    B. blocking the reuptake of dopamine
    C. blocking dopamine receptors
    D. none of the above

85. Which of the following drugs is indicated for bipolar disorder?
    A. Librium
    B. Luminal
    C. Lithium
    D. Levodopa

86. Pharmacological therapy for Parkinson's disease is aimed at
    A. decreasing dopamine stimulation
    B. restoring the balance between norepinephrine and acetylcholine
    C. increasing acetylcholine stimulation
    D. blocking dopamine receptors

87. The space between two nerve cells is called a
    A. neuroeffector junction
    B. neurotransmitter junction
    C. synapse
    D. neuron

Match the neurotransmitters with their respective uses:

88. ____ Sympathetic preganglionic
89. ____ Sympathetic postganglionic
90. ____ Parasympathetic preganglionic
91. ____ Parasympathetic postganglionic

 A. Acetylcholine
 B. Norepinephrine

92. The parasympathetic nervous system is responsible for
    A. custodial functions
    B. resting heart rate
    C. digestion
    D. all of the above

93. The parasympathetic nervous system exerts its control via
    A. several cranial nerves
    B. three thoracic nerves
    C. some lumbar nerves
    D. all of the above

94. When stimulated, parasympathetic receptors cause
    A. decreased salivation
    B. pupil dilation
    C. increased heart rate
    D. none of the above

95. Medications that stimulate the parasympathetic nervous system are called
    A. anticholinergics
    B. parasympatholytics
    C. parasympathomimetics
    D. cholinergic antagonists

96. Classic effects of cholinergic medications include
    A. increased salivation
    B. decreased gastric motility
    C. dry mucous membranes
    D. constipation

97. Acetylcholine is degraded by
    A. monoamine oxidase
    B. cholinesterase
    C. neostigmine
    D. cholinesterase inhibitors

98. Which of the following drugs is a direct acting cholinergic?
    A. Physostigmine (Antilirium)
    B. Neostigmine (Prostigmine)
    C. Echothiophate (Phospholine Iodide)
    D. Bethanechol (Urecholine)

99. Which of the following drugs is a reversible cholinesterase inhibitor?

    A. Physostigmine (Antilirium)
    B. Sarin
    C. Echothiophate (Phospholine Iodide)
    D. Bethanechol (Urecholine)

100. Treatment for toxic cholinergic exposure, such as nerve gas, includes
    A. atropine
    B. pralidoxime
    C. Protopam
    D. all of the above

101. Atropine is classified as a
    A. nicotinic agonist
    B. nicotinic antagonist
    C. muscarinic agonist
    D. muscarinic antagonist

102. Ipratropium bromide (Atrovent) is an anticholinergic medication used to treat
    A. emesis
    B. asthma
    C. anxiety
    D. delirium tremons

103. Succinylcholine is classified as a _____ neuromuscular blocker.
    A. depolarizing
    B. nondepolarizing

104. The sympathetic nervous system is responsible for
    A. vegetative functions
    B. custodial functions
    C. "feeding and breeding"
    D. the stress response

105. Sympathetic fibers arise from
    A. several sacral nerves
    B. T1–L2
    C. cranial nerves III–X
    D. the midbrain

106. When stimulated, the sympathetic nervous system causes all of the following physiological responses EXCEPT
   A. pupil dilation
   B. peripheral vasodilation
   C. increased cardiac contractions
   D. increased heart rate

Match the following adrenergic receptors with their respective functions:

107. _____ Alpha 1
108. _____ Alpha 2
109. _____ Beta 1
110. _____ Beta 2
111. _____ Dopaminergic

   A. Renal artery dilator
   B. Arteriole and bronchial dilator
   C. Peripheral vasoconstrictor
   D. Increased chronotropy and inotropy
   E. Presynaptic inhibition

112. An alpha 1 agonist works by
   A. dilating bronchial smooth muscle
   B. dilating arterioles
   C. causing massive fluid shifts
   D. constricting peripheral vessels

113. Which of the following drugs is classified as an alpha 1 antagonist?
   A. Epinephrine
   B. Prazosin (Minipress)
   C. Propranolol (Inderal)
   D. Dantrolene (Dantrium)

114. Which of the following drugs is classified as a beta 1 selective antagonist?
   A. Propranolol (Inderal)
   B. Atenolol (Tenormin)
   C. Albuterol (Proventil)
   D. Diltiazem (Cardizem)

115. Class I antidysrhythmics such as lidocaine, procainamide, and flecainide work by blocking
   A. calcium channels
   B. beta 1 receptors
   C. potassium channels
   D. sodium channels

116. Propranolol (Inderal), a class II antidysrhythmic, works by blocking
   A. calcium channels
   B. beta 1 receptors
   C. potassium channels
   D. sodium channels

117. Verapamil, diltiazem, and nifedipine are classified as
   A. beta blockers
   B. sympathomimetics
   C. calcium channel blockers
   D. none of the above

118. Which of the following statements is true regarding digoxin?
   A. Its side effects include every type of dysrhythmia
   B. It has a very narrow therapeutic index
   C. It is a negative chronotrope and a positive inotrope
   D. All of the above

119. Which of the following diuretics works in the loop of Henle?
   A. Furosemide (Lasix)
   B. Hydrochlorothiazide (HydroDIURIL)
   C. Spironolactone (Aldactone)
   D. Mannitol (Osmitrol)

120. Which of the following is a side effect of administering furosemide too quickly?
   A. Vasoconstriction
   B. Reflex bradycardia
   C. Tinnitis and deafness
   D. Hyperkalemia

121. Clonodine (Catapres) and methyldopa (Aldomet) both reduce blood pressure by
    A. blocking beta 2 receptors
    B. causing direct vasodilation
    C. inhibiting sympathetic stimulation in CNS
    D. blocking angiotension conversion

122. An alpha 1 antagonist reduces blood pressure by
    A. causing direct vasoconstriction
    B. reducing peripheral vascular resistance
    C. reducing the intrinsic firing rate of the SA node
    D. increasing angiotension conversion

123. ACE inhibitors captopril (Capoten) and enalapril (Vasotec) reduce blood pressure by preventing the conversion of angiotensin I to
    A. angiotensin II
    B. renin
    C. aldosterone
    D. angiotensinogen

124. Losartan (Cozaar) is classified as a/an
    A. ACE inhibitor
    B. direct vasodilator
    C. angiotensin II blocker
    D. alpha antagonist

125. Which of the following calcium channel blockers does not exert its effect on the heart?
    A. Verapamil
    B. Diltiazem
    C. Nifedipine
    D. Calan

126. Sodium nitroprusside (Nipride) is a drug that
    A. reduces blood pressure by vasodilation
    B. raises cardiac output by increasing stroke volume
    C. increases preload
    D. stabilizes the cardiac rhythm

127. Nitroglycerine is administered to patients suffering from angina because it
    A. lowers the heart rate
    B. increases preload
    C. dilates coronary arteries
    D. all of the above

128. Aspirin is classified as a/an
    A. antiplatelet
    B. anticoagulant
    C. antihyperlipidemic
    D. thrombolytic

129. Warfarin (Coumadin) is classified as a/an
    A. antiplatelet
    B. anticoagulant
    C. antihyperlipidemic
    D. thrombolytic

130. Streptokinase (Streptase) and alteplase (tPA) are classified as
    A. antiplatelets
    B. anticoagulants
    C. antihyperlipidemics
    D. thrombolytics

131. Simvastatin (Zocor) works by
    A. raising blood levels of HDLs
    B. lowering blood levels of LDLs
    C. decreasing LDL receptors in the liver
    D. none of the above

Match the following asthma medications with their respective classes:

132. _____ Epinephrine
133. _____ Albuterol (Proventil)
134. _____ Theophylline (Theo-Dur)
135. _____ Ipratropium (Atrovent)
136. _____ Beclomethasone (Beclovent)

137. ____ Zafirlukast (Accolate)

138. ____ Cromolyn sodium (Intal)

A. Beta 2 selective agonist
B. Leukotriene antagonist
C. Mast cell stabilizer
D. Beta agonist
E. Glucocorticoid
F. Methylxanthine
G. Anticholinergic

139. The main ingredient used in nasal decongestants is a/an
A. beta 1 agonist
B. alpha 2 antagonist
C. beta 2 antagonist
D. alpha 1 agonist

140. Antihistamines work by
A. blocking the release of histamine from mast cells
B. interrupting the inflammatory cascade
C. competing for histamine receptor sites
D. none of the above

141. An antitussive works by
A. increasing cough production
B. making mucus more watery
C. suppressing the cough mechanism
D. dilating the airways

142. Which of the following medication classes is NOT an approach to treating peptic ulcer disease?
A. Cholinergics
B. Proton pump inhibitors
C. H$_2$ receptor antagonists
D. Antacids

143. Which of the following is NOT a type of laxative?
A. Surfactant
B. Bulk-forming

C. Osmotic
D. Compazine

144. Which of the following drug classes is NOT used to treat emesis?
A. Serotonin antagonists
B. Phenothiazines
C. Cannabinoids
D. Cholinergics

145. Antiglaucoma medications work by
A. dilating the pupils
B. reducing intraoccular pressure
C. paralyzing the ciliary muscles
D. decreasing pain and sensation

146. Your patient takes gentamicin sulfate otic solution (Garamycin). Why?
A. He has an otitis
B. He has excessive cerumin
C. He has swimmer's ear
D. He has tinnitis

147. Which of the following is NOT an effect of vasopressin (Pitressin)?
A. Peripheral vasoconstriction
B. Less concentrated urine
C. Increased water reabsorption
D. Decreased blood pressure

148. Your patient takes levothyroxine (Synthroid) for which disease?
A. Hypothyroidism
B. Hyperthyroidism
C. Thyroid storm
D. Graves' disease

149. Which of the following is NOT a hormone secreted by the adrenal cortex?
A. Androgen
B. Glucagon
C. Mineralocorticoid
D. Glucocorticoid

150. Which of the following hormones promotes both glycogenolysis and gluconeogenesis?
    A. Glucagon
    B. Insulin
    C. NPH
    D. Somatostatin

151. The major advantage of human insulin over animal insulin is that
    A. it has a longer duration of action
    B. it does not cause allergic reactions
    C. dosing is not as strictly regulated
    D. none of the above

152. Which of the following oral hypoglycemic agents works by delaying carbohydrate metabolism?
    A. Tolbutamide (Orinase)
    B. Metformin (Glucophage)
    C. Acarbose (Precose)
    D. Troglitazone (Rezulin)

153. Antineoplastic agents are used to treat
    A. asthma
    B. hypercholesterolemia
    C. inflammation
    D. cancer

154. Penicillins and cephalosporins work by
    A. blocking receptor sites
    B. inhibiting cell wall synthesis
    C. preventing the bacteria from replicating
    D. inhibiting protein synthesis

155. Pain-relieving drugs such as aspirin, ibuprofen, and naproxen are commonly known as
    A. NSAIDs
    B. NIDDMs
    C. TCAs
    D. SSRIs

156. Uricosuric drugs are used to treat
    A. gout
    B. bladder infections
    C. urinary blockage
    D. malaria

answers & rationales

1.

D. Furosemide, diazepam, and meperidine are examples of generic names. The generic name is the name usually given to a drug by its first manufacturer and is an abbreviated version of the chemical name. (PCPP 1–277   EPC 341)

2.

A. Lasix®, Valium®, and Demerol® are examples of trade names. The trade name is a name given to a drug by each manufacturer. A medication may appear under several trade names if it is made by a number of manufacturers. (PCPP 1–277   EPC 341)

3.

A. Atropine and digitalis are examples of drugs derived from plants. (PCPP 1–277   EPC 341)

4.

C. Insulin and Pitocin are examples of drugs derived from animals. (PCPP 1–277   EPC 341)

5.

B. Calcium chloride and magnesium sulfate are examples of drugs derived from minerals. (PCPP 1–277   EPC 341)

6.

B. In an effort to regulate and eliminate "snake-oil salesmen," Congress enacted the Pure Food and Drug Act in 1906 and named the U.S. Pharmacopoeia as the country's official source for drug information. (PCPP 1–279   EPC 343)

7.

A. The Federal Food, Drug, and Cosmetic Act of 1938 requires the names of all ingredients of foods and medications to be placed on the product label. It also requires that the labels state whether the ingredients are habit forming and what percentages of those drugs are present. (PCPP 1–279   EPC 343)

8.

B. The Harrison Narcotic Act of 1915 regulates the sale, importation, and manufacture of the opium plant and its derivatives. (PCPP 1–279   EPC 343)

9.

D. Since 1970, the government has regulated addictive medications through the Controlled Substances Act. This act classifies addictive medications into five schedules, prohibits the refilling of prescriptions for Schedule II drugs, and requires that the original prescription be filled within 72 hours. (PCPP 1–279   EPC 343)

10.

B. Schedule I drugs have a high abuse potential, and their use may lead to severe dependence. They have no accepted medical indications and are used for research, analysis, or instruction only. Examples include heroin, LSD, and mescaline. (PCPP 1–279   EPC 343)

11.

C. Schedule II drugs have a high abuse potential, and their use may lead to severe dependence. However, they have accepted medical indications. Examples include opium, cocaine, morphine, codeine, oxycodone, methadone, and secobarbital. (PCPP 1–279   EPC 343)

12.

A. Schedule III drugs have less abuse potential than Schedule I and II drugs, and their use may lead to moderate or low physical or high psychological dependence. However, they have accepted medical indications. Examples include limited opioid amounts combined with noncontrolled substances, such as Vicodin and Tylenol with codeine. (PCPP 1–279   EPC 343)

13.

B. Schedule IV drugs have a low abuse potential compared to Schedule III drugs, and their use causes limited physical and psychological dependence. They have accepted medical indications. Examples include diazepam, lorazepam, and phenobarbital. (PCPP 1–279   EPC 343)

14.

B. Over-the-counter (OTC) medications are usually available in lower doses than their prescribed counterparts and present a lower risk for patients taking them. Most EMS systems require EMS providers to obtain a physician's order (written, verbal, or standing) to administer OTC drugs. (PCPP 1–280 EPC 344)

15.

C. A drug's pharmacokinetics refer to its absorption, distribution, metabolism, and excretion. Paramedics should be familiar with this information for all drugs they administer. For example, by knowing that adenosine is metabolized rapidly en route to the heart, you know you need to administer it rapidly into a vein close to the heart and flush the line immediately. (PCPP 1–280   EPC 348)

16.

B., D., C., A.   The Food and Drug Administration (FDA) has a rigid process for approving new drugs. Following animal studies, the human component takes place in four phases. In phase 1, the drug is administered to healthy adults to determine its pharmacokinetics, toxicity, and safe dose. In phase 2, it is tested on a limited number of diseased adults to reevaluate and redefine its therapeutic level, toxicity, and side effects. In phase 3, double-blind studies are performed on a large patient population to collect data on side effects. Finally, phase 4 testing analyzes the drug during its conditional approval period. (PCPP 1–281)

17.

C. Thalidomide, an antiemetic, was prescribed by physicians to pregnant women to treat their nausea. No one could have predicted the horrible birth de-

fects caused by this drug because it was not tested on women and children. (PCPP 1–282)

18.

D. Administering any drug to a pregnant woman is risky to both the mother and her unborn child. Even after birth, if she is nursing, she can transfer the drug's effects to her infant. There are, however, circumstances that demand the use of drugs for the health of the baby and mother. These include diabetes, hypertension, and seizure disorders. (PCPP 1–284   EPC 346)

19.

A. Some drugs bind to plasma proteins in the blood. But not all the drug molecules bind. The ones that do not are available in the body to cause the desired or undesired effects. This is known as free drug availability. Since children under 1 year old have diminished plasma protein concentrations, these drugs have higher free drug availability. Because of this, you can expect to reach therapeutic and toxic effects at lower doses. (PCPP 1–284   EPC 346)

20.

A. Most drugs are metabolized, or biotransformed, in the liver. If your patient has depressed liver function because of the aging process or a disease such as cirrhosis or hepatitis, you can expect drug action to be prolonged. (PCPP 1–285   EPC 351)

21.

C. During the shock state, blood flow to the peripheral blood vessels in the skin is blocked in order to preserve circulation to the vital organs. Administering a drug into the subcutaneous tissue during the shock state may result in decreased, if any, absorption. In severe anaphylaxis, epinephrine may be administered at a lower concentration (1:10,000) directly into a vein. (PCPP 1–287   EPC 350)

22.

D. How well a drug is absorbed is determined by a number of factors. These include its concentration, pH, ionization, and solubility; the nature of the absorbing surface; and blood flow through the administration area. (PCPP 1–287   EPC 349)

23.

B. A loading dose is administered to raise the blood levels of a drug quickly to a therapeutic level. A maintenance dose is administered to keep the blood levels in the therapeutic range. You would load your patient (in stable ventricular tachycardia) until the rhythm converts to sinus rhythm and then begin the drip to prevent a sudden recurrence. (PCPP 1–288 EPC 350)

24.

C. A high pH encourages protein binding. Protein-bound drugs cannot exert their effects on the target cells. One treatment for patients overdosed on tricyclic antidepressants, which strongly bind to proteins, is to raise the pH to encourage protein binding. This reduces the effects of the drug on the cells. (PCPP 1–288 EPC 350)

25.

D. Warfarin is highly protein bound. In fact, 99% of it is unavailable for the cells. Yet, the 1% that is available is therapeutic in most adults. Aspirin displaces warfarin on the plasma proteins, raising the blood levels of free warfarin. This can result in life-threatening hemorrhage. (PCPP 1–289 EPC 350)

26.

B. For a drug to cross the blood-brain barrier or the placenta barrier, it should be non-ionized, lipid soluble, and non-protein bound. (PCPP 1–289 EPC 351)

27.

A. Most drugs are metabolized, or biotransformed, in the liver. Patients with preexisting liver disease can be expected to develop toxic blood levels of drugs at lower doses than do those with healthy livers. A good example of this is lidocaine. If you suspect your patient has an impaired liver, consider administering a reduced dose. (PCPP 1–289 EPC 351)

28.

D. Most drugs are excreted in the urine. Conditions that affect renal elimination include glomerular filtration, which is affected by blood pressure and blood flow; urine pH; and drugs that affect the ATP pumps. (PCPP 1–290 EPC 352)

29.

C. Enteral routes deliver medications by absorption through the GI tract. These include oral (PO), orogastric tube (OG), nasogastric tube (NG), sublingual (SL), buccal, and rectal (PR). (PCPP 1–291 EPC 353)

Matching (PCPP 1–292 EPC 354)

30. **C**	Tincture	**A.** Alcohol and water
31. **E**	Suspension	solvent with flavorings
32. **D**	Emulsion	**B.** Volatile drug in alcohol
33. **B**	Spirit	**C.** Extracted with alcohol
34. **A**	Elixir	**D.** Oily solvent
		E. Preparation that precipitates when left alone

35.

C. Affinity is the force of attraction between a drug or other substance and a receptor. For example, the carbon monoxide molecule has an affinity for hemoglobin that is 210 times greater than the affinity of the oxygen molecule. The same holds true for drugs. The greater the affinity, the stronger the bond. (PCPP 1–293 EPC 355)

36.

D. Efficacy describes a drug's ability to produce a response. It is different from its ability to bind with the receptor. One drug may bind more easily, but another may cause a stronger response when bound. (PCPP 1–293 EPC 355)

37.

D. Drugs are not magical. They cannot alter a cell's function qualitatively, only quantitatively. They can either stimulate or inhibit a cell's normal physiological function. For example, acetylcholine will stimulate a smooth muscle cell to constrict, while albuterol will inhibit constriction (resulting in dilation). (PCPP 1–293 EPC 355)

38.

B. Drugs that bind to a receptor and produce a response are known as agonists. An example is epinephrine, which stimulates the alpha and beta receptors in the heart, blood vessels, and lower airways. (PCPP 1–294 EPC 356)

39.

A. Drugs that bind to a receptor and block a response are known as antagonists. An example is naloxone, which blocks the narcotic receptor sites. (PCPP 1–294 EPC 356)

40.

C. Morphine is an opiate agonist. Naloxone is an opiate antagonist. Together they compete for the same opiate receptor sites. Whichever drug binds to the site either stimulates the opiate effect (morphine) or blocks it (naloxone). (PCPP 1–294 EPC 356)

41.
C. Repeating boluses of lidocaine until the desired effect is reached is an example of cumulative action. This occurs when a drug is administered in several doses, causing an increasing effect that is usually due to a build-up of the drug in the blood. (PCPP 1–296 EPC 358)

42.
B. The enhancing effect of taking promethazine with morphine is an example of potentiation. Potentiation is the enhancement of one drug's effects by another. (PCPP 1–296 EPC 358)

43.
B. A patient who requires a higher dose of the same medication to reach the desired effect is an example of tolerance. In order to produce the desired effect, you must increase the dose. (PCPP 1–295 EPC 357)

44.
B. An idiosyncrasy is an individual reaction to a drug that is unusually different from that normally seen. For example, antibiotics normally cause gastrointestinal distress. If antibiotics turn your hair green, this is an idiosyncrasy. (PCPP 1–295 EPC 357)

45.
D. Drugs with a low therapeutic index are difficult to titrate because they have a narrow therapeutic range. It is very easy to overdose patients on these types of drugs. (PCPP 1–296 EPC 358)

True or False   (PCPP 1–297   EPC 359)

46.   _T_   Infants and elderly patients are susceptible to having an altered response to drugs.

47.   _T_   A given amount of drug will have a lower concentration in a person with lower body mass.

48.   _T_   Fat distribution alters drug concentration.

49.   _T_   A patient's environment may alter the physiological or psychological response to drugs.

50.   _T_   An empty stomach can aid in drug absorption.

51.   _F_   Renal failure may increase drug elimination.

52.   _T_   Liver failure may decrease drug metabolism.

53.   _T_   Derangements in acid-base may alter absorption and elimination of drugs.

54.   _F_   A patient's mental state has no effect on the drug response.

55.   _T_   A patient's genetics may alter drug absorption and biotransformation.

56.
B. Analgesics are drugs that relieve the sensation of pain. There are basically two types of analgesics—narcotic analgesics (from the opioid plant) and non-narcotic analgesics. (PCPP 1–300 EPC 362)

57.
A. Morphine is a narcotic agonist. It stimulates the release of pain-reducing peptides called endorphins, which reduce the sensation of pain. (PCPP 1–300 EPC 362)

58.
C. Morphine is prescribed for moderate to severe pain. In addition, its vasodilatory effects are beneficial in reducing the workload of the heart by causing venous pooling in the extremities. This effect helps rid the lungs of excess fluid in patients with pulmonary edema. (PCPP 1–300 EPC 362)

59.
D. Ibuprofen is classified as a nonopioid analgesic with antipyretic (fever-reducing) properties. It is in a subclass known as nonsteroidal anti-inflammatory drugs (NSAIDs). (PCPP 1–300 EPC 362)

60.
C. Heroin is an opioid agonist. When overdosed, it causes severe respiratory depression, unconsciousness, and pinpoint pupils. To treat a heroin overdose, administer naloxone, a competitive opioid antagonist. The naloxone will compete with the heroin for the receptor sites and block the effects of the opioid—namely, respiratory depression. (PCPP 1–300 EPC 362)

61.
A. Sometimes drugs such as diazepam, lorazepam, midazolam, and promethazine are administered

concurrently with analgesics to prolong or intensify the effects. (PCPP 1–301   EPC 362)

62.

D. Drugs like nalbuphine (Nubain), pentazocine (Talwin), and butorphanol (Stadol) are examples of agonist/antagonist drugs. These drugs exert an agonist effect (reduce pain) and an antagonist effect (fewer side effects and respiratory depression). (PCPP 1–301   EPC 363)

63.

A. Anesthetics are drugs that induce a loss of the sensation of touch or pain. They are used during unpleasant procedures, such as suturing and electrical cardioversion. Some anesthetics allow the patient to remain conscious during the procedure but induce amnesia so that they will not remember how unpleasant it was. (PCPP 1–301 EPC 363)

64.

D. Epinephrine is a potent alpha1 agent. When administered into a wound, it causes vasoconstriction, which reduces bleeding and systemic absorption of the lidocaine. This prolongs the anesthetic effect of lidocaine. (PCPP 1–302   EPC 364)

65.

B. Since it was introduced in 1884, cocaine has been used as a topical anesthetic for the eye. (PCPP 1–302   EPC 364)

66.

D. Sedative-hypnotic drugs are used to induce sleep and relieve anxiety. The two main pharmacological classes of such drugs are benzodiazepines and barbiturates. (PCPP 1–302   EPC 364)

67.

C. Benzodiazepines and barbiturates both work by increasing the GABA response. GABA is the chief inhibitory neurotransmitter in the central nervous system. By increasing GABA, you hyperpolarize the inside of the cell, making it difficult to depolarize. This results in sedation and reduced anxiety at low doses and in induced sleep and anesthesia at higher doses. They are also useful in treating seizures. (PCPP 1–302   EPC 364)

68.

B. Flumazenil (Romazicon) competitively binds with benzodiazepine receptors and in the GABA receptorchloride ion channel complex. This reverses the sedative effects of the benzodiazepine. (PCPP 1–302   EPC 364)

Matching   (PCPP 1–303   EPC 365)

69. C	Carbamazepine (Tegretol)	**A.**	Inhibits calcium channel influx
70. C	Phenytoin (Dilantin)	**B.**	Increases GABA response
71. A	Valproic acid (Depakote)	**C.**	Inhibits sodium channel influx
72. B	Diazepam (Valium)		
73. B	Phenobarbital (Luminal)		

74.

C. Central nervous stimulants work either by increasing the release or effectiveness of excitatory neurotransmitters or by decreasing the release or effectiveness of inhibitory neurotransmitters. They are used to treat fatigue, drowsiness, narcolepsy, obesity, and attention deficit hyperactivity disorder. (PCPP 1–303   EPC 365)

75.

A. Dexedrine is an amphetamine that increases the release of excitatory neurotransmitters (dopamine and norepinephrine). Its uses include treating drowsiness and fatigue and suppressing the appetite. (PCPP 1–304   EPC 366)

76.

A. As strange as it may sound, treatment for the hyperactive disorder known as attention deficit hyperactivity disorder (ADHD) is methylphenidate, a drug that increases the release of excitatory neurotransmitters. The stimulant effects of Ritalin increase the patient's ability to concentrate. (PCPP 1–304   EPC 366)

77.

D. While their mechanism of action is unclear, methylxanthines appear to inhibit the effects of excitatory impulses. Examples include caffeine, chocolate, colas, and the drugs aminophylline and theophylline. They are used to dilate the airways in asthma and chronic obstructive pulmonary disease (COPD). (PCPP 1–304   EPC 366)

78.

A. Psychotherapeutic drugs are used to treat mental dysfunction. They work by regulating the excitatory and inhibitory neurotransmitters (especially norepinephrine, dopamine, and serotonin) in the brain. Some block dopamine receptors (to treat schizophrenia), while others stimulate neurotransmitter release (to treat depression). (PCPP 1–305   EPC 367)

79.

B. Common side effects of antipsychotic medications include muscle tremors and Parkinson-like effects, also known as extrapyramidal symptoms (EPS). (PCPP 1–305   EPC 367)

80.

C. Treatment for EPS's acute dystonic reactions includes the antihistamine diphenhydramine (Benadryl) because it also contains anticholinergic properties. (PCPP 1–305   EPC 367)

81.

D. There are three drug classes used to treat clinical depression: selective serotonin reuptake inhibitors (SSRIs), monoamine oxidase (MAO) inhibitors, and tricyclic antidepressants (TCAs). (PCPP 1–306   EPC 368)

82.

B. TCAs work by blocking the reuptake of norepinephrine and serotonin, which prolongs their effects. Because of their cardiotoxic side effects, they are becoming less popular. Overdose is treated with sodium bicarbonate to alkalinize the urine and hasten excretion. (PCPP 1–306   EPC 368)

83.

A. As the name suggests, SSRIs selectively block the reuptake of serotonin but do not affect dopamine or norepinephrine. Also, because they do not block histamine or cholinergic receptors, they lack many of the side effects of the tricyclics. (PCPP 1–306 EPC 368)

84.

A. MAO inhibitors work by promoting the release of norepinephrine. These drugs have lost their popularity due to the risk of hypertensive crisis and other unwanted side effects. (PCPP 1–307   EPC 369)

85.

C. Bipolar disorder, also known as manic-depressive disorder, is treated with the mood stabilizer lithium. Its exact mechanism of action is not clearly understood. (PCPP 1–307   EPC 369)

86.

B. Pharmacological therapy for Parkinson's disease is aimed at restoring the balance between norepinephrine and acetylcholine. This is done either by increasing the stimulation of dopamine receptors (dopaminergic effects) or by decreasing the stimulation of acetylcholine receptors (anticholinergic effects). (PCPP 1–308   EPC 370)

87.

C. There is no physical connection between two nerve cells. Instead there is a space called a synapse. The space between a nerve cell and the target organ it innervates is called a neuroeffector junction. A neurotransmitter is a chemical that conducts a nervous impulse across a synapse or neuroeffector junction. (PCPP 1–311   EPC 372)

Matching   (PCPP 1–311   EPC 372)

88. A	Sympathetic preganglionic	**A.** Acetylcholine
89. B	Sympathetic postganglionic	**B.** Norepinephrine
90. A	Parasympathetic preganglionic	
91. A	Parasympathetic postganglionic	

92.

D. The parasympathetic nervous system primarily controls custodial or vegetative functions, such as digestion of food and resting heart rate. It is often referred to as the "feed or breed" aspect of the autonomic nervous system. (PCPP 1–309   EPC 371)

93.

D. The parasympathetic nervous system exerts its control via cranial nerves III (occulomotor), VII (facial), IX (glossopharyngeal), and X (vagus) and via sacral nerves S_2–S_4. (PCPP 1–310)

94.

D. When stimulated, the parasympathetic nervous system decreases the heart rate, promotes increased salivation, and causes pupillary constriction. (PCPP 1–311   EPC 376)

95.

C. Drugs that stimulate the parasympathetic nervous system are called parasympathomimetics. Drugs that antagonize the parasympathetic nervous system are called parasympatholytics or anticholinergics. (PCPP 1–314   EPC 372)

96.

A. A helpful mnemonic for remembering the side effects of cholinergic medications is "SLUDGE." SLUDGE stands for salivation, lacrimation, urination, defecation, gastric motility, and emesis. (PCPP 1–314   EPC 372)

97.

B. Acetylcholine is biodegraded by the enzyme cholinesterase. One of the common ways to prolong cholinergic effects is to administer drugs that inhibit the breakdown of acetylcholine by cholinesterase. (PCPP 1–314   EPC 372)

98.

D. Bethanechol (Urecholine) is the prototype cholinergic medication that acts directly on ACh receptors, much like acetylcholine, except that it is not biodegraded by cholinesterase, resulting in a longer duration of action. (PCPP 1–314   EPC 372)

99.

A. The two common reversible cholinesterase inhibitors are physostigmine (Antilirium) and neostigmine (Prostigmine). Physostigmine (short acting) is used to treat anticholinergic overdoses. Neostigmine (long acting) is used to treat myasthenia gravis. Both inhibit the breakdown of acetylcholine by cholinesterase. (PCPP 1–315   EPC 373)

100.

D. Treatment for toxic cholinergic overdose, such as nerve gas or organophosphate insecticides, includes large doses of atropine and pralidoxime (Protopam, 2-Pam). Atropine competes for ACh receptor sites, while pralidixome encourages cholinesterase release. (PCPP 1–315   EPC 373)

101.

D. Atropine is the prototype muscarinic antagonist. It binds with ACh receptors and blocks the effects of ACh on muscarinic sites. It is most often used to increase the heart rate in symptomatic bradycardia. (PCPP 1–315   EPC 374)

102.

B. Ipratropium bromide (Atrovent) is an aerosolized anticholinergic medication used to treat asthma because of its ability to dilate bronchial smooth muscle. It is often combined with an inhaled beta agonist. (PCPP 1–316   EPC 374)

103.

A. Succinylcholine is a depolarizing neuromuscular blocker. It binds with ACh receptor sites (nicotinic) and depolarizes them, causing brief muscular contraction. But since it does not freely separate from the receptor site, it remains bound, preventing repolarization. Thus, the patient becomes paralyzed. It is biodegraded by its own enzyme, pseudocholinesterase, and has a short duration of action. (PCPP 1–317   EPC 375)

104.

D. In contrast to the parasympathetic, the sympathetic nervous system is our body's defense against extreme stress. Also known as the "fight or flight" response, the sympathetic storm readies our bodies to withstand perceived threats. (PCPP 1–317   EPC 375)

105.

B. Sympathetic nerve fibers arise from the spinal cord at the levels of T1 through L2 and run along each side of the spinal column in special ganglionic "chains." In addition, collateral ganglia that innervate the abdominal organs are located in the abdominal cavity. (PCPP 1–317)

106.

B. When stimulated, the sympathetic nervous system causes pupillary dilation, an increase in heart rate, an increase in the force of cardiac contractions, peripheral vasoconstriction, and an increase in metabolic rate. All these reactions are designed to help us meet the challenge of a severe physical or psychological stressor. (PCPP 1–347   EPC 375)

Matching (PCPP 1–321   EPC 376)

107. C Alpha 1	**A.** Renal artery dilator
108. E Alpha 2	**B.** Arteriole and bronchial dilator
109. D Beta 1	
110. B Beta 2	**C.** Peripheral vasoconstrictor
111. A Dopaminergic	**D.** Increased chronotropy and inotropy
	E. Presynaptic inhibition

112.

D. Alpha 1 agonists cause peripheral vasoconstriction and mild bronchoconstriction. Drugs in this class include epinephrine, norepinephrine, phenylephrine, and ephedrine. They are used to raise blood pressure and decrease nasal congestion, and they are combined with local anesthetics to decrease systemic absorption. (PCPP 1–322 EPC 376)

113.

B. Prazosin (Minipress) is an alpha 1 antagonist. By blocking alpha 1 stimulation, it dilates the peripheral blood vessels. Its main use is controlling hypertension. (PCPP 1–322 EPC 377)

114.

B. Drugs such as atenolol (Tenormin) and metoprolol (Lopressor) selectively block beta 1 receptor sites and have little or no effect on the beta 2 receptors in the lungs. They are prescribed to decrease the cardiac rate and contractility in patients with reactive airway disease (COPD, asthma) because they do not block the beta 2 bronchodilation effects. (PCPP 1–323 EPC 378)

115.

D. Class I antidysrhythmics inhibit the influx of sodium in phases 0 and 4 of fast potentials. This slows conduction down the specialized conduction system of the atria and ventricles. Drugs in this class include procainamide (IA), lidocaine (IB), and flecainide. (PCPP 1–328 EPC 379)

116.

B. Propranolol (Inderal) is a class II antidysrhythmic. A nonselective beta blocker, propranolol competes for all beta 1 receptors in the heart and beta 2 receptors in the lungs and vasculature. Drugs such as atenolol and metoprolol are beta 1 selective beta blockers that do not affect the lungs. (PCPP 1–330 EPC 380)

117.

C. Verapamil, diltiazem, and nifedipine, all class III antidysrhythmics, work by inhibiting the slow influx of calcium. They slow conduction through the AV node and are prescribed for angina, hypertension, and tachycardia. (PCPP 1–330 EPC 330)

118.

D. Digoxin is a paradoxical drug. It decreases the intrinsic firing rate of the SA node (negative chronotrope), while it strengthens the force of contractions (positive inotrope). It also is a common cause of various types of dysrhythmia, especially bradycardias and ventricular ectopy. It has an extremely narrow therapeutic range, so always suspect digoxin toxicity. (PCPP 1–330 EPC 381)

119.

A. Loop diuretics block sodium reabsorption in the ascending loop of Henle, increasing the excretion of water. The most popular loop diuretic is furosemide (Lasix). (PCPP 1–332 EPC 382)

120.

C. Administering furosemide too rapidly may cause ototoxicity, resulting in tinnitis or deafness. (PCPP 1–332 EPC 382)

121.

C. Clonodine (Catapres) and methyldopa (Aldomet) are both alpha 2 blockers. They reduce blood pressure by inhibiting central nervous system (CNS) stimulation of the sympathetic receptors (alpha 1, beta 1, beta 2). (PCPP 1–333 EPC 383)

122.

B. Alpha 1 receptors are located in the peripheral blood vessels. When stimulated, they cause profound vasoconstriction. When blocked, they reduce peripheral vascular resistance and lower the blood pressure. (PCPP 1–334 EPC 383)

123.

A. ACE inhibitors block the conversion of angiotensin I to angiotensin II, a powerful vasoconstrictor. They work primarily in the lungs. (PCPP 1–334 EPC 384)

124.

C. A new class of drugs, angiotensin II blockers, achieves the same effects as ACE inhibitors without the side effect of coughing or angioedema. These drugs allow the conversion of angiotensin I to angiotensin II but block the angiotensin II receptor sites. The prototype is losartan (Cozaar). (PCPP 1–335   EPC 385)

125.

C. Verapamil and diltiazem are the only two calcium channel blockers that work on the heart. Nifedipine works on the smooth muscle of the arterioles and causes dilation. It is prescribed mainly for hypertension. (PCPP 1–335   EPC 385)

126.

A. Nitrates cause smooth muscle relaxation, especially in the blood vessels. Sodium nitroprusside is used to reduce blood pressure in hypertensive emergencies by causing direct vasodilation. (PCPP 1–336   EPC 387)

127.

C. People with angina take nitroglycerine to cause vasodilation and to cause venous pooling. This reduces preload and the workload of the heart. It also dilates the coronary arteries, allowing more oxygenated blood to reach the myocardium. (PCPP 1–337   EPC 387)

128.

A. Aspirin is the prototype antiplatelet drug. It decreases the formation of platelet plugs by inhibiting cyclooxygenase, the enzyme needed for platelet aggregation. (PCPP 1–338   EPC 388)

129.

B. Warfarin (Coumadin), first developed as a rat poison, is an anticoagulant because it interrupts the clotting cascade by antagonizing the effects of vitamin K. Vitamin K is essential for the clotting cascade. (PCPP 1–339   EPC 388)

130.

D. Thrombolytics are drugs that act directly on thrombi to break them down. They are used to treat most myocardial infarctions and some strokes. The most popular thrombolytics are streptokinase (Streptase), alteplase (tPA), reteplase (Retavase), and anistreplase (Eminase). (PCPP 1–339   EPC 389)

131.

B. Antihyperlipidemics are used to treat high blood cholesterol by reducing blood levels of LDLs (low density lipoproteins), which cause atherosclerosis and coronary artery disease. Lovastatin (Mevacor) and simvastatin (Zocor) are popular drugs in this class. (PCPP 1–340   EPC 389)

Matching   (PCPP 1–341   EPC 391)

132. D	Epinephrine	**A.** Beta 2 selective agonist
133. A	Albuterol (Proventil)	**B.** Leukotriene antagonist
134. F	Theophylline (Theo-Dur)	**C.** Mast cell stabilizer
135. G	Ipratropium (Atrovent)	**D.** Beta agonist
136. E	Beclomethasone (Beclovent)	**E.** Glucocorticoid
137. B	Zafirlukast (Accolate)	**F.** Methylxanthine
138. C	Cromolyn sodium (Intal)	**G.** Anticholinergic

139.

D. Nasal congestion is caused by dilated and engorged capillaries. By administering an alpha 1 agonist, you vasoconstrict the tissue beds, reducing the tissue size and relieving the congested nasal passages. Common decongestants contain pseudoephedrine, phenylephrine, or phenylpropanolamine and are administered in drops or nasal spray. (PCPP 1–343 EPC 393)

140.

C. Antihistamines compete for histamine receptor sites in the blood vessels, airways, and GI tract. The effects of histamine include vasodilation and capillary leaking, bronchoconstriction and increased mucus production, and abdominal cramping. (PCPP 1–343   EPC 393)

141.

C. An antitussive medication suppresses the cough stimulus in the central nervous system. Dextromethorphan is the leading drug in this class and is present in many over-the-counter cough and cold preparations. (PCPP 1–344   EPC 394)

142.

A. Peptic ulcer disease is treated by a combination of medications that kill bacteria (antibiotics), reduce acid secretion (proton pump inhibitors, H_2 receptor blockers, anticholinergics), and reduce the stomach's pH (antacids). (PCPP 1–346 EPC 395)

143.

D. Laxatives come in four varieties based on their mechanism of action. Surfactant laxatives, such as docusate (Colace), decrease surface tension and increase water absorption into the feces. Bulk-forming laxatives, such as psyllium (Metamucil), contain fiber, which absorbs water into the stool. Osmotic laxatives, such as Milk of Magnesia, increase osmotic pressure in the feces, drawing water. Stimulant laxatives, such as phenolphthalein (Ex-Lax), increase intestinal motility. (PCPP 1–346 EPC 396)

144.

D. Antiemetics are medications used to control vomiting. Serotonin antagonists, such as ondansetron (Zofran), block the chemoreceptor trigger zone (CTZ) in the medulla. Phenothiazines, such as prochlorperazine (Compazine), block dopamine receptors in the CTZ. Cannabinoids, such as tetrahydrocannabinol (THC), are used to treat chemotherapy-induced nausea and vomiting. (PCPP 1–347 EPC 397)

145.

B. All antiglaucoma medications work by decreasing intraoccular pressure. These medications include beta blockers, such as timolol (Timoptic), and cholinergics, such as pilocarpine (Isopto-Carpine). (PCPP 1–348 EPC 398)

146.

A. A patient using gentamicin sulfate otic solution has otitis, an ear infection. (PCPP 1–348 EPC 399)

147.

B. Vasopressin is an analog to antidiuretic hormone (ADH). When administered, it causes increased water reabsorption in the kidneys, creating more concentrated urine. At high doses, it causes peripheral vasoconstriction and increased blood pressure. (PCPP 1–350 EPC 399)

148.

A. Hypothyroidism is manifested by a decreased metabolic rate, weight gain, fatigue, and bradycardia. The treatment is thyroid hormone replacement therapy. The prototype is levothyroxine (Synthroid). (PCPP 1–351 EPC 399)

149.

B. The adrenal cortex secretes three classes of hormones: androgens (sex hormones), glucocorticoids (cortisol), and mineralocorticoids (aldosterone). (PCPP 1–351 EPC 400)

150.

A. Glucagon is secreted by the alpha cells in the pancreas. It causes both gluconeogenesis (synthesis of glucose) and glycogenolysis (glycogen breakdown into glucose). It is secreted when blood glucose levels fall. Paramedics administer it to hypoglycemic patients to increase blood glucose levels. It is also given for severe beta blocker overdose because it raises intracellular levels of cyclic AMP, which increases automaticity. (PCPP 1–352 EPC 401)

151.

B. Insulin preparations derived from beef or pork, as well as the Lentes, may lead to allergic reactions. Natural human insulin does not have this effect. (PCPP 1–353 EPC 401)

152.

C. There are four types of oral hypoglycemic agents, all aimed at decreasing blood levels of glucose. Sulfonylureas, such as tolbutamide (Orinase) and glyburide (Micronase), stimulate the pancreas to secrete insulin. Biguanides, such as metformin (Glucophage), decrease glucose synthesis and increase glucose uptake. Alpha-glucosidase inhibitors, such as acarbose (Precose), delay carbohydrate metabolism. Thiazolidinediones, such as troglitazone (Rezulin), promote tissue response to insulin. (PCPP 1–354 EPC 402)

153.

D. Antineoplastic agents are drugs used to treat cancer. Chemotherapy is aimed at destroying cancerous cells. Unfortunately the drugs cannot differentiate between cancerous cells and healthy cells and often cause horrible side effects. There are many types, classified according to their mechanism of action. Paramedics may be called to manage the common side effects of nausea and vomiting. (PCPP 1–356   EPC 405)

154.

B. Drugs in the penicillin and cephalosporin classes inhibit cell wall synthesis, which allows an osmotic shift of water into the cell until the cell ruptures, killing the bacteria. Other antibiotic classes inhibit protein synthesis and prevent bacteria from spreading to other cells and thus spreading the infection. (PCPP 1–357   EPC 406)

155.

A. Aspirin, ibuprofen, and naproxen are known as nonsteroidal anti-inflammatory drugs (NSAIDs). They work by interfering with the production of prostaglandins and the inflammatory process. These popular over-the-counter medications are used to relieve pain. (PCPP 1–358   EPC 407)

156.

A. Gout is an inflammatory disease caused by an altered metabolism of uric acid and marked by an elevated level of uric acid in the blood. Uricosuric drugs, such as colchicine and allopurinol (Zyloprim), are used to manage the pain and swelling of the joints caused by gout. (PCPP 1–358   EPC 408)

10 Medication Administration

DIRECTIONS Each of the questions or incomplete statements below is followed by suggested answers or completions. Select the **one answer** that is best in each case.

1. Which of the following would you use to clean the skin prior to starting an IV?
   A. An antiseptic solution
   B. A disinfectant solution
   C. Neither A nor B
   D. Either A or B

2. Nitroglycerine patches are examples of _____ medications.
   A. intradermal
   B. transtracheal
   C. subcutaneous
   D. transdermal

Match the following percutaneous medication routes with their respective definitions:

3. _____ Sublingual
4. _____ Buccal
5. _____ Ocular
6. _____ Aural
7. _____ Nasal

A. Through the mucous membranes of the eye
B. Through the nares
C. Into the ear canal
D. Between the cheek and gums
E. Under the tongue

8. Your mother's eye drop prescription reads 2 gtts o.s. What does this mean?
   A. 2 drops each day
   B. 2 drops each eye
   C. 2 drops right eye
   D. 2 drops left eye

9. When setting up a nebulizer treatment, set the oxygen source at _____ liters/minute.
   A. 2–4
   B. 5–8

C. 9–12
D. 15

10. For patients with decreased tidal volumes, how would you administer a nebulized medication?
    A. Connect the nebulizer to a bag-valve-mask
    B. Inject the medication down the ET tube
    C. Spray the medication into the oral cavity
    D. None of the above

11. Which of the following drugs can be administered directly down an endotracheal tube?
    A. Sodium bicarbonate
    B. Atropine
    C. Diazepam (Valium)
    D. Dopamine

12. Which of the following devices facilitates the use of a metered dose inhaler?
    A. Endotracheal tube
    B. Bag-valve-mask
    C. Nebulizer
    D. Spacer

13. Where do you measure the amount of liquid in a medicine cup?
    A. At the sides
    B. At the center
    C. At the highest level
    D. None of the above

14. A teaspoon holds _____ ml of liquid.
    A. 1
    B. 3
    C. 5
    D. 10

15. After administering a medication orally, follow it with at least _____ ounces

of water to push the medication into the stomach.

A. 4–8

B. 10–15

C. 1–3

D. 16–20

16. Which of the following may **NOT** be administered via an orogastric tube?

A. Crushed time-released capsules

B. Crushed pills

C. Crushed tablets

D. Liquids

17. Which of the following statements regarding rectal administration is true?

A. Absorption is usually slow

B. The drug is subject to hepatic alteration

C. The drug will not pass through the liver

D. Absorption time is unpredictable

18. You are preparing to administer 3 cc of medication. Which size syringe would be most appropriate?

A. 5 cc

B. 3 cc

C. 10 cc

D. 20 cc

19. Which of the following is the largest bore hypodermic needle?

A. 27 gauge

B. 25 gauge

C. 19 gauge

D. 18 gauge

20. You hold a glass vial containing a medication that reads 250 mg in 10 ml. What is the concentration?

A. 4/1

B. 10/1

C. 25/1

D. None of the above

21. An intradermal injection is administered at a _____ angle to the skin.

A. 45°

B. 90°

C. 180°

D. 10°

22. A subcutaneous injection is administered at a _____ angle to the skin.

A. 45°

B. 90°

C. 180°

D. 15°

23. An intramuscular injection is administered at a _____ angle to the skin.

A. 45°

B. 90°

C. 180°

D. 55°

24. You are ordered to administer 5 ml of a medication IM. You can safely administer this medication into all of the following muscles **EXCEPT**

A. vastus lateralis

B. rectus femoris

C. deltoid

D. dorsal gluteal

25. It is important to aspirate for blood return when administering medications via the IM route to ensure

A. the airway is patent

B. the needle is in a vein

C. the needle is in the artery

D. the needle is not in a blood vessel

26. Which of the following is **NOT** an indication for starting an IV?

A. Replacing fluid and blood

B. Administering a drug

C. Meeting a CME requirement

D. Obtaining blood samples for lab analysis

27. Which of the following is considered a peripheral vein?
    A. Internal jugular
    B. Subclavian
    C. Femoral
    D. External jugular

28. Which of the following statements is true regarding the use of peripheral veins?
    A. They tend to roll and elude IV placement
    B. They collapse in hypovolemic patients
    C. They are often fragile in the elderly
    D. All of the above

29. A PICC line is
    A. a peripheral line started in a central vein
    B. a central line started in a peripheral vein
    C. a multilumen central line
    D. another name for a Swan-Ganz catheter

30. Which of the following solutions is a crystalloid?
    A. Plasmanate
    B. Dextran
    C. Hetastarch
    D. None of the above

31. Which type of IV solution will remain in the bloodstream initially and not cause a shift in water?
    A. Hypotonic
    B. Hypertonic
    C. Isotonic
    D. Hyperlipid

32. Which type of IV solution will rapidly leave the intravascular space?
    A. Hypotonic
    B. Hypertonic
    C. Isotonic
    D. Hyperlipid

33. Which type of IV solution will draw water into the vascular space?
    A. Hypotonic
    B. Hypertonic
    C. Isotonic
    D. Hyperlipid

34. Lactated Ringer's contains all of the following EXCEPT
    A. proteins
    B. potassium chloride
    C. calcium chloride
    D. sodium lactate

35. You have infused 2 liters of 0.9% sodium chloride into your hypovolemic trauma patient. In one hour, how much will be lost to the intravascular space?
    A. 1 liter
    B. 2 liters
    C. 660 ml
    D. 1320 ml

36. In a microdrip solution set, _____ drops equal 1 ml.
    A. 10
    B. 15
    C. 30
    D. 60

37. The main difference between normal IV tubing and blood tubing is
    A. the width of the tubing
    B. the presence of an administration port
    C. a filter to prevent an embolism
    D. the absence of a flow clamp

38. Through which of the following catheters can you deliver the most rapid fluid challenge?
    A. 12 gauge, 4 inch
    B. 12 gauge, 1 inch
    C. 24 gauge, 4 inch
    D. 24 gauge, 1 inch

39. Chills, fever, nausea, and vomiting following IV insertion indicate
    A. an inadvertent arterial puncture
    B. a pyrogenic reaction
    C. thrombophlebitis
    D. an air embolism

40. In this case, you should immediately
    A. place the patient head down on his left side
    B. place warm packs on the IV site
    C. stop the IV
    D. clear the IV line of any air

41. A Huber needle is used with
    A. a venous access device
    B. an infusion controller
    C. an infusion pump
    D. blood tubes

42. Which of the following IV devices delivers fluids and medications under positive pressure?
    A. The Huber device
    B. An infusion controller
    C. An infusion pump
    D. The Hickman device

Match the following blood tube color tops with their respective anticoagulants:

43. ____ Red
44. ____ Blue
45. ____ Green
46. ____ Purple
47. ____ Gray

    A. EDTA
    B. None
    C. Fluoride
    D. Citrate
    E. Heparin

48. If you leave the constricting band on your patient's arm too long prior to drawing a venous blood sample, what might be the result?
    A. Hemoconcentration
    B. Hemolysis
    C. Hemophilia
    D. A and B

49. Generally you will use the intraosseous route for pediatric patients in what age group?
    A. 3–7
    B. 5–10
    C. Newborn–10
    D. Newborn–5

50. When inserting an IO needle, you must be careful not to
    A. infuse crystalloids
    B. damage the epiphyseal plate
    C. enter the medullary canal
    D. use the medial tibial plateau

51. For the adult or geriatric patient, you should insert an IO needle
    A. into the proximal tibia
    B. into the distal tibia
    C. superior to the medial malleolus
    D. B and C

52. When inserting an IO needle, you stop when you
    A. feel an increase in resistance
    B. feel a "pop"
    C. hear a "whoosh"
    D. see a bone marrow return

53. Which of the following is a contraindication to IO insertion?
    A. Fracture to the tibia
    B. Fracture to the ipsilateral femur
    C. Osteogenesis imperfecta
    D. All of the above

Make the following conversions:

54.	3 kilograms	= _____	grams
55.	2.5 grams	= _____	milligrams
56.	8 milligrams	= _____	micrograms
57.	3000 milliliters	= _____	liters
58.	22 pounds	= _____	kilograms
59.	800 micrograms	= _____	milligrams
60.	3 liters	= _____	milliliters
61.	500 milligrams	= _____	grams
62.	5 grams	= _____	micrograms

Calculate the following drug orders:

	Drug Order	Patient Weight	Administer
63.	1 mg/kg	176 lbs.	_____ mg
64.	10 mg/kg	220 lbs.	_____ mg
65.	20 ml/kg	55 lbs.	_____ ml
66.	5 mcg/kg/min	110 lbs.	_____ mcg/min
67.	0.1 mg/kg	22 lbs.	_____ mg

Determine the following drug concentrations:

68.	100 mg/10 ml	_____/ml
69.	50 mg/2 ml	_____/ml
70.	250 mg/20 ml	_____/ml
71.	1 gram/10 ml	_____/ml
72.	1 mg/1 ml	_____/ml

Calculate the following drug administrations:

	Drug on Hand	MD Order	Administer
73.	100 mg/5 ml	75 mg	_____ ml
74.	1 mg/1 ml	0.25 mg	_____ ml
75.	50 mg/2 ml	25 mg	_____ ml

76.	200 mg/5 ml	50 mg	_____ ml
77.	1 mg/10 ml	0.5 mg	_____ ml
78.	500 mg/10 ml	5 mg/kg (198 lbs.)	_____ ml
79.	100 mg/10 ml	1 mg/kg (187 lbs.)	_____ ml
80.	2 mg/1 ml	10 mg	_____ ml
81.	40 mg/10 ml	120 mg	_____ ml
82.	400 mg/20 ml	80 mg	_____ ml

Calculate the following drip rates using microdrip solution sets (60 drops/ml):

	Drug	Solution	MD Order	Drip Rate
83.	1 gram	250 ml	3 mg/min	___ drops/min
84.	2 grams	500 ml	2 mg/min	___ drops/min
85.	1 mg	250 ml	4 mcg/min	___ drops/min
86.	400 mg	500 ml	5 mcg/kg/min (176 lbs.)	___ drops/min
87.	1 gram	500 ml	2 mg/min	___ drops/min

Calculate the following fluid infusion rates:

	Volume	Infusion Set	Time	
88.	300 ml	10 gtts/ml	60 minutes	___ drops/min
89.	200 ml	15 gtts/ml	60 minutes	___ drops/min
90.	20 ml	60 gtts/ml	20 minutes	___ drops/min

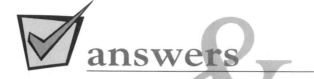

answers & rationales

1.

A. A disinfectant is toxic to human tissue. An antiseptic is not. Therefore, use an antiseptic solution or wipe to cleanse the skin prior to injection. (PCPP 1–372 EPC 415)

2.

D. Nitroglycerine patches, some hypertension medications, and hormones are examples of medications given transdermally. A transdermal medication is absorbed through the skin into the circulatory system. (PCPP 1–374 EPC 417)

Matching (PCPP 1–375 EPC 418)

3.	**E**	Sublingual	**A.**	Through the mucous membranes of the eye
4.	**D**	Buccal		
5.	**A**	Ocular	**B.**	Through the nares
6.	**C**	Aural	**C.**	Into the ear canal
7.	**B**	Nasal	**D.**	Between the cheek and gums
			E.	Under the tongue

8.

D. Refer to the following Latin abbreviations with regard to the eye drop prescription: (PCPP 1–377 EPC 419)

o.d. (oculus dexter)   right eye
o.s. (oculus sinister)   left eye
o.u. (oculus uterque)   both eyes

9.

B. When setting up a nebulizer—as with albuterol, for example—set the oxygen source at 5–8 liters/minute. Any lower setting will not create enough pressure to aerosolize the medication. A setting greater than 8 will create too much pressure and damage the delivery system at its weakest point. (PCPP 1–380 EPC 422)

10.

A. If your patient has a decreased tidal volume, the medication may not reach the lower lungs. In this case, attach the nebulizer to a bag-valve-mask, and perform intermittent positive pressure ventilation with the nebulizer running. (PCPP 1–380 EPC 422)

11.

B. In the emergency setting, atropine, lidocaine (Xylocaine), naloxone (Narcan), and epinephrine may be administered safely down the endotracheal tube when vascular access cannot be obtained. (PCPP 1–383 EPC 425)

12.

D. It is very difficult for the untrained person to use a metered dose inhaler effectively because it requires a great deal of coordination and rarely do patients receive proper training. The spacer was invented to help patients use the inhaler. As they simply have to breathe in and out of the device, its operation requires little coordination or training. (PCPP 1–381 EPC 423)

13.

B. When you pour a liquid medication into a medicine cup, it does not form a flat surface. Instead it clings to the sides at a higher level. Therefore, always measure the liquid at the center, at the lowest point. (PCPP 1–385 EPC 427)

14.

C. A measured teaspoon holds 5 milliliters of liquid. Since household spoons are notoriously inaccurate, always use a measured spoon or syringe. (PCPP 1–385 EPC 427)

15.

A. After administering an oral medication, you should follow it with at least 4–8 ounces of water or other fluid to help transport it to the stomach. (PCPP 1–386 EPC 428)

16.

A. Because it would alter the slow-release mechanism, you should never administer time-release capsules or enteric coated tablets through an orogastric tube. (PCPP 1–386 EPC 428)

17.

C. Drugs administered per rectum (PR) are rapidly absorbed through the rich capillary beds of the rectum and do not make a first pass through the liver; thus, hepatic alteration is avoided. (PCPP 1–388 EPC 430)

18.

A. The size of the syringe (the barrel) should be slightly larger than the amount of medication you are going to deliver. Thus, for a 3 cc delivery, select a 5 cc syringe. (PCPP 1–390 EPC 432)

19.

D. A needle's gauge describes its diameter. The numbers are in reverse order of their sizes. For example, an 18 gauge is larger than a 27 gauge. (PCPP 1–391 EPC 433)

20.

C. To calculate a drug's concentration, simply divide the amount of drug (250 mg) by the amount of fluid (10 cc). In this case, the concentration is 250 mg/10 ml or 25/1. (PCPP 1–392 EPC 434)

21.

D. An intradermal injection is administered at a 10–15° angle to the skin. (PCPP 1–398 EPC 440)

22.

A. A subcutaneous injection is administered at a 45° angle to the skin. (PCPP 1–399 EPC 441)

23.

B. An intramuscular injection is administered at a 90° angle to the skin. (PCPP 1–403 EPC 444)

24.

C. You can safely administer 5 ml of medication into the vastus lateralis (lateral thigh), the rectus femoris (anterior thigh), and the dorsal gluteal (buttock). You should administer only up to 2 ml into the deltoid muscle of the lateral shoulder. (PCPP 1–405 EPC 446)

25.

D. It is important to aspirate for blood return when administering medications via the IM (intramuscular) route to ensure that the needle is not in a blood vessel. Administering an IM medication directly into the bloodstream (IV) could be fatal. (PCPP 1–405 EPC 446)

26.

C. There are three reasons for starting an IV: to replace fluid or blood, to administer drugs, and to obtain venous blood samples for laboratory analysis. Never start one just because you need the CME credit. (PCPP 1–407 EPC 448)

27.

D. The external jugular is considered a peripheral vein. The subclavian, internal jugular, and femoral are all considered central veins. (PCPP 1–408 EPC 449)

28.

D. Peripheral veins are the easiest to cannulate during an emergency because of their accessibility. Unfortunately, they often collapse during hypovolemia or circulatory failure, roll and hide during IV placement, and can be extremely fragile in elderly patients. (PCPP 1–408 EPC 449)

29.

B. A PICC (peripherally inserted central catheter) line is a central line started in a peripheral vein. It is smaller than a normal central line and is used primarily for infants and children requiring long-term care. (PCPP 1–409 EPC 450)

30.

D. Crystalloids contain water and electrolytes but lack the proteins and larger molecules of the colloids.

Examples of crystalloids include normal saline, lactated Ringer's, and D₅W. (PCPP 1–410   EPC 451)

31.

C. An isotonic solution has the same concentration (tonicity) on both sides of a semipermeable membrane (the vein). Because of this, there is no gradient (pulling force) created and no resulting water shift initially. (PCPP 1–410   EPC 451)

32.

A. A hypotonic solution has a lower solute concentration on one side of the semipermeable membrane (vein). Because of this, a pulling force (an osmotic gradient) is created, and water is "pulled" from the vein into the interstitial space. Examples include D₅W and 0.45% normal saline (one-half NS). (PCPP 1–410   EPC 451)

33.

B. A hypertonic solution has a higher solute concentration on one side of the semipermeable membrane and creates a gradient that pulls water into the vein. Examples include D₅₀W, mannitol, and the colloids. (PCPP 1–410   EPC 451)

34.

A. The isotonic solution named after Sidney Ringer contains sodium chloride, potassium chloride, calcium chloride, sodium lactate, and water. (PCPP 1–410   EPC 451)

35.

D. Two-thirds of an isotonic solution, such as normal saline (0.9% sodium chloride), will leave the intravascular space within 1 hour. (PCPP 1–411 EPC 451)

36.

D. In a microdrip solution set, 60 drops equal 1 ml. (PCPP 1–413   EPC 452)

37.

C. Blood tubing contains a filter to prevent clots or other debris from entering the patient. If a clot or debris enters the bloodstream, it could travel, as an embolus; lodge in a narrowed vessel; and occlude all blood flow distal to the occlusion. (PCPP 1–415 EPC 455)

38.

B. In order to infuse the most fluid the most rapidly, use the largest diameter cannula with the shortest possible needle length. (PCPP 1–419   EPC 458)

39.

B. A pyrogenic reaction occurs when pyrogens, "foreign particles capable of producing fever," are present in the administration set or intravenous solution. It is characterized by the abrupt onset of fever, chills, backache, headache, nausea, and vomiting. Cardiovascular collapse may also result. (PCPP 1–427   EPC 465)

40.

C. In a case of pyrogenic reaction, terminate the IV immediately and establish another IV in the other arm, using a new administration set and solution. (PCPP 1–427   EPC 1500)

41.

A. A Huber needle has an opening on the side of the shaft instead of at the tip. It is used with venous access devices to inject medications or fluid. Every venous access device has its own specialized needle. (PCPP 1–435   EPC 473)

42.

C. An infusion pump is a device that delivers fluids and medications under positive pressure rather than gravity. The major disadvantage of these devices is that you may cause more complications if the vein is infiltrated because of the positive pressure. (PCPP 1–437   EPC 475)

Matching   (PCPP 1–439   EPC 477)

43.	**B**	Red		**A.**	EDTA
44.	**D**	Blue		**B.**	None
45.	**E**	Green		**C.**	Fluoride
46.	**A**	Purple		**D.**	Citrate
47.	**C**	Gray		**E.**	Heparin

48.

D. If you leave the constricting band on too long prior to drawing a venous blood sample, you run the risk of causing hemoconcentration (elevated numbers of red and white blood cells) and hemolysis (destruction of red blood cells). Both will render the results of the blood sample inaccurate and unusable. (PCPP 1–442   EPC 480)

49.

D. As a rule, you can use the intraosseous (IO) route for rapid venous access in critical patients less than 5 years of age. (PCPP 1–442   EPC 480)

50.

B. At the proximal end of the tibial shaft lies the epiphyseal (or growth) plate. If damaged, it can cause long-term growth complications or abnormalities. Always select an insertion site that is below the tibial tuberosity and on the medial tibial plateau. (PCPP 1–443   EPC 481)

51.

D. For the adult or geriatric patient, you may insert an IO needle into the distal tibia, just superior to the medial malleolus. (PCPP 1–444   EPC 482)

52.

B. When inserting an IO needle with a twisting motion, you should stop pushing when you feel a sudden decrease in resistance, or a "pop." Remember, one pop is good (you are in). Two pops are bad (you have gone through the other side). (PCPP 1–445 EPC 483)

53.

D. Do not attempt an IO line if your patient has a fractured tibia, has a fractured femur on the same side, or has osteogenesis imperfecta, a congenital bone disease that causes fragile bones. (PCPP 1–449 EPC 486)

The conversions are based on the following metric system table:
1 gram = 1000 milligrams = 1,000,000 micrograms
1000 grams = 1 kilogram
1 kilogram = 2.2 pounds
1 liter = 1000 milliliters

Math Problems (PCPP 1–450–1–458   EPC 487–495)

54. 1 kilogram = 1000 grams; 3 kilograms = 3000 grams

55. 1 gram = 1000 milligrams; 2.5 grams = 2500 milligrams

56. 1 milligram = 1000 micrograms; 8 milligrams = 8000 micrograms

57. 1000 milliliters = 1 liter; 3000 milliliters = 3 liters

58. 2.2 pounds = 1 kilogram; 22 pounds = 10 kilograms

59. 1000 micrograms = 1 milligram; 800 micrograms = 0.8 milligram

60. 1 liter = 1000 milliliters; 3 liters = 3000 milliliters

61. 1000 milligrams = 1 gram; 500 milligrams = 0.5 gram

62. 1 gram = 1,000,000 micrograms; 5 grams = 5,000,000 micrograms

63.

The patient weighs 176 lbs. $176 \div 2.2 = 80$ kg
$1 \text{ mg} \times 80 \text{ kg} = 80$ mg (PCPP 1–451)

64.

Patient weighs 220 lbs. $220 \div 2.2 = 100$ kg
$10 \text{ mg} \times 100 \text{ kg} = 1000$ mg

65.

Patient weighs 55 lbs. $55 \div 2.2 = 25$ kg   20 ml
$\times 25 \text{ kg} = 500$ ml

66.

Patient weighs 110 lbs. $110 \div 2.2 = 50$ kg
$50 \text{ kg} \times 5 \text{ mcg/kg/min} = 250$ mcg/min

67.

Patient weighs 22 lbs. $22 \div 2.2 = 10$ kg   10 kg
$\times 0.1 \text{ mg/kg} = 1.0$ mg

68.

$100 \text{ mg} \div 10 \text{ ml} = 10$ mg/ml

69.

$50 \text{ mg} \div 2 \text{ ml} = 25$ mg/ml

70.

$250 \text{ mg} \div 20 \text{ ml} = 12.5$ mg/ml

71.

1 gram (1000 mg) $\div 10 \text{ ml} = 100$ mg/ml

72.

$1 \text{ mg} \div 1 \text{ ml} = 1 \text{ mg/ml}$

The following calculations are based on the formula:

$$X = \frac{\text{Volume on hand} \times \text{Desired dose (MD order)}}{\text{Drug on hand}}$$

73.

$$X = \frac{5 \text{ ml} \times 75 \text{ mg}}{100 \text{ mg}} \quad X = \frac{375}{100} \quad X = 3.75 \text{ ml}$$

74.

$$X = \frac{1 \text{ ml} \times 0.25 \text{ mg}}{1 \text{ mg}} \quad X = \frac{0.25}{1} \quad X = 0.25 \text{ ml}$$

75.

$$X = \frac{2 \text{ ml} \times 25 \text{ mg}}{50 \text{ mg}} \quad X = \frac{50}{50} \quad X = 1 \text{ ml}$$

76.

$$X = \frac{5 \text{ ml} \times 50 \text{ mg}}{200 \text{ mg}} \quad X = \frac{250}{200} \quad X = 1.25 \text{ ml}$$

77.

$$X = \frac{10 \text{ ml} \times 0.5 \text{ mg}}{1 \text{ mg}} \quad X = \frac{5.0}{1} \quad X = 5.0 \text{ ml}$$

78.

Patient weighs 198 lbs. $198 \div 2.2 = 90 \text{ kg}$
MD order is 5 mg/kg $90 \text{ kg} \times 5 \text{ mg} = 450 \text{ mg}$

$$X = \frac{10 \text{ ml} \times 450 \text{ mg}}{500 \text{ mg}} \quad X = \frac{4500}{500} \quad X = 9 \text{ ml}$$

79.

Patient weighs 187 lbs. $187 \div 2.2 = 85 \text{ kg}$
MD order is 1 mg/kg $85 \text{ kg} \times 1 \text{ mg} = 85 \text{ mg}$

$$X = \frac{10 \text{ ml} \times 85 \text{ mg}}{100 \text{ mg}} \quad X = \frac{850}{100} \quad X = 8.5 \text{ ml}$$

80.

$$X = \frac{1 \text{ ml} \times 10 \text{ mg}}{2 \text{ mg}} \quad X = \frac{10}{2} \quad X = 5 \text{ ml}$$

81.

$$X = \frac{10 \text{ ml} \times 120 \text{ mg}}{40 \text{ mg}} \quad X = \frac{1200}{40} \quad X = 30 \text{ ml}$$

82.

$$X = \frac{20 \text{ ml} \times 80 \text{ mg}}{400 \text{ mg}} \quad X = \frac{1600}{400} \quad X = 4 \text{ ml}$$

The following drip rate calculations are based on the formula:

$$X = \frac{\text{Solution volume} \times \text{Dose/min} \times \text{Drops/ml in solution set}}{\text{Drug in solution}}$$

83.

$$X = \frac{250 \text{ ml} \times 3 \text{ mg/min} \times 60 \text{ drops/ml}}{1000 \text{ mg}}$$

$$X = \frac{750 \times 60}{1000} \quad X = \frac{45,000}{1000} \quad X = 45 \text{ drops/min}$$

84.

$$X = \frac{500 \text{ ml} \times 2 \text{ mg/min} \times 60 \text{ drops/ml}}{2000 \text{ mg}}$$

$$X = \frac{1000 \times 60}{2000} \quad X = \frac{60,000}{2000} \quad X = 30 \text{ drops/min}$$

85.

$$X = \frac{250 \text{ ml} \times 4 \text{ mcg/min} \times 60 \text{ drops/ml}}{1 \text{ mg} (1000 \text{ mcg})}$$

$$X = \frac{1000 \times 60}{1000} \quad X = \frac{60,000}{1000} \quad X = 60 \text{ drops/min}$$

86.

Patient weighs 176 lbs. $176 \div 2.2 = 80 \text{ kg}$
MD order is 5 mcg/kg $80 \times 5 = 400 \text{ mcg}$

$$X = \frac{500 \text{ ml} \times 400 \text{ mcg} \times 60 \text{ drops/ml}}{400 \text{ mg} (400,000 \text{ mcg})}$$

$$X = \frac{200,000 \times 60}{400,000} \quad X = \frac{12,000,000}{400,000} \quad X = 30 \text{ drops/min}$$

87.

$$X = \frac{500 \text{ ml} \times 2 \text{ mg/min} \times 60 \text{ drops/ml}}{1000 \text{ mg}}$$

$$X = \frac{1000 \times 60}{1000} \quad X = \frac{60,000}{1000} \quad X = 60 \text{ drops/min}$$

The following drip rate calculations are based on the formula:

$$\frac{\text{Volume} \times \text{Infusion set}}{\text{Time}}$$

88.

$$\frac{300 \text{ ml} \times 10 \text{ drops per ml}}{60 \text{ min}} = \frac{3000 \text{ drops}}{60 \text{ min}} = 50 \text{ drops per min}$$

89.

$$\frac{200 \text{ ml} \times 15 \text{ drops per ml}}{60 \text{ min}} = \frac{3000 \text{ drops}}{60 \text{ min}} = 50 \text{ drops per min}$$

90.

$$\frac{20 \text{ ml} \times 60 \text{ drops per ml}}{20 \text{ min}} = \frac{1200 \text{ drops}}{20 \text{ min}} = 60 \text{ drops per min}$$

11 Therapeutic Communications

1. Being able to identify with and understand another person's situation or feelings is known as
   A. encoding
   B. decoding
   C. empathy
   D. sympathy

2. To decode means to
   A. send a message
   B. receive a message
   C. create a message
   D. respond to a message

3. Which of the following examples demonstrates a failure to communicate?
   A. Lacking concern about your patient's injuries following a drunk driving incident
   B. Not obtaining a true menstrual history from your 15-year-old patient with her parents present
   C. Being unable to hear your patient's answer due to a loud stereo in the living room
   D. All of the above

4. All of the following are methods to build trust and rapport with your patient EXCEPT
   A. using the patient's name or "honey"
   B. modulating your voice as appropriate to the situation
   C. using a calm, kind facial expression
   D. explaining what you are doing and why

5. A person's "personal space" is considered to be
   A. <18 inches
   B. >12 feet
   C. 4–12 feet
   D. 1.5–4 feet

6. You are attending to a small, frightened child. You place yourself below her eye level. This indicates to her that
   A. you are in charge
   B. you are the authority figure
   C. you are allowing her to have some control of the situation
   D. none of the above

7. A closed stance means that you are
   A. open to discussion
   B. uncomfortable
   C. warm and compassionate
   D. attentive

8. The social distance is best for
   A. conducting an impersonal business transaction
   B. obtaining a history
   C. performing a physical exam
   D. assessing breath sounds

9. Which of the following is an example of an open-ended question?
   A. Did you eat breakfast today?
   B. Is your chest pain sharp?
   C. What time did your back start hurting?
   D. Would you describe your chest discomfort to me?

10. Your patient says he has had ear pain and a "ball in his throat" for 2 days. You ask, "What exactly do you mean by a 'ball' in your throat?" This is an example of
    A. reflection
    B. confrontation
    C. facilitation
    D. clarification

11. Active listening techniques include all of the following EXCEPT
    A. confrontation
    B. reflection
    C. evocation
    D. clarification

12. All of the following are effective ways to communicate with children EXCEPT
    A. telling them a painful procedure will hurt
    B. telling them what you are about to do
    C. allowing them to handle your equipment
    D. placing yourself above their eye level

13. John, an experienced paramedic, is an ethnocentric person. This means that he
    A. always tries to empathize with his patient's situation
    B. tries to accept the philosophy of others
    C. always thinks his way is the best way
    D. none of the above

14. If your patient is hostile, you should
    A. approach him in a firm, but cautious, manner
    B. leave him alone
    C. never make a show of force
    D. always have a clear exit

15. You are assessing a febrile Southeast Asian child and notice round welts on her body. The parents claim they practiced "coining" prior to calling 911 because they believe this practice helps reduce fever. You should
    A. accept this as their custom and proceed
    B. report them for child abuse
    C. explain to them the errors of their harmful ways
    D. have the child immediately placed in protective custody

answers & rationales

1.

C. Empathy is the ability to identify with and understand another person's point of view, while remaining true to yourself. Empathy is a powerful communication trait. The great educator Dale Carnegie believed that seeing the world through another person's eyes was one of the keys to "winning friends and influencing people." (PCPP 1–463 EPC 575)

2.

B. To decode a message means to interpret it with the same meaning the sender (encoder) intended to convey. When communicating with another person, it is important to encode your message in such a way that the receiver (decoder) can understand it. (PCPP 1–463 EPC 575)

3.

D. Failure to communicate happens for a variety of reasons. Prejudice, lack of privacy, and external and internal distractions can all result in a complete or partial failure to communicate. (PCPP 1–463 EPC 575)

4.

A. Just as there are ways to communicate ineffectively, there are things you can do to build trust and patient rapport, both of which enhance communication. These include using your patient's name appropriately, modulating your voice, and using calm, kind facial expressions. It is always best to describe what you are doing and why you are doing it. Never lie, especially to children. (PCPP 1–465 EPC 576)

5.

A. In the United States, "personal space" is within 18 inches. Always keep in mind that you are invited into your patient's personal space. In order to stay there, you need to build trust and maintain a good rapport. (PCPP 1–466 EPC 578)

6.

C. Placing yourself below the eye level of your patient indicates that you are allowing the patient to have some control of the situation. This is an effective way to communicate with children and the elderly. (PCPP 1–466 EPC 578)

7.

B. A closed stance is any posture that is tense and suggests negativity, discomfort, fear, disgust, or anger. Use an open stance instead if you want to build a trust with your patient. (PCPP 1–466 EPC 578)

8.

A. Social distance (4–12 feet) is used when strangers conduct business or when you have a patient with whom you have not yet established a rapport. The wise paramedic will maintain this space when confronted with an unruly, hostile, possibly violent patient. (PCPP 1–466 EPC 578)

9.

D. Closed-ended questions call for a quick, one- or two-word answer. They are good for clarifying factual information from patients who ramble or who are having difficulty breathing. Open-ended questions provide the patient with the opportunity to explain in his own words his symptoms. Both are effective when used at the proper times. (PCPP 1–469 EPC 580)

10.

D. Often patients will tell you things about which you are unclear. Asking them to describe their symptoms in a different way is an example of clarification and is an excellent active listening technique. (PCPP 1–470 EPC 582)

11.

C. Active listening is an effective way to provide the feedback loop to your patients and to encourage them to speak freely and share important, sometimes intimate, information with you. The techniques of active listening include silence, reflection, facilitation, empathy, clarification, confrontation, interpretation, explanation, and summarization. (PCPP 1–470   EPC 582)

12.

D. Communicating with strange children is a challenging proposition. You can encourage a positive interaction by explaining what you are doing, warning them that an important procedure will probably hurt, allowing them to handle your equipment, and placing yourself below their eye level. (PCPP 1–472   EPC 584)

13.

C. An ethnocentric person views his own life as the most desirable and acts in a superior manner with regard to another culture's way of life. Cultural differences can create communication problems, especially during an emergency. Try at all times to practice empathy and accept your patient's different view of life. (PCPP 1–475   EPC 586)

14.

D. If you are confronted with an obviously hostile patient, always maintain a safe exit pathway. Never allow him to stand between you and the exit. If necessary, make a show of force to prevent a bad situation from getting worse. Watch him closely and do not leave him unguarded. (PCPP 1–476 EPC 587)

15.

A. Often the customs of foreign cultures may seem very strange, even harmful. We mistrust what we do not understand. When confronted with unusual circumstances, consider that major cultural differences may exist. (PCPP 1–475   EPC 587)

12

Life-Span Development

DIRECTIONS Each of the questions or incomplete statements below is followed by suggested answers or completions. Select the **one answer** that is best in each case.

1. During the pediatric years, you expect a person's pulse rate to _____, the blood pressure to _____, and the respiratory rate to _____.
   A. increase, increase, increase
   B. decrease, decrease, decrease
   C. decrease, increase, decrease
   D. increase, decrease, increase

2. An infant's head is equal to _____ % of his total body weight.
   A. 10
   B. 25
   C. 33
   D. 45

3. Immediately after birth, the _____ constricts, causing a change in blood pressure that forces the foramen ovale to close.
   A. ductus arteriosus
   B. ligamentum teres
   C. ductus venosum
   D. foramen arteriosum

4. Which of the following statements is true regarding the infant's pulmonary system?
   A. Infants are primarily mouth breathers
   B. Surfactant is not continuously produced until the second week of life
   C. Infants are primarily diaphragmatic breathers
   D. Normal respiratory rates can exceed 60 breaths per minute, even in the healthy infant

5. Normal birth weight of an infant is usually between
   A. 4 and 6 lbs.
   B. 3 and 3.5 kg
   C. 7 and 9 kg
   D. 4 and 6 kg

6. To best count respirations in the infant, watch for
   A. the rise and fall of the chest
   B. abdominal movement
   C. nasal flaring
   D. "puffing" of the mouth

7. Which of the following statements best describes a newborn's renal function?
   A. Newborns cannot produce concentrated urine
   B. Newborns excrete a diluted fluid
   C. Newborns are prone to electrolyte imbalances
   D. All of the above

8. Control for such things as blinking, sucking, and swallowing arises from
   A. cranial nerves
   B. cervical nerves
   C. sympathetic ganglionic nerves
   D. a reflex arc

9. The Moro reflex is best described as an infant
   A. turning his head when a hand touches his cheek
   B. grasping a finger placed in his palm
   C. throwing his arms wide and trying to grab at things
   D. sucking when something is placed in his mouth

10. The anterior fontanelle closes within
    A. 3–9 months
    B. 9–18 months
    C. 18–24 months
    D. none of the above

11. The epiphyseal plates are
    A. points of attachment for tendons
    B. bone-forming centers

C. nerve-containing outer layers for flat bones

D. another name for the meniscus

True or False—Identify whether the following statements about children are true or false:

12. ____ The capillary beds can assist in thermoregulation of the body.
13. ____ Hemoglobin levels are still far below those of adults.
14. ____ The muscles of respiration are still underdeveloped.
15. ____ The kidneys produce concentrated urine similar to that of adults.
16. ____ Passive acquired immunity is lost.
17. ____ Fine motor skills begin to develop.
18. ____ Hearing reaches maturity at 3 to 4 years.
19. ____ Toilet training should begin by 15 months.
20. ____ Separation anxiety usually develops between 18 and 24 months.
21. ____ You can learn about a child's true feelings and frustrations by watching him play.
22. ____ Authoritarian parents usually raise children with low self-esteem and low competence.
23. ____ Authoritative parents usually raise children who are self-assertive, independent, friendly, and cooperative.
24. ____ Permissive parents usually raise children who have low self-reliance, low self-control, and low maturity and who lack responsible behavior.
25. ____ Children often blame themselves for their parents' divorce.

Place the following stages of reasoning development in chronological order:

26. ____ Stage 1
27. ____ Stage 2
28. ____ Stage 3
29. ____ Stage 4
30. ____ Stage 5
31. ____ Stage 6

A. Serves own self-interest
B. Is concerned about community needs and rights
C. Does one's duty
D. Does what is morally right and wrong
E. Obeys the rules to avoid punishment
F. Seeks approval of others

32. Gonadotropin promotes the production of
    A. testosterone
    B. estrogen
    C. progesterone
    D. all of the above

33. Depression and suicide are more common during which of the following age groups?
    A. Late adulthood
    B. Early adulthood
    C. Middle adulthood
    D. Adolescence

34. Which of the following statements is true regarding the vascular system of people in their late adulthood years?
    A. The walls of blood vessels become thinner
    B. Peripheral vascular resistance decreases
    C. Baroreceptor sensitivity increases
    D. Blood vessel elasticity decreases

35. Which of the following factors increases the likelihood for older adults to develop lung disease?
    A. Smoking
    B. Increased lung elasticity
    C. Increased alveolar surface area
    D. All of the above

36. Which of the following statements is true regarding endocrine system function in the elderly?
    A. There is an overall decrease in endocrine function

B. Insulin production increases, while glucose metabolism decreases

C. The pituitary gland overrides deficient glands

D. None of the above

37. All of the following statements are true regarding the gastrointestinal system in the elderly EXCEPT

A. acid secretion decreases

B. gastric emptying is faster

C. the swallowing mechanism is slower

D. peristalsis is decreased

38. Presbycusis is best described as

A. a type of hearing loss

B. decreased kidney function

C. advanced pituitary dysfunction

D. a loss of visual acuity

39. At what age does ill health become the major cause of death?

A. 18

B. 40

C. 60

D. 80

40. Which of the following makes up the single poorest group in the United States?

A. Clergy

B. Hispanics

C. Older women

D. Amish

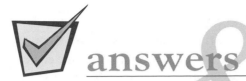

answers & rationales

1.

C. The greatest changes in the range of vital signs occur during the pediatric years. As a child grows, his pulse and respiratory rates decrease, while his blood pressure increases. As a paramedic, you need to be aware of vital sign norms per age. (PCPP 1–481   EPC 321)

2.

B. An infant's head is equal to 25% of his total body weight. Always support an infant's head because his neck muscles are not developed enough to support such a relatively heavy weight. (PCPP 1–482 EPC 322)

3.

C. Immediately following birth, the blood vessel that connects the umbilical vein with the inferior vena cava (the ductus venosum) constricts. This causes a change in blood pressure that closes the opening between the right and left atria (the foramen ovale). (PCPP 1–482   EPC 322)

4.

C. Infants are primarily nose breathers who use their diaphragms to generate the negative pressure necessary to ventilate their lungs. They produce surfactant continuously from birth. Remember the rule of 60s: In the pediatric patient, the respiratory rate should never rise above 60, and the heart rate and blood pressure should never fall below 60. (PCPP 1–482   EPC 322)

5.

B. Normal birth weight is between 3 and 3.5 kg (6.6 and 7.7 lbs.). It will drop by 5–10% in the first week due to fluid loss but exceed the birth weight by the second week. (PCPP 1–482   EPC 322)

6.

B. Because their chest walls are less rigid than those of adults, infants primarily use their diaphragm to breathe. The most effective way to evaluate an infant's respiratory rate is to observe the rise and fall of his abdomen. (PCPP 1–483   EPC 323)

7.

D. A newborn's kidneys are not able to produce concentrated urine, so they excrete a diluted fluid, which makes them susceptible to water and electrolyte imbalance. (PCPP 1–483   EPC 323)

8.

A. An infant's cranial nerves control such things as blinking, swallowing, sucking, and the gag reflex, so you can expect them to have strong, well-developed abilities in these movements. (PCPP 1–483   EPC 323)

9.

C. The Moro, or startle, reflex occurs when an infant is startled. The arms are thrown wide, the fingers spread, and a grabbing motion follows. An asymmetric Moro reflex suggests unilateral paralysis or weakness. (PCPP 1–483   EPC 323)

10.

B. The anterior fontanelle closes between 9 and 18 months. The anterior fontanelle is used to estimate an infant's state of hydration. A sunken fontanelle suggests dehydration. A bulging fontanelle suggests increased intracranial pressure. (PCPP 1–484 EPC 324)

11.

B. Epiphyseal plates are bone-forming centers in long bones. As the epiphysis grows, it becomes a part of the larger bone. The tibial epiphyseal plate is an important landmark that you must avoid during intraosseous needle insertion. Damaging the growth plate may interfere with long bone growth. (PCPP 1–484   EPC 324)

True or False

12. __T__ The capillary beds can assist in thermoregulation of the body.
13. __F__ Hemoglobin levels are still far below those of adults.
14. __T__ The muscles of respiration are still underdeveloped.
15. __F__ The kidneys produce concentrated urine similar to that of adults.
16. __T__ Passive acquired immunity is lost.
17. __T__ Fine motor skills begin to develop.
18. __T__ Hearing reaches maturity at 3 to 4 years.
19. __F__ Toilet training should begin by 15 months.
20. __T__ Separation anxiety usually develops between 18 and 24 months.
21. __T__ You can learn about a child's true feelings and frustrations by watching him play.
22. __T__ Authoritarian parents usually raise children with low self-esteem and low competence.
23. __T__ Authoritative parents usually raise children who are self-assertive, independent, friendly, and cooperative.
24. __T__ Permissive parents usually raise children who have low self-reliance, low self-control, and low maturity and who lack responsible behavior.
25. __T__ Children often blame themselves for their parents' divorce. (PCPP 1–486–1–489 EPC 326–329)

Matching

26. **E** Stage 1
27. **A** Stage 2
28. **F** Stage 3
29. **C** Stage 4
30. **B** Stage 5
31. **D** Stage 6
A. Serves own self-interest
B. Is concerned about community needs and rights
C. Does one's duty
D. Does what is morally right and wrong
E. Obeys the rules to avoid punishment
F. Seeks approval of others (PCPP 1–490   EPC 330)

32.
D. During adolescence, the endocrine system works overtime and causes the characteristic physical and psychological changes associated with teenagers. Gonadotropin hormone promotes the production of estrogen, progesterone, and testosterone. (PCPP 1–490   EPC 330)

33.
D. Depression and suicide are more common in adolescence than in any other age group. The great number of physical and psychological changes that occur during this age, the increasing demands of becoming an adult, and their unrealistic and naive outlook on life, combined with immature coping mechanisms, make teenagers an easy target for antisocial and destructive behavior. (PCPP 1–491 EPC 331)

34.
D. The cardiovascular system undergoes many changes in the later years. Blood vessel walls thicken and lose their elasticity, raising peripheral vascular resistance. Baroreceptor sensitivity also decreases, which lessens the ability to recognize changes in blood pressure and initiate compensatory mechanisms. (PCPP 1–494   EPC 333)

35.
A. A number of factors increase the likelihood for older adults to develop lung disease. These include decreased alveolar surface area, decreased elasticity, stiffening of the chest wall, metabolic changes, decreased diffusion from a lifetime of inhaling pollutants, and an ineffective cough mechanism. However, the greatest amount of disability is produced by smoking. (PCPP 1–494   EPC 333)

36.
A. As we enter the late adult years (>60 years), there is an overall decrease in endocrine system function. (PCPP 1–494   EPC 333)

37.
B. The gastrointestinal system undergoes many changes as we enter the late adult years. These include a reduced ability to chew, reduced taste sensation, slower swallowing, prolonged gastric emptying, decreased peristalsis, and less gastric secretion. (PCPP 1–495   EPC 334)

38.

A. Hearing loss for pure tones increases with age, and higher frequencies become less audible than lower frequencies. This is known as presbycusis. (PCPP 1–496 EPC 335)

39.

B. When adults reach 40, ill health becomes the major cause of death rather than accidents, suicide, and homicide. Heart disease is the major killer after the age of 40 in all age, sex, and racial groups. (PCPP 1–497 EPC 336)

40.

C. In the United States, older women make up the single poorest group in our society. In this highly sophisticated country of increasing technological marvels, more than 50% of all single women over the age of 60 live at or below the poverty level. (PCPP 1–498 EPC 337)

13

Airway Management and Ventilation

DIRECTIONS Each of the questions or incomplete statements below is followed by suggested answers or completions. Select the **one answer** that is best in each case.

1. Which of the following is a responsibility of the nasal cavity?
   A. Filter the incoming air
   B. Humidify the incoming air
   C. Warm the incoming air
   D. All of the above

2. What purpose do the conchae serve?
   A. They secrete mucus into the nasal cavity
   B. They propel foreign particles into the pharynx
   C. They cause air flow turbulence
   D. They stimulate the cilia

3. Which of the following is NOT a function of the sinus cavities?
   A. They help trap bacteria
   B. They help cool the inhaled air
   C. They reduce the weight of the head
   D. They help moisten and purify the inhaled air

4. The eustachian tube connects the nasal cavity with the
   A. ear
   B. larynx
   C. pharynx
   D. esophagus

5. The muscular tube that extends from the back of the soft palate to the esophagus is the
   A. trachea
   B. larynx
   C. pharynx
   D. eustachian tube

6. A leaf-shaped cartilage that prevents food from entering the larynx during swallowing is the

   A. arytenoid
   B. cricoids
   C. epiglottis
   D. hyoid

7. The depression between the epiglottis and the base of the tongue is the
   A. eustachian tube
   B. vallecula
   C. hyoid
   D. pyriform fossa

8. The narrowest part of the adult upper airway is at the level of the
   A. vocal cords
   B. cricoid cartilage
   C. cricothyroid membrane
   D. hyoid bone

9. The space between the vocal cords is known as the
   A. eustachian tube
   B. hyoid process
   C. cricothyroid membrane
   D. glottis

10. The trachea divides into the right and left mainstem bronchi at the
    A. hyoid bone
    B. carina
    C. vallecula
    D. parenchyma

11. An endotracheal tube inserted too far will most likely rest in the
    A. right mainstem bronchus
    B. left mainstem bronchus
    C. lung parenchyma
    D. carina

12. Most gas exchange occurs in the
    A. respiratory bronchioles
    B. alveoli
    C. alveolar ducts
    D. bronchioles

13. The _____ pleura covers the lungs.
    A. visceral
    B. parietal
    C. pulmonary
    D. respiratory

14. Which of the following statements is true regarding the pediatric respiratory system?
    A. The cricoid cartilage is the narrowest part of the airway
    B. The tongue is relatively smaller
    C. The ribs and cartilage are stiff and non-pliable
    D. Children rely on their intercostals for breathing

15. During inspiration, air enters the lungs because of a/an _____ in intrathoracic pressure.
    A. increase
    B. decrease

16. The lungs receive deoxygenated blood from the
    A. right heart
    B. left heart
    C. pulmonary veins
    D. bronchial arteries

17. The normal PaO_2 for a healthy adult breathing room air is _____ torr.
    A. 60
    B. 80–100
    C. 35–45
    D. 40

18. The normal $PaCO_2$ for a healthy adult breathing room air is _____ torr.

    A. 60–80
    B. 80–100
    C. 35–45
    D. 7.35–7.45

19. Oxygen molecules move from the alveoli into the pulmonary capillary because of a process known as
    A. osmosis
    B. ventilation/perfusion mismatch
    C. atelectasis
    D. diffusion

20. Ninety-seven percent of the oxygen that enters the bloodstream
    A. is dissolved in plasma
    B. binds with hemoglobin
    C. is transported as bicarbonate
    D. is exhaled into the atmosphere

21. In which of the following cases will the oxygen saturation and partial pressure be high, yet the patient will die of hypoxia?
    A. Carbon monoxide poisoning
    B. Hypothermia
    C. Hypovolemia
    D. All of the above

22. Which of the following conditions might cause a ventilation/perfusion mismatch?
    A. Pneumothorax
    B. Hemothorax
    C. Pulmonary embolism
    D. All of the above

23. The FiO_2 of room air is
    A. 80–100 torr
    B. 21%
    C. 100%
    D. 40 torr

24. When it enters the bloodstream, the majority of carbon dioxide

A. is dissolved in the plasma

B. binds with hemoglobin

C. is transported as bicarbonate

D. combines with carbon monoxide

25. Which of the following would **NOT** increase a patient's $PaCO_2$?

A. Hyperventilation

B. Hypoventilation

C. Airway obstruction

D. Muscle exertion

26. The main respiratory center lies in the

A. apneustic center

B. pneumotaxic center

C. stretch receptors

D. medulla

27. The Hering-Breuer reflex is a process that

A. ensures rhythmic inspiration

B. monitors for changes in $PaCO_2$

C. prevents overinflation of the lungs

D. controls hypoxic drive

28. Chemoreceptors are stimulated by which of the following?

A. Increased PaO_2

B. Increased $PaCO_2$

C. Increased pH

D. None of the above

29. Patients with hypoxic drive are stimulated to breathe by

A. increases in PaO_2

B. decreases in $PaCO_2$

C. increases in pH

D. none of the above

Match the following modified forms of respiration with their respective descriptions:

30. ____ Coughing

31. ____ Sneezing

32. ____ Hiccoughing

33. ____ Sighing

34. ____ Grunting

A. Prolonged exhalation

B. Respiratory distress sign in infants

C. Protective airway function

D. Caused by nasal irritation

E. Diaphragmatic spasm

35. The average volume of gas inhaled in one respiratory cycle is known as

A. minute volume

B. tidal volume

C. alveolar volume

D. none of the above

36. Maximum lung capacity in the average adult male is approximately

A. 4500 ml

B. 350 ml

C. 6000 ml

D. 500 ml

37. The average tidal volume in the healthy adult male is approximately

A. 150 ml

B. 500 ml

C. 350 ml

D. 6000 ml

38. Minute volume is calculated as

A. respiratory rate + dead air space

B. tidal volume − dead air space

C. alveolar volume ÷ dead air space

D. tidal volume × respiratory rate

39. The stiffness or flexibility of the lungs is known as

A. capnography

B. compliance

C. saturation

D. atelectasis

Match the following types of breathing with their respective definitions:

40. _____ Eupnea

41. _____ Dyspnea

42. _____ Tachypnea

43. _____ Bradypnea

44. _____ Hyperpnea

45. _____ Apnea

46. _____ Orthopnea

A. Absence of breathing

B. Slow breathing

C. Deep breathing

D. Fast breathing

E. Difficulty breathing

F. Difficulty breathing lying down

G. Normal breathing

47. Grunting in children and pursed-lip breathing in adults are both manifestations of patients trying to
   A. draw air into the lungs
   B. create back pressure to help expel air from the lungs
   C. increase the respiratory rate
   D. dislodge a foreign body

48. A patient with pulsus paradoxus has
   A. an increase in heart rate during inhalation
   B. a decrease in heart rate during exhalation
   C. an increase in blood pressure during exhalation
   D. a decrease in blood pressure during inhalation

49. Normal SaO_2 should be
   A. under 95%
   B. 95–99%
   C. 90–100%
   D. 80–100%

50. Which of the following could cause an inaccurate SaO_2 reading?
   A. Severe anemia
   B. Hypovolemia
   C. CO poisoning
   D. All of the above

51. Immediately following endotracheal intubation you apply the esophageal detector device and notice that there is a free, effortless return of air after you squeeze the bulb device. This indicates that
   A. you have intubated the esophagus
   B. you have entered the left mainstem bronchus
   C. you have intubated the trachea
   D. none of the above

52. Your patient is semiconscious with a gag reflex. Which of the following airway adjuncts is indicated?
   A. Oropharyngeal airway
   B. Nasopharyngeal airway
   C. Endotracheal tube
   D. Esophageal obturator airway

53. The major advantage of using a nasopharyngeal airway is that
   A. it isolates the trachea
   B. it is easy to suction through
   C. it can be used in the presence of a gag reflex
   D. none of the above

54. Noncuffed endotracheal tubes are recommended for children under the age of
   A. 5 years
   B. 8 years
   C. 10 years
   D. 12 years

55. Endotracheal intubation may be attempted in all of the following situations **EXCEPT**

A. a patient without a gag reflex

B. anaphylaxis

C. respiratory burns

D. epiglottitis

56. Which of the following drugs may NOT be administered down the endotracheal tube?

A. Epinephrine

B. Atropine

C. Lidocaine

D. Diazepam

57. Each endotracheal intubation attempt should be limited to _____ seconds.

A. 10

B. 15

C. 30

D. 60

58. Which of the following indicates an esophageal intubation?

A. Phonation

B. Absence of breath sounds

C. Gurgling sounds heard over the epigastrium

D. All of the above

59. The proper position of the head and neck for endotracheal intubation in the nontrauma patient is the _____ position.

A. neutral

B. hyperextended

C. sniffing

D. flexed

60. The curved, or Macintosh, blade is designed to

A. lift the epiglottis

B. spread the vocal cords

C. fit into the vallecula

D. none of the above

61. If your intubated patient has breath sounds only over the right chest, you should

A. remove the tube immediately

B. secure the tube in place

C. bring the tube back a few centimeters and recheck

D. push the tube in a few centimeters and recheck

62. You have successfully intubated your patient and your partner has been performing bag-valve-mask ventilation for the past few minutes when he tells you that the bag is becoming harder to squeeze. You notice distended jugular veins and cyanosis. Upon auscultation, the right chest is silent, and the left has diminished sounds. What do you do immediately?

A. Insert an oropharyngeal airway as a bite block

B. Extubate the patient

C. Decompress the right chest with a large-bore catheter

D. Perform a cricothyrotomy

63. Which of the following drugs is used for rapid sequence intubation?

A. Midazolam

B. Succinylcholine

C. Lidocaine or atropine

D. All of the above

64. Which of the following statements is true regarding pediatric intubation?

A. The curved blade is the preferred device

B. ETT size = (Age in years + 4)/8

C. They have greater vagal tone than the adult

D. All of the above

65. Which of the following is an indication for performing blind nasotracheal intubation?

A. Apneic patient

B. Suspected basilar skull fracture

C. Breathing patient with spinal injury

D. Unresponsive patient

66. The esophageal tracheal combitube (ETCT) and the pharyngo-tracheal lumen (PTL) airways are similar in that
    A. both are inserted blindly
    B. both depend on accurate placement assessment
    C. neither requires maneuvering the head and neck
    D. All of the above

67. Which of the following is an advantage of using the laryngeal mask airway (LMA)?
    A. It isolates the trachea
    B. It protects against regurgitation and aspiration
    C. It can be used in a patient with a gag reflex
    D. None of the above

68. Which of the following is NOT a contraindication for using the esophageal obturator airway (EOA)?
    A. Age less than 16 years
    B. Height over 6 feet
    C. Ingestion of caustic substance
    D. History of alcoholism

69. Which of the following is true regarding suctioning?
    A. Limit the suctioning to 30 seconds
    B. Apply suction during insertion and during removal
    C. Hyperventilate the patient before and after suctioning
    D. All of the above

70. When you arrive on the scene of a patient in respiratory arrest, you notice that personnel are performing bag-valve-mask ventilation. You also notice that the patient's abdomen is extremely distended. After you intubate the patient, you notice resistance when you squeeze the bag. Lung sounds are diminished bilaterally, neck veins are normal, and the trachea is midline. What should you do?
    A. Insert a nasogastric tube
    B. Pull back the tube 2 cm
    C. Perform a cricothyrotomy
    D. Decompress both sides of the chest

71. The nasal cannula delivers oxygen concentrations in the range of
    A. 10–50%
    B. 50–100%
    C. 24–44%
    D. 40–60%

72. Nasal cannula flow rates should not exceed _____ liters/minute.
    A. 3
    B. 6
    C. 8
    D. 10

73. The simple face mask delivers oxygen concentrations in the range of
    A. 20–40%
    B. 40–60%
    C. 60–80%
    D. 80–100%

74. Simple face mask flow rates should never fall below _____ liters/minute.
    A. 3
    B. 6
    C. 8
    D. 10

75. The non-rebreather mask delivers oxygen concentrations in the range of
    A. 20–40%
    B. 40–60%
    C. 60–80%
    D. 80–100%

76. To deliver the above oxygen concentration, the non-rebreather mask flow rate should be _____ liters/minute.
    A. 6
    B. 8
    C. 10
    D. 15

77. The Venturi system delivers oxygen concentrations in the range of
    A. 24–40%
    B. 40–60%
    C. 60–80%
    D. 80–100%

78. Which of the following statements is true regarding the use of a bag-valve-mask?
    A. Always engage the pop-off valve
    B. Use an oxygen reservoir whenever possible
    C. Reusable BVMs are acceptable
    D. Adult BVMs are unacceptable for pediatric patients

79. Using a pocket mask without supplemental oxygen delivers oxygen in the range of
    A. 16–17%
    B. 21–22 %
    C. 20–50%
    D. 90–100%

80. A bag-valve-mask device with an oxygen reservoir can deliver up to _____ of oxygen with flow rates at 10–15 liters/minute.
    A. 50%
    B. 60%
    C. 80%
    D. 95%

81. Using a bag-valve-mask without supplemental oxygen delivers _____ oxygen.

    A. 17%
    B. 21%
    C. 50%
    D. 90%

82. A demand valve resuscitator will deliver up to _____ oxygen at its highest flow rates.
    A. 50%
    B. 60%
    C. 80%
    D. 100%

83. Which of the following complications is associated with demand valve use?
    A. Pneumothorax
    B. Subcutaneous emphysema
    C. Gastric distention
    D. All of the above

84. Which of the following is true regarding the use of an automatic ventilator?
    A. It delivers higher minute volumes than the bag-valve-mask
    B. Most units deliver controlled ventilation only
    C. It can be used safely in all age groups
    D. The pop-off valves should be disengaged

85. In which of the following cases might higher airway pressures be necessary to ventilate the lungs?
    A. Cardiogenic pulmonary edema
    B. Adult respiratory distress syndrome
    C. Bronchospasm
    D. All of the above

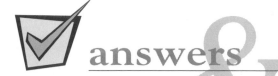

answers & rationales

1.

D. The nasal cavity is responsible for filtering, humidifying, and warming the incoming air. (PCPP 1–505   EPC 227)

2.

C. The conchae or turbinates are shelf-like structures that cause turbulent airflow. This turbulence helps deposit any airborne particles onto the mucous membrane that lines the nasal cavity. (PCPP 1–505 EPC 227)

3.

B. The sinuses (ethmoid, maxillary, frontal, sphenoid) are air-filled, mucus-lined cavities that help moisten, purify, and warm the air we breathe. They also reduce the weight of the head. (PCPP 1–504   EPC 227)

4.

A. The Eustachian, or auditory, tube connects the nasal cavity (nasopharynx) with the ear. This tube is flat in children, providing an easy route for the spread of bacteria to the ear canal (otitis media). (PCPP 1–504   EPC 227)

5.

C. The pharynx, or throat, is a muscular tube that extends vertically from the back of the soft palate to the upper end of the esophagus. It allows the flow of air into and out of the respiratory tract and the passage of foods and liquids into the digestive system. (PCPP 1–506   EPC 228)

6.

C. The epiglottis is a leaf-shaped cartilage that prevents food from entering the respiratory tract during the act of swallowing. (PCPP 1–506   EPC 228)

7.

B. The depression between the epiglottis and the base of the tongue is known as the vallecula. This landmark is significant because, during intubation, you insert the curved blade into this crevice. (PCPP 1–506   EPC 228)

8.

A. In adults, the portion of the thyroid cartilage housing the vocal cords is the narrowest part of the upper airway. (PCPP 1–507   EPC 229)

9.

D. The glottis is the slit-like opening between the vocal cords, also known as the glottic opening. (PCPP 1–507   EPC 229)

10.

B. The carina is the point at which the trachea bifurcates into the right and left mainstem bronchi. (PCPP 1–509   EPC 230)

11.

A. The right mainstem bronchus is almost straight with a slight curve, while the left main stem bronchus angles more acutely to the left. An endotracheal tube inserted too far will most likely rest in the right mainstem bronchus for that reason. (PCPP 1–509   EPC 229)

12.

B. A limited gas exchange may occur in the alveolar ducts and respiratory bronchioles. Most gas exchange takes place in the alveoli. The alveoli comprise the key functional unit of the respiratory system. (PCPP 1–509   EPC 231)

13.

A. Lungs are covered by connective tissue called pleura. The pleura consists of two layers, the visceral pleura (covers the lungs) and the parietal pleura (lines the inner chest wall). (PCPP 1–510   EPC 232)

14.

A. Children are not just small adults. Their respiratory anatomy and physiology are different. For example, their jaws are smaller, while their tongues are relatively larger. Their epiglottis is floppy, round, and more anterior. The cricoid cartilage is the narrowest part of the airway. Children's ribs and cartilage are soft and pliable, and they rely more on their diaphragms for breathing. (PCPP 1–510   EPC 232)

15.

B. During inspiration, the size of the thoracic cavity is made larger by contracting the diaphragm and the intercostal muscles. This causes a great and instant decrease in the intrathoracic pressure. This decrease in intrathoracic pressure causes air to rush into the lungs. (PCPP 1–512   EPC 233)

16.

A. The lungs receive deoxygenated blood from the right side of the heart through the pulmonary artery. The pulmonary artery is the only artery in the body that carries deoxygenated blood. (PCPP 1–513   EPC 235)

17.

B. The normal PaO_2 for a healthy adult breathing room air is 80–100 torr. (PCPP 1–514   EPC 236)

18.

C. The normal $PaCO_2$ for a healthy adult breathing room air is 35–45 torr. (PCPP 1–514   EPC 236)

19.

D. Diffusion is the movement of gas from an area of higher partial pressure concentration to an area of lower partial pressure concentration. This process allows oxygen molecules to move from the alveoli into the pulmonary capillary. (PCPP 1–515   EPC 236)

20.

B. Of the oxygen that enters the bloodstream, 97% of it binds with the hemoglobin molecule on the red blood cells; 3% is dissolved in plasma. (PCPP 1–515   EPC 236)

21.

A. Consider the patient with carbon monoxide poisoning. Since carbon monoxide has a greater affinity for the hemoglobin molecule than oxygen does, it will replace it, if present. That means that most of the oxygen inhaled will be dissolved in plasma. If arterial blood gas samples are taken, they will reveal a normal or high PaO_2 because the PaO_2 measures the freely dissolved oxygen in the bloodstream. The pulse oximeter measures the saturation of the hemoglobin molecule. In this case, it is saturated not with oxygen but with carbon monoxide. Both measurements will read high, yet the patient will die of hypoxia. It is the hemoglobin that transports oxygen to the peripheral tissues. (PCPP 1–515   EPC 236)

22.

D. Ideally each milliliter of air we inhale should meet up with 1 ml of blood. When it does not, a ventilation/perfusion mismatch occurs. This can be caused by a problem with ventilation or a problem with circulation. Ventilation-perfusion mismatches are the most common cause of respiratory distress. (PCPP 1–516   EPC 237)

23.

B. The FiO_2 is a measurement of the concentration of oxygen in the inspired air. The FiO_2 of room air is approximately .21 (21%). (PCPP 1–516   EPC 237)

24.

C. Carbon dioxide is transported mainly in the form of bicarbonate. Approximately 66% is transported in this manner, while 33% binds with and is transported with hemoglobin. Less than 1% is dissolved in the plasma. (PCPP 1–516 EPC 236)

25.

A. Carbon dioxide concentrations in the blood are influenced by increases and decreases in CO_2 production and/or elimination. $PaCO_2$ would be increased by hypoventilation, airway obstruction, or muscle exertion. (PCPP 1–516   EPC 236)

26.

D. The respiratory center lies in the medulla, located in the brain stem. (PCPP 1–517   EPC 238)

27.

C. The Hering-Breuer reflex is a process that prevents overexpansion of the lungs. During inspiration, the lungs become distended, activating what are known as stretch receptors. As the degree of stretch increases, these receptors fire more frequently, sending a message to the brain stem to inhibit the respiratory inspiration. (PCPP 1–517 EPC 238)

28.

B. Receptors are located in the carotid bodies, the aortic arch, and the medulla. In the normal person, these chemoreceptors are stimulated by decreased PaO_2, increased $PaCO_2$, and a decreased pH. (PCPP 1–517   EPC 238)

29.

D. People with chronic respiratory disease, such as emphysema and chronic bronchitis, tend to retain carbon dioxide and often develop a condition known as hypoxic drive. These patients are stimulated to breath by decreases in PaO_2. (PCPP 1–517 EPC 239)

Matching (PCPP 1–524   EPC 502)

30. **C**   Coughing
31. **D**   Sneezing
32. **E**   Hiccoughing
33. **A**   Sighing
34. **B**   Grunting

A. Prolonged exhalation
B. Respiratory distress sign in infants
C. Protective airway function
D. Caused by nasal irritation
E. Diaphragmatic spasm

35.

B. Tidal volume is the average volume of gas inhaled or exhaled in one respiratory cycle. (PCPP 1–518 EPC 239)

36.

C. Total lung capacity in the average adult male is approximately 6 liters. (PCPP 1–518   EPC 239)

37.

B. The average tidal volume in a healthy adult male is approximately 500 ml. (PCPP 1–518   EPC 239)

38.

D. Minute volume is the amount of gas moved in and out of the respiratory tract in 1 minute. It is measured by multiplying the tidal volume times the respiratory rate. (PCPP 1–518   EPC 240)

39.

B. Compliance refers to the stiffness or flexibility of the lung tissue. It is determined by how easily air flows into the lungs. When compliance is good, airflow occurs with a minimal amount of resistance. Poor compliance means that ventilation is harder to achieve. It is often poor in patients with diseased lungs, chest wall injuries, or tension pneumothorax. (PCPP 1–527   EPC 505)

Matching (PCPP 1–524)

40. **G**   Eupnea
41. **E**   Dyspnea
42. **D**   Tachypnea
43. **B**   Bradypnea
44. **C**   Hyperpnea
45. **A**   Apnea
46. **F**   Orthopnea

A. Absence of breathing
B. Slow breathing
C. Deep breathing
D. Fast breathing
E. Difficulty breathing
F. Difficulty breathing lying down
G. Normal breathing

47.

B. Infants grunt and adults purse their lips during exhalation to create a back pressure that maintains open airways so that they can expel air from their lungs. They are both indicative of respiratory distress caused by an inability to exhale normally. (PCPP 1–525   EPC 503)

48.

D. During pulsus paradoxus, the patient's blood pressure drops at least 10 torr during inspiration due to an increase in intrathoracic pressure. This is usually a sign of severe obstructive lung disease, such as asthma or COPD. (PCPP 1–525   EPC 503)

49.

B. Normal SaO_2 should be between 95% and 99%. (PCPP 1–528   EPC 505)

50.

D. Hypovolemia, CO poisoning, severe anemia, high-intensity lighting, certain hemoglobin abnormalities, and an absent pulse can result in a false SaO_2 reading. Always use pulse oximetry as ONE of your assessment tools. (PCPP 1–528   EPC 506)

51.

C. If there is a free flow of air after you squeeze the bulb device, you are in the wide, uncollapsible trachea. If the bulb does not refill, you are in a collapsed esophagus. (PCPP 1–531   EPC 509)

52.

B. In the semiconscious patient with a gag reflex, the nasopharyngeal airway is an excellent initial airway adjunct. (PCPP 1–536   EPC 512)

53.

C. The major advantage of using the nasopharyngeal airway is that it can be used in the presence of the gag reflex. (PCPP 1–536   EPC 512)

54.

B. Noncuffed endotracheal tubes are recommended for children under the age of 8. In these children, the cricoid cartilage acts as an anatomical cuff, since it is the narrowest part of the pediatric airway. (PCPP 1–565   EPC 541)

55.

D. Tracheal intubation should never be attempted in patients suspected of having epiglottitis. Any unnecessary agitation of the patient can cause immediate laryngospasm and subsequent respiratory arrest. (PCPP 1–545   EPC 521)

56.

D. The following medications can be administered down the endotracheal tube: oxygen, naloxone, atropine, epinephrine, and lidocaine. (PCPP 1–546   EPC 522)

57.

C. Endotracheal intubation attempts should be limited to 30 seconds to prevent hypoxia. (PCPP 1–547   EPC 523)

58.

D. Signs of an esophageal intubation include an absence of chest rise and breath sounds with ventilatory support, gurgling sounds heard over the epigastrium, the absence of breath condensation in the endotracheal tube, a persistent air leak despite inflation of the distal cuff, cyanosis, progressive worsening of the patient's condition, and phonation. (PCPP 1–547   EPC 523)

59.

C. The proper position of the head and neck for endotracheal intubation in the nontrauma patient is the sniffing position. This is accomplished by flexing the neck forward and the head backward or by inserting a rolled towel under the patient's shoulders or the back of the head. (PCPP 1–550   EPC 526)

60.

C. The curved, or Macintosh, blade is designed to fit into the vallecula. The vallecula is the space between the base of the tongue and the epiglottis. (PCPP 1–541   EPC 517)

61.

C. If your intubated patient has breath sounds heard only over the right chest, you should assume a right mainstem bronchus intubation. In this case, withdraw the tube a few centimeters and recheck placement. (PCPP 1–548   EPC 528)

62.

C. The most common cause of tension pneumothorax is positive pressure ventilation. This includes over-aggressive bag-valve-mask ventilation. Classic signs include increasing difficulty using the bag, distended jugular veins, absent breath sounds on the affected side, and diminished sounds on the opposite side. Treatment is immediate decompression with a large-bore catheter on the affected side—second intercostal space, midclavicular line. (PCPP 1–548   EPC 524)

63.

D. To perform rapid sequence intubation, you will need a sedative, such as midazolam; a neuromuscular blocker, such as succinylcholine; and premedication with atropine or lidocaine. (PCPP 1–563   EPC 537)

64.

C. Intubating an infant or young child is a challenging proposition. The mouth is smaller, the tongue is larger, the larynx is more anterior, and the epiglottis is elongated and floppy. Infants and young children also have greater vagal tone than do adults. (PCPP 1–565   EPC 540)

65.

C. Indications for performing blind nasotracheal intubation include a breathing patient with a spinal injury, and a patient with clenched teeth, oral fractures, significant angioedema, obesity, or arthritis preventing placement in the sniffing position. (PCPP 1–568   EPC 544)

66.

D. The ETCT and the PTL airways are similar in that they are both inserted blindly, they both depend on the accurate assessment of their placement, and neither requires movement of the head and neck. (PCPP 1–572   EPC 547)

67.

D. The LMA does not isolate the trachea or protect the lung against regurgitation and aspiration. It cannot be used for people with a gag reflex. (PCPP 1–573 EPC 549)

68.

B. Contraindications for using the EOA or EGTA include age less than 16 years, height over 6 feet 7 inches or less than 5 feet, possible ingestion of caustic poisons, and a history of alcoholism or esophageal disease. (PCPP 1–576   EPC 552)

69.

C. Suctioning should always be limited to 10 seconds. You should hyperventilate the patient before and after all suctioning attempts and always apply suction during removal. (PCPP 1–587   EPC 564)

70.

A. Often performing ventilation on an unintubated patient causes gastric distention. The distention puts pressure on the diaphragm, making ventilation more difficult. In these cases, decompress the stomach by inserting a nasogastric tube. (PCPP 1–589   EPC 565)

71.

C. The nasal cannula delivers oxygen concentrations in the range of 24–44%, depending on the liter flow. (PCPP 1–592   EPC 567)

72.

B. Nasal cannula flow rates should not exceed 6 liters/minute, as this will dry the mucous membrane and cause headaches. (PCPP 1–592   EPC 567)

73.

B. The simple face mask delivers oxygen concentrations in the range of 40–60%. Oxygen is delivered through the bottom of the mask via its oxygen inlet port. (PCPP 1–592   EPC 567)

74.

B. No fewer than 6 liters/minute should be administered through this device, as expired carbon dioxide can otherwise accumulate in the mask. (PCPP 1–592   EPC 567)

75.

D. The non-rebreather mask consists of oxygen tubing and a face mask with an attached reservoir bag. When the patient inhales, 100% oxygen contained in the reservoir is drawn into the mask and the patient's respiratory passageways. The non-rebreather mask delivers the highest concentration of oxygen. Once applied, a flow rate of 10–15 liters/minute can deliver an 80–100% oxygen concentration. (PCPP 1–592   EPC 567)

76.

D. In order to deliver an oxygen concentration of 80–95%, the flow meter should be set at 15 liters/minute. (PCPP 1–592   EPC 567)

77.

A. The Venturi system is a high flow device including oxygen tubing, a face mask, and the Venturi system. As oxygen passes through a jet port in the base of the mask, it entrains room air. Depending on the device used, oxygen concentrations can be delivered in the range of 24–40%. (PCPP 1–592   EPC 567)

78.

B. Proper use of a bag-valve-mask (BVM) device includes disengaging the pop-off valve (to prevent underventilation), using disposable devices only, watching for chest rise (to prevent overventilation, especially in the pediatric patient), and always using an oxygen reservoir (to deliver maximum FiO$_2$). (PCPP 1–594   EPC 569)

79.

A. Using a pocket mask without supplemental oxygen delivers the oxygen in the range of 16–17%—in other words, your own expired FiO$_2$. (PCPP 1–593 EPC 568)

80.

D. A bag-valve-mask device with an oxygen reservoir can deliver up to 95% of oxygen with flow rates at 15 liters/minute. (PCPP 1–594   EPC 569)

81.

B. Using a BVM without supplemental oxygen delivers 21% FiO$_2$—in other words, room air. (PCPP 1–594   EPC 569)

82.

D. A demand valve resuscitator will deliver up to 100% oxygen at its highest flow rates. (PCPP 1–596   EPC 571)

83.

D. Using a demand valve has its disadvantages. Some of these include creating a pneumothorax, subcutaneous emphysema, or gastric distention. (PCPP 1–596   EPC 571)

84.

A. Automatic ventilators deliver higher minute volumes than the bag-valve-mask. (PCPP 1–597 EPC 572)

85.

D. In cases such as cardiogenic pulmonary edema, adult respiratory distress syndrome, and bronchospasm, higher airway pressures may be necessary to ventilate the lungs. (PCPP 1–597   EPC 572)

14 The History

1. Which of the following is an effective method for establishing a positive rapport with your patient when you first meet him?
   A. Stand over him when you introduce yourself
   B. Avoid eye contact initially
   C. Introduce yourself and offer a handshake
   D. Use a firm voice to gain control of the situation

2. You arrive at the nursing home of an elderly woman whose name is Helen Smith. How should you address her until told otherwise by her?
   A. Honey
   B. Helen
   C. Mrs. Smith
   D. Any of the above

3. Which of the following is an open-ended question?
   A. Would you please describe your chest pain?
   B. Does your chest hurt?
   C. Are you having any difficulty breathing?
   D. Do you take insulin everyday?

4. Your patient tells you about his chest pain. As he relates his story, you maintain sincere eye contact and repeat things like "Mm-hmm," and "Go on." This is an example of
   A. clarification
   B. reflection
   C. confrontation
   D. facilitation

5. Your patient denies chest pain but keeps rubbing his chest. You say to him, "You say your chest doesn't hurt but I notice you keep rubbing it." This is an example of
   A. facilitation
   B. confrontation
   C. clarification
   D. reflection

6. The pain, discomfort, or dysfunction that caused your patient to request help is known as the
   A. primary problem
   B. nature of the illness
   C. differential diagnosis
   D. chief complaint

Match the following elements of the present illness of the patient with a chief complaint of chest pain with their respective examples:

7. _____ O
8. _____ P
9. _____ Q
10. _____ R
11. _____ S
12. _____ T
13. _____ AS
14. _____ PN

A. Pain is 6 on a scale of 1–10
B. Patient also complains of shortness of breath and nausea
C. Sudden onset
D. Pain began 2 hours ago
E. Pain worsens while lying down
F. Patient denies dizziness
G. Pain goes through to the back
H. Pain is heavy and vise-like

15. Cardiac chest pain is commonly felt in the jaw and down the left arm. This is known as
   A. sympathetic pain
   B. tenderness
   C. referred pain
   D. associated pain

16. A person with PND may have orthopnea. You would have elicited this information during which part of your History of Present Illness?
    A. R
    B. AS
    C. P
    D. Q

17. Which of the following is NOT a component of the Past History?
    A. Adult diseases
    B. Medications
    C. Surgeries
    D. Accidents

18. Which of the following would NOT be included when eliciting current medications?
    A. Illegal substances
    B. Prescribed medications
    C. Over-the-counter medications
    D. Home remedies

19. Your patient has smoked 2 packs of cigarettes each day for the past 35 years. He is a _____ pack/year smoker.
    A. 35
    B. 70
    C. 730
    D. 25,550

20. The CAGE questionnaire is used as an evaluation tool to assess
    A. alcoholism
    B. lung disease
    C. allergies
    D. pregnancy

21. Which of the following statements is true regarding the Review of Systems?
    A. The questions asked cover sleep patterns and family history
    B. You should begin your history with the Review of Systems

C. The questions will be determined by your patient's chief complaint, condition, and clinical status
D. It is important to use the entire Review of Systems with each patient

22. The mnemonic GPAL is used to evaluate
    A. alcoholism
    B. allergies
    C. pregnancy history
    D. endocrine dysfunction

23. Which of the following is a valid reason why your patient suddenly became silent?
    A. Organic brain syndrome
    B. Clinical depression
    C. Your insensitivity
    D. All of the above

24. A mood disorder characterized by hopelessness and malaise is known as
    A. dementia
    B. dysmenorrhea
    C. delirium
    D. depression

25. You ask your patient when his headaches began, and he answers, "My head feels like a squirrel." His problem may be due to
    A. psychosis
    B. organic disease
    C. head injury
    D. all of the above

Match the following components of the comprehensive history with their respective categories:

26. _____ Pertinent negatives
27. _____ Tobacco use
28. _____ Current medications
29. _____ HEENT
30. _____ Exercise and leisure activities
31. _____ Religious beliefs
32. _____ Onset

33. _____ Allergies

34. _____ Adult diseases

35. _____ Cardiac

36. _____ Diet

37. _____ Endocrine

38. _____ Provocation

39. _____ Injuries

40. _____ CAGE

41. _____ Family history

42. _____ Skin

43. _____ Surgeries

44. _____ Time

45. _____ Region/radiation

46. _____ Urinary

47. _____ Sleep patterns

48. _____ Substance abuse

49. _____ GPAL

50. _____ Respiratory

A. History of Present Illness

B. Past History

C. Current Health Status

D. Review of Systems

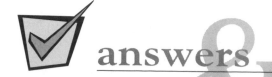

answers & rationales

1.

C. You get only one chance to make a good first impression, and your patient will form an impression of you in the first few moments. A positive, caring, professional impression will put your patient at ease and facilitate your assessment. Make sincere eye contact at eye level, introduce yourself, and offer a handshake or comforting touch. Always remain calm, regardless of how your patient presents. (PCPP 2–6   EPC 577)

2.

C. Proper respect for your elders dictates that you use the formal Mrs. Smith until you are told otherwise by your patient. Respect begets respect. (PCPP 2–7 EPC 577)

3.

A. Open-ended questions allow your patient to answer in detail. Closed-ended questions elicit one-word answers, such as "yes" or "no." Used appropriately, both types are effective methods of conducting a patient interview. (PCPP 2–8   EPC 580)

4.

D. Facilitation is a simple method of practicing active listening. You maintain eye contact, listen intently, and follow up his statements with phrases such as "Mm-hmm" or "I'm listening" to let your patient know you are indeed listening. (PCPP 2–9 EPC 582)

5.

B. Sometimes your patients will try to hide the truth. If you suspect they are, you might try confronting them with the discrepancy between what they say and what you see. It may help them open up. (PCPP 2–10   EPC 582)

6.

D. The pain, discomfort, or dysfunction that caused your patient to request help is known as the chief complaint. Elicit the chief complaint with an open-ended question, such as "Why did you call us today?" or "What seems to be the problem?" Document the chief complaint in the patient's own words. (PCPP 2–11   EPC 580)

Matching   (PCPP 2–12   EPC 595)

7. C   O
8. E   P
9. H   Q
10. G   R
11. A   S
12. D   T
13. B   AS
14. F   PN

A. Pain is 6 on a scale of 1–10
B. Patient also complains of shortness of breath and nausea
C. Sudden onset
D. Pain began 2 hours ago
E. Pain worsens while lying down
F. Patient denies dizziness
G. Pain goes through to the back
H. Pain is heavy and vise-like

15.

C. Referred pain is pain that is felt at a location away from its source. For example, cardiac chest pain is referred to the left arm and jaw, gallbladder pain is referred to the right shoulder, and splenic pain is referred to the left shoulder and testicles. (PCPP 2–13   EPC 596)

16.

C. The "P" in the mnemonic OPQRST–ASPN stands for "provocative" (things that worsen) and "palliative" (things that relieve) factors. PND stands for paroxysmal nocturnal dyspnea, which is sudden shortness of breath while sleeping. It usually indicates orthopnea from congestive heart failure and is a provocative factor. (PCPP 2–12   EPC 595)

17.

B. The components of the Past History include general state of health, childhood diseases, adult diseases, psychiatric diseases, accidents or injuries, and surgeries or hospitalizations. (PCPP 2–14   EPC 597)

18.

A. Your patient's current medications include prescriptions, over-the-counter drugs, home remedies, vitamins, and minerals. Always ask your patient to describe any reactions he may have had to any medications. (PCPP 2–15   EPC 598)

19.

B. The number of pack/years is calculated as packs/day times years. Your patient is a 70 pack/year smoker. Anything over 30 pack/years is considered significant. Members of the "Century Club" (100 pk/yrs) can be expected to exhibit significant lung disease. (PCPP 2–15   EPC 598)

20.

A. The CAGE questionnaire is used to evaluate the presence of alcoholism. The CAGE questionnaire is as follows:

C Have you ever felt the need to **C**ut down on your drinking?

A Have you ever felt **A**nnoyed by criticism of your drinking?

G Have you ever felt **G**uilty about your drinking?

E Have you ever taken a drink as an **E**ye opener?

Two or more "yes" answers suggest alcoholism and further inquiry. (PCPP 2–15   EPC 598)

21.

C. The Review of Systems is a series of questions designed to identify problems your patient has not already mentioned. The list is categorized by body system and is more comprehensive than the basic history. Your patient's chief complaint, condition, and clinical status will determine how much of the Review of Systems to use. (PCPP 2–17   EPC 600)

22.

C. The mnemonic GPAL is used to evaluate the pregnancy history. It stands for

Gravida   How many pregnancies?
Para   How many viable births?
Abortions   How many abortions?
Living   How many living children? (PCPP 2–18   EPC 601)

23.

D. A patient who becomes silent can be a challenge to even the most experienced paramedic. He may have a pathological problem (organic brain disease or dysarthria), he may be upset or scared, or you may have caused the silence by your behavior. If your patient suddenly becomes silent, try to determine why, what is happening, and what you can do about it. (PCPP 2–19   EPC 602)

24.

D. Depression is a mood disorder characterized by hopelessness and malaise. Depression is potentially lethal, so you must recognize its signs and evaluate its severity. (PCPP 2–21   EPC 604)

25.

D. When your patient's answers do not seem to make any sense, it may be due to psychosis (mental illness), organic disease (dementia or delirium), head injury, or a stroke. (PCPP 2–21   EPC 605)

Matching   (PCPP 2–12 through 2–19 EPC 595–602)

26. A Pertinent negatives
27. C Tobacco use
28. C Current medications
29. D HEENT
30. C Exercise and leisure activities
31. C Religious beliefs
32. A Onset
33. C Allergies
34. B Adult diseases
35. D Cardiac
36. C Diet
37. D Endocrine
38. A Provocation
39. B Injuries
40. C CAGE
41. C Family history
42. D Skin

43. B   Surgeries
44. A   Time
45. B   Region/radiation
46. D   Urinary
47. C   Sleep patterns
48. C   Substance abuse

49. D   GPAL
50. D   Respiratory
   A. History of Present Illness
   B. Past History
   C. Current Health Status
   D. Review of Systems

15 Physical Exam Techniques

DIRECTIONS Each of the questions or incomplete statements below is followed by suggested answers or completions. Select the **one answer** that is best in each case.

1. Which of the following is NOT a physical exam technique?
   A. Inspection
   B. Palpitation
   C. Percussion
   D. Auscultation

2. Which of the following should be used to palpate lymph nodes or rib fractures?
   A. The pads of the fingers
   B. The tips of the fingers
   C. The back of the hand
   D. The palm of the hand

3. Which of the following should be used to assess tactile fremitus?
   A. The pads of the fingers
   B. The tips of the fingers
   C. The back of the hand
   D. The palm of the hand

4. Which of the following statements is true regarding abdominal palpation?
   A. Always perform deep palpation first
   B. Observe your patient's face during the procedure
   C. Use the heel of one hand to perform deep palpation
   D. Always palpate the painful area first

5. A hollow and vibrating resonance heard when percussing the chest indicates the presence of
   A. air
   B. blood
   C. pleural fluid
   D. pus

6. When reporting and recording lung sounds, you should note the
   A. abnormal sound
   B. location
   C. timing during the respiratory cycle
   D. all of the above

7. You will usually perform auscultation last except in which of the following situations?
   A. Acute pulmonary edema
   B. Acute abdomen
   C. Acute myocardial infarction
   D. Arterial bruits

8. A healthy adult's pulse rate at rest should be between _____ and _____ beats per minute.
   A. 50, 90
   B. 60, 90
   C. 50, 100
   D. 60, 100

9. A weak, thready pulse is a common finding in a patient with
   A. circulatory collapse
   B. high blood pressure
   C. heat stroke
   D. increasing intracranial pressure

Match the following respiratory patterns with their respective definitions:

10. ____ Eupnea
11. ____ Tachypnea
12. ____ Bradypnea
13. ____ Apnea
14. ____ Hyperpnea
15. ____ Cheyne-Stokes
16. ____ Biot's
17. ____ Kussmaul's
18. ____ Apneustic

A. Normal rate, but deeper
B. Prolonged inspiration, shortened expiration

C. Normal rate and depth

D. Rapid and deep

E. Rapid rate

F. Increases, decreases, absence

G. Slow rate

H. Rapid, deep gasps with periods of apnea

I. Absence of breathing

19. The amount of air you breathe in and out of your lungs in one breath is known as

A. minute volume

B. respiratory output

C. stroke volume

D. tidal volume

20. Korotkoff sounds are generated by

A. the heart valves closing

B. the heart valves opening

C. blood hitting the arterial walls

D. blockage in the carotid arteries

21. A patient with a blood pressure of 150/80 has a pulse pressure of _____ mmHg.

A. 230

B. 70

C. 100

D. none of the above

22. A rising pulse pressure indicates

A. increasing intracranial pressure

B. pericardial tamponade

C. tension pneumothorax

D. decompensated shock

23. Hypertension in adults is defined as a blood pressure higher than

A. 100/70

B. 120/80

C. 140/90

D. 150/100

24. If your supine patient's pulse rate rises 10–20 beats per minute or his blood pressure drops

10–20 mmHg when you sit him up, what should you suspect?

A. Congestive heart failure

B. Significant blood loss

C. Severe hypertension

D. Coronary artery disease

25. At which body temperature will brain cells die and seizures become imminent?

A. 102° F

B. 103° F

C. 104° F

D. 105° F

26. The preferred device for measuring temperature in children younger than 6 years old is

A. rectal

B. oral

C. tympanic

D. axillary

27. You should use the diaphragm of your stethoscope to auscultate

A. heart sounds

B. lung sounds

C. bowel sounds

D. all of the above

28. Which of the following statements is true regarding stethoscopes?

A. Thin, flexible tubing transmits sound better

B. Longer tubing minimizes distortion

C. Angle the earpiece toward the nose

D. Use a flexible diaphragm cover

29. To visualize the tympanic membrane, you would use a/an

A. otoscope

B. ophthalmoscope

C. sphygmomanometer

D. sterile tongue blade

30. A specialized hammer is used to assess your patient's
    A. cranial nerves
    B. deep tendon reflexes
    C. range of motion
    D. vibration sense

31. A Broselow tape is used to
    A. calculate infant blood pressure
    B. measure an infant patient's length
    C. estimate your patient's weight
    D. secure an endotracheal tube

32. If your patient wears shoes that have been altered with slits, holes, or open laces, you might suspect he is suffering from
    A. gout
    B. bunions
    C. edema
    D. all of the above

33. Your patient presents with a bitter almond odor on his breath. This may suggest
    A. hypercarbia
    B. hypocalcemia
    C. cyanide poisoning
    D. methanol overdose

34. Which is the most reliable location for obtaining an accurate pulse rate on an infant?
    A. Apical
    B. Carotid
    C. Radial
    D. Brachial

35. If you are unsuccessful in obtaining a blood pressure, you should wait _____ until trying it again in the same arm.
    A. 15 seconds
    B. 30 seconds
    C. 1 minute
    D. 5 minutes

36. Normal SaO_2 at sea level on room air should be
    A. 80–100%
    B. 90–120%
    C. 96–100%
    D. 90–95%

37. Your patient is suspected of having carbon monoxide poisoning, yet his SaO_2 is 98%. How is this possible?
    A. The pulse oximeter is inaccurate
    B. His hemoglobin is saturated with CO
    C. His hematocrit is below 25%
    D. He is bleeding out somewhere

38. Which of the following information is NOT obtained by cardiac monitoring?
    A. Cardiac output
    B. Heart rate
    C. Cardiac cycle measurement
    D. Identification of dysrhythmias

39. If your patient's skin color is cyanotic, you should suspect
    A. hypocarbia
    B. deoxyhemoglobin
    C. DNA abnormalities
    D. hypovolemia

40. Your patient presents with a yellowish tint only to the palms of his hands, the soles of his feet, and his face. He is most likely suffering from
    A. liver failure
    B. cirrhosis
    C. carotanemia
    D. none of the above

Match the following skin conditions with their respective causes:

41. ____ Oily skin
42. ____ Localized warmth
43. ____ Generalized coolness

44. ____ Thick skin

45. ____ Poor turgor

46. ____ Decreased mobility

A. Scleroderma
B. Dehydration
C. Hypothermia
D. Hyperthyroidism
E. Bleeding
F. Eczema

47. You are evaluating a mass that appears to be a tumor and note that it is affixed to your patient's rib and is immobile. This usually suggests
A. a malignancy
B. a benign cyst
C. an aneurysm
D. a petechial wheal

48. Hirsutism is defined as
A. male pattern baldness
B. severe dandruff
C. abnormal facial hair growth in women
D. transverse depressions in the nail beds

49. You can differentiate nits (lice eggs) from dandruff by
A. the color
B. how easily they flake off the hair
C. movement
D. the formation of clumps

50. Periorbital ecchymosis and mastoid process discoloration are classic signs of
A. increased intracranial pressure
B. basilar skull fracture
C. orbital injury
D. TMJ dislocation

51. Placing the tip of your finger into the depression just anterior to the tragus and asking your patient to open his mouth is the procedure for assessing his

A. gag reflex
B. cranial nerve IX
C. TMJ
D. ability to swallow

52. To test visual acuity with a pocket card, have your patient hold the card _____ inches from his face.
A. 8
B. 14
C. 24
D. 30

53. You test your patient's pupillary response to light by shining your light directly into one eye and watching its response. When you observe the other eye's reaction, you are testing its _____ response.
A. indirect
B. sympathetic
C. corneal
D. consensual

Match the following direct pupillary responses to their respective causes:

54. ____ Unilateral sluggish pupil

55. ____ Bilateral sluggishness

56. ____ Constricted pupil

57. ____ Fixed and dilated pupil

A. Brain death
B. Opiate poisoning
C. Global hypoxia
D. Increased intracranial pressure

58. You ask your patient to focus on an object in the distance. Then you ask him to focus on an object right in front of him. What should normally happen?
A. Both pupils should constrict
B. Both pupils should dilate
C. Both pupils should remain the same size
D. None of the above

59. The "H" test evaluates
    A. eyelid opening
    B. peripheral vision
    C. extraoccular muscles
    D. the corneal reflex

60. To assess for papilledema and retinal hemorrhaging, you will use a/an
    A. otoscope
    B. ophthalmoscope
    C. penlight
    D. slit lamp

61. As you press on your patient's tragus, he complains of tenderness. This could suggest _____ and further inspection with a/an _____.
    A. pharyngitis, tongue blade and penlight
    B. retinal occlusion, ophthalmoscope
    C. deviated septum, otoscope
    D. otitis, otoscope

62. Your patient presents with a watery, clear rhinitis and a cobblestone appearance to his conjunctiva. These are usually caused by
    A. bacterial infection
    B. viral infection
    C. septal defect
    D. allergies

63. Pressing underneath the zygomatic arches evaluates the _____ sinuses.
    A. frontal
    B. ethmoid
    C. sphenoid
    D. maxillary

64. You are evaluating a patient in his late 50s who smokes cigarettes, chews tobacco, and drinks alcohol. Where should you specifically look in the mouth for signs of malignancies?
    A. Under the tongue

    B. On the sides of the mouth
    C. On the hard palate
    D. Just anterior to the uvula

65. While you are palpating your patient's thyroid gland, ask him to
    A. take a deep breath
    B. turn his head to each side
    C. swallow
    D. cough

Match the following lymph nodes with their respective locations:

66. ____ Posterior auricular
67. ____ Preauricular
68. ____ Occipital
69. ____ Supraclavicular
70. ____ Posterior cervical
71. ____ Anterior cervical
72. ____ Deep cervical
73. ____ Submental
74. ____ Submandibular

    A. Under the chin
    B. Anterior to the tragus
    C. Just above the clavicle
    D. Anterior to the sternocleidomastoid
    E. Under the lateral jaw
    F. At the base of the skull
    G. Posterior to the sternocleidomastoid
    H. Deep to the sternocleidomastoid
    I. Behind the ear

75. Which of the following is **NOT** a chest wall abnormality?
    A. Barrel chest
    B. Pigeon chest
    C. Funnel chest
    D. Squirrel chest

76. You are performing tactile fremitus and note that your patient has increased fremitus over

the area of the left lower lobe only. A probable cause of this is

A. acute pulmonary edema

B. pneumothorax

C. emphysema

D. pneumonia

77. A hyperresonant percussion sound in the right chest only might indicate

A. pneumonia

B. acute pulmonary edema

C. pneumothorax

D. hemothorax

78. As you evaluate for diaphragmatic excursion, you note asymmetrical findings. Which of the following is a possible cause for this phenomenon?

A. Lower airway obstruction

B. C6 fracture and cord disruption

C. Paralyzed phrenic nerve

D. C2 fracture and cord disruption

79. At which point of the respiratory cycle will wheezes originate?

A. Beginning of inspiration

B. End of inspiration

C. Beginning of exhalation

D. End of exhalation

80. Which of the following assessment techniques would you perform on a patient suspected of having a lower respiratory infection?

A. Whispered pectoriloquoy

B. Egophony

C. Bronchophony

D. All of the above

81. When palpating the carotid arteries, you notice a left-sided thrill, or humming. Which procedure should you perform next?

A. Auscultate for bruits

B. Percuss for dullness

C. Carotid sinus massage

D. Egophony

82. Which of the following structures is found at the PMI?

A. The upper border of the kidney

B. The apex of the heart

C. The diaphragmatic pouch

D. The carina

83. Where do you auscultate for S_1?

A. Second intercostal space, left sternal border, PMI

B. Second intercostal space, right and left sternal borders

C. Fifth intercostal space, left sternal border, PMI

D. Fifth intercostal space, right sternal border, PMI

84. Where do you auscultate for S_2?

A. Second intercostal space, left sternal border, PMI

B. Second intercostal space, right and left sternal borders

C. Fifth intercostal space, left sternal border, PMI

D. Fifth intercostal space, right sternal border, PMI

85. To make an abdominal exam easier for you and more comfortable for your patient, have him

A. place a pillow under his pelvis

B. place his hands above his head

C. empty his bladder prior to the exam

D. lay laterally recumbent

86. Cullen's sign and Grey-Turner's sign are classic findings in

A. peritonitis

B. intra-abdominal hemorrhage

C. appendicitis

D. hernias in males

87. A suprapubic bulge suggests a
    A. hernia
    B. pregnant uterus
    C. distended bladder
    D. B and C

88. Which of the following signs suggests an intestinal obstruction?
    A. Absent bowel sounds
    B. Decreased bowel sounds
    C. Increased bowel sounds
    D. Bruits

89. Rebound tenderness is a classic sign of
    A. bowel obstruction
    B. abdominal aortic aneurysm
    C. peritonitis
    D. hernia

90. The presence of ascites is a classic sign of
    A. congestive heart failure
    B. bowel obstruction
    C. paralytic ileus
    D. hernia

91. You are examining the external genitalia of your female patient and notice a yellow discharge from the urethral opening and a foul-smelling odor. You suspect
    A. candidiasis
    B. gonorrhea
    C. a fungal infection
    D. herpes simplex

Match the following joints with their respective ranges of motion (select all that apply):

92. _____ DIP, PIP, MCP
93. _____ Wrist
94. _____ Elbow
95. _____ Shoulder
96. _____ Ankle
97. _____ Knee

98. _____ Hip
99. _____ Spine
    A. Flexion/extension
    B. Abduction/adduction
    C. Supination/pronation
    D. internal/external rotation
    E. Lateral bending
    F. Rotation
    G. Deviation
    H. Inversion/eversion

100. Your patient complains of increasing pain in her left elbow and increasing immobility. You inspect and palpate the joint and notice redness, swelling, and warmth. During the range of motion exam, she has difficulty with both active and passive movements. You suspect
    A. a nerve disorder
    B. arthritis
    C. a weakened muscle
    D. a subluxation

101. Your patient complains of nontraumatic left-hand pain and numbness. Following a physical exam, you make a field diagnosis of carpal tunnel syndrome. This involves inflammation of the _____ nerve.
    A. radial
    B. ulnar
    C. median
    D. biceps brachii

102. Inflammation of the lateral or medial epicondyles of the elbow suggests
    A. tendonitis
    B. bursitis
    C. subluxation
    D. arthritis

103. Lateral ankle sprains are more common than medial sprains because the lateral ligaments are smaller and weaker. You should expect

severe pain during which range of motion movements?

A. Eversion and dorsiflexion

B. Inversion and dorsiflexion

C. Inversion and plantar flexion

D. Eversion and plantar flexion

104. You will use the drawer test to evaluate the

A. medial and collateral cruciate ligaments

B. patellar and quadriceps tendons

C. rotator cuff

D. anterior and posterior cruciate ligaments

105. Exaggerated lumbar concavity (swayback) is known as

A. kyphosis

B. scoliosis

C. lordosis

D. lumbago

106. You are reading a patient's chart during your ICU rotation and notice a notation that reads radial pulse 1+. This means that the pulse is

A. normal

B. bounding

C. weak and thready

D. absent

107. When assessing the extremities, unilateral coldness suggests

A. an environmental problem

B. an arterial occlusion

C. a venous occlusion

D. shock

108. After assessing for pitting edema, you note that you can create a pit that is greater than 1 inch deep. You would record this as _____ pitting.

A. 1+

B. 2+

C. 3+

D. 4+

109. Your patient complains of a swollen, painful lower leg. Upon palpation, you note a tender femoral vein and calf tenderness. These are both classic signs of a/an

A. DVT

B. arterial occlusion

C. aneurysm

D. varicose vein

110. Manic behavior is best described as a state of

A. hopelessness and slowed pace

B. restlessness and tense posture

C. extreme agitation

D. overexuberance and expansive movements

111. Your patient has dysarthria. This is best described as a speech defect caused by

A. vocal cord problems

B. damage to the cortex

C. motor deficits

D. psychotic disorder

Match the following thought and perception abnormalities with their respective descriptions:

112. ____ Loose associations

113. ____ Flight of ideas

114. ____ Incoherence

115. ____ Confabulation

116. ____ Compulsion

117. ____ Obsession

118. ____ Feelings of unreality

119. ____ Delusions

120. ____ Illusions

121. ____ Hallucinations

A. Makes up facts and events

B. Sees things that are not real

C. Often shifts to unrelated topics

D. Has recurrent, uncontrollable feeling of doom

E. Misinterprets what is real

F. Rambles in related areas with no real conclusion

G. Senses things in environment are strange

H. Has false personal beliefs not shared by group

I. Is driven to prevent some unrealistic future event

J. Rambles on with unrelated, illogical thoughts

122. Your patient believes that there are bugs crawling all over him. This type of behavior suggests

A. psychedelic drug ingestion

B. alcohol withdrawal

C. acute psychosis

D. obsessive-compulsive disorder

123. Digit span, serial sevens, and backward spelling all evaluate your patient's

A. orientation

B. concentration

C. immediate memory

D. remote memory

124. To assess your patient's recent memory, ask him to

A. repeat several unrelated words

B. describe his boyhood neighborhood

C. describe his last meal

D. give you his social security number

125. Assessing the pupils for their response to light is testing which two cranial nerves?

A. Optic (CN-II) and occulomotor (CN-III)

B. Occulomotor (CN-III) and trochlear (CN-IV)

C. Olfactory (CN-I) and optic (CN-II)

D. Trochlear (CN-IV) and optic (CN-II)

126. To evaluate the function of the extraoccular muscles, you are assessing the integrity of which cranial nerve(s)?

A. Occulomotor (CN-III)

B. Occulomotor (CN-III) and trochlear (CN-IV)

C. Optic (CN-II), occulomotor (CN-III), and trochlear (CN-IV)

D. Occulomotor (CN-III), trochlear (CN-IV), and abducens (CN-VI)

127. Asking your patient to clench his teeth while you palpate his temporal and masseter muscles is assessing for which cranial nerve?

A. Trochlear (CN-IV)

B. Facial (CN-VII)

C. Trigeminal (CN-V)

D. Glossopharyngeal (CN-IX)

128. Your patient has Bell's palsy. Because of this, the entire left side of his face droops. Bell's palsy is an inflammation of which cranial nerve?

A. Facial (CN-VII)

B. Trigeminal (CN-V)

C. Glossopharyngeal (CN-IX)

D. Abducens (CN-VI)

129. Ask your patient to stand and close his eyes to test his balance. If he becomes dizzy, it could suggest a problem with which cranial nerve?

A. Vagus (CN-X)

B. Hypoglossal (CN-XII)

C. Accessory (CN-XI)

D. Acoustic (CN-VIII)

130. Which two cranial nerves are responsible for the gag reflex?

A. Glossopharyngeal (CN-IX) and vagus (CN-X)

B. Vagus (CN-X) and accessory (CN-XI)

C. Accessory (CN-XI) and hypoglossal (CN-XII)

D. Facial (CN-VII) and glossopharyngeal (CN-IX)

131. You ask your patient to open his mouth and say "aaaahhhhh." You note that his uvula deviates toward the left side. This suggests a lesion to his _____ nerve.

A. right glossopharyngeal (CN-IX)

B. left glossopharyngeal (CN-IX)

C. right vagus (CN-X)

D. left vagus (CN-X)

132. You ask your patient to stick out his tongue. You note that the tongue projects midline. This indicates a functioning _____ nerve.

A. glossopharyngeal (CN-IX)

B. vagus (CN-X)

C. hypoglossal (CN-XII)

D. accessory (CN-XI)

133. Your patient's hands begin to twitch when he tries to sign the run sheet. The probable diagnosis for this condition is

A. chronic psychosis

B. chronic neurosis

C. Parkinson's

D. postural tremors

134. You put your patient through a range of motion exam. During the exam, you notice he exhibits resistance in a ratchet-like fashion. This jerky resistance is known as cog-wheel rigidity. Which of the following is the most likely reason?

A. He has advanced Parkinson's disease

B. He has a lower neuron disease

C. He is faking his symptoms

D. He has paratonia

135. You are reading a patient's chart at the orthopedic clinic and notice a score of 3 for the range of motion exam on his shoulder. A score of 3 means

A. barely palpable muscle contraction without movement

B. active movement against gravity

C. active movement against some resistance

D. active movement with gravity removed

136. Cerebellar function is assessed by which of the following tests?

A. Romberg

B. Pronator drift

C. Rapid alternating movements

D. All of the above

137. Placing a familiar object such as a key into your patient's hand and asking him to identify it is known as

A. position sense

B. discrimination

C. vibration sense

D. spinothalamic testing

138. You are perusing your patient's chart further and notice the notation for deep tendon reflexes. You read that for the biceps and triceps, his grade is ++. This score means

A. below normal

B. normal

C. brisker than normal

D. hyperactive

139. To assess the biceps tendon reflex, place the arm in a _____ position.

A. slightly flexed

B. fully flexed

C. fully extended

D. none of the above

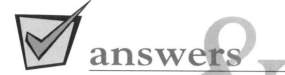

answers & rationales

1.

B. The four basic physical exam techniques are inspection, palpation, auscultation, and percussion. (PCPP 2–29 EPC 610)

2.

A. The pads of the fingers are more sensitive than the tips for detecting masses, fluid, position, consistency, size, and crepitus. (PCPP 2–31 EPC 611)

3.

D. To detect vibrations, such as fremitus, you should use the palm of your hand because the skin is thinner and more sensitive. (PCPP 2–31 EPC 612)

4.

B. When palpating your patient's abdomen, observe how your patient responds with facial expressions while you palpate tender areas. Even if he is unconscious, he may respond to pain with facial expressions or movement. (PCPP 2–31 EPC 612)

5.

A. Percussion evaluates the surface and the tissue beneath by sending a vibration through it. A hollow and vibrating resonance heard when percussing the chest indicates the presence of air. (PCPP 2–31 EPC 612)

6.

D. When reporting and recording lung sounds, you should note the abnormal sound you hear (crackles, wheezes, rhonchi), the location (bilateral, right lower lobe, bases), and the timing during the respiratory cycle (inspiratory, end-expiratory). (PCPP 2–32 EPC 613)

7.

B. Generally auscultate after you have used other assessment techniques. The only exception to this rule is the abdomen, which you should auscultate before palpating and percussing. (PCPP 2–32 EPC 613)

8.

D. A healthy adult should have a resting heart rate between 60 and 100 beats per minute. (PCPP 2–34 EPC 614)

9.

A. A weak, thready pulse is a common finding in a patient in circulatory collapse, such as in shock. (PCPP 2–34 EPC 615)

Matching (PCPP 2–36 EPC 617)

10. C Eupnea
11. E Tachypnea
12. G Bradypnea
13. I Apnea
14. A Hyperpnea
15. F Cheyne-Stokes
16. H Biot's
17. D Kussmaul's
18. B Apneustic

A. Normal rate, but deeper
B. Prolonged inspiration, shortened expiration
C. Normal rate and depth
D. Rapid and deep
E. Rapid rate
F. Increases, decreases, absence
G. Slow rate
H. Rapid, deep gasps with periods of apnea
I. Absence of breathing

19.

D. Tidal volume is the amount of air a person breathes in and out of the lungs in one breath. A healthy adult at rest breathes approximately 500 ml of air each breath, just enough to make the chest rise. (PCPP 2–35 EPC 616)

20.

C. Korotkoff sounds are the sounds of blood hitting the arterial walls that you auscultate when you take your patient's blood pressure. (PCPP 2–35   EPC 616)

21.

B. Pulse pressure is the difference between the systolic and diastolic pressures. A patient with a BP of 150/80 has a pulse pressure of 70 mmHg. (PCPP 2–36   EPC 617)

22.

A. The pulse pressure rises in a patient with increasing intracranial pressure in the body's attempt to perfuse the brain. A narrowing pulse pressure suggests tamponade, tension pneumothorax, or hypovolemic shock. (PCPP 2–36   EPC 617)

23.

C. Blood pressure higher than 140/90 in adults is considered hypertension. (PCPP 2–36   EPC 617)

24.

B. If your supine patient's pulse rate rises more than 10–20 beats per minute or his blood pressure drops 10–20 mmHg when you sit him up, you should suspect a significant blood loss. This is known as a positive "tilt test," or orthostatic hypotension. (PCPP 2–36   EPC 617)

25.

D. At temperatures above 105° F (41° C), brain cells die and seizures may occur. (PCPP 2–37   EPC 618)

26.

A. A rectal thermometer is the preferred method for measuring temperature in children younger than 6 years old. (PCPP 2–37   EPC 618)

27.

A. To maximize your ability to auscultate blood pressure, heart sounds, or arterial bruits, use the diaphragm side of your stethoscope. To hear lung or bowel sounds, the bell side is recommended. (PCPP 2–37   EPC 618)

28.

C. To maximize your ability to auscultate sound, use a rigid diaphragm cover and thick, heavy, short tubing; always angle the earpiece toward the nose. (PCPP 2–38   EPC 619)

29.

A. An otoscope is used to visualize the tympanic membrane (eardrum). It has a light source, a speculum, and a magnifying glass that you insert into the ear canal. (PCPP 2–39   EPC 620)

30.

B. A reflex hammer is used to assess your patient's deep tendon reflexes, a component of a comprehensive neurological exam. (PCPP 2–40   EPC 621)

31.

B. A Broselow tape is a measuring device used to provide you with information regarding airway equipment, drug dosages, and IV calculations based on your patient's height. You simply measure your patient from the feet to the top of the head and use the color-coded information provided. (PCPP 2–42 EPC 623)

32.

D. Look at your patient's shoes. If they have been altered with slits, holes, or open laces, he may be compensating for a painful foot condition, such as gout, edema, or bunions. (PCPP 2–42   EPC 623)

33.

C. Your patient's breath sometimes can provide important clues that aid you in forming your field diagnosis. The smell of bitter almonds is a classic finding in cyanide poisoning. (PCPP 2–42   EPC 623)

34.

D. When assessing the pulse rate in an infant, use the brachial pulse, located just medial to the biceps tendon. Auscultating the apical pulse provides the sounds of the cardiac valves closing but tells you nothing about the quality of the pulse wave generated. (PCPP 2–43   EPC 624)

35.

B. If you do not obtain a reading, wait 30 seconds to allow the blood pressure to normalize before inflating the cuff again. Failure to wait will render an inaccurate reading. (PCPP 2–46   EPC 625)

36.

C. A pulse oximeter measures the oxygen saturation of the blood. At sea level on room air, your oxygen saturation should be between 96 and 100%. This means that 96 100% of your hemoglobin is saturated—preferably with oxygen. (PCPP 2–46 EPC 625)

37.

B. This patient's hemoglobin is saturated with carbon monoxide because the CO molecule binds 200 times more easily with hemoglobin than oxygen does. Therefore, the pulse oximeter reads that 96% of the hemoglobin is indeed saturated and does not distinguish between CO and O_2. (PCPP 2–47 EPC 628)

38.

A. Cardiac monitoring is an effective assessment tool for patients requiring advanced life support. It tells you the heart rate, measures the cardiac cycle, and allows you to identify cardiac dysrhythmias. It cannot, however, provide hemodynamic information (i.e., whether the heart is pumping effectively, or at all). Always correlate what you see on the monitor with your clinical assessment (taking a pulse and BP). (PCPP 2–48 EPC 629)

39.

B. Bright red oxyhemoglobin gives the skin a pink color. As the hemoglobin loses its oxygen to the tissues, it changes color to the darker blue deoxyhemoglobin. Increased deoxyhemoglobin causes cyanosis, a bluish skin color, and signifies decreased oxygen at the tissue level. Cyanosis = hypoxia. (PCPP 2–50 EPC 630)

40.

C. Only your patient's palms, soles, and face appear yellow—he probably has carotanemia, a harmless nutritional condition caused by eating a diet high in carrots and yellow vegetables or fruits. Jaundice, a yellow color that first appears in the sclera and then all over the body, indicates severe liver disease. (PCPP 2–50 EPC 630)

Matching (PCPP 2–51 EPC 630)

41. **D** Oily skin
42. **E** Localized warmth
43. **C** Generalized coolness
44. **F** Thick skin
45. **B** Poor turgor
46. **A** Decreased mobility

A. Scleroderma
B. Dehydration
C. Hypothermia
D. Hyperthyroidism
E. Bleeding
F. Eczema

47.

A. If you palpate a mass and it is affixed to a specific structure and immobile, suspect a malignancy. Also note its color and border. An irregular border and dark color also suggest a malignancy. (PCPP 2–52 EPC 631)

48.

C. Hirsutism is abnormal facial hair growth in women caused by a hormonal imbalance. (PCPP 2–54 EPC 633)

49.

B. To differentiate dandruff from nits (lice eggs), see how easily they flake off the hair. The nits cling firmly to the hair shaft, while dandruff flakes off easily. (PCPP 2–54 EPC 634)

50.

B. Periorbital ecchymosis (raccoon eyes) and discoloration at the mastoid process (Battle's sign) are classic signs of a basilar skull fracture. Sinuses in the skull allow blood to pool in the soft tissues around the eyes and behind the ears following a fracture of the base of the skull. (PCPP 2–59 EPC 636)

51.

C. To evaluate your patient's temporomandibular joint (TMJ), place your finger tip into the depression just in front of the tragus and ask him to open his mouth. As he opens his mouth, your finger should drop into the joint space. Palpate it for tenderness, crepitus, swelling, and range of motion. (PCPP 2–59 EPC 636)

52.

B. Using a pocket visual acuity card is a simple process. Have your patient hold the card 14 inches from his face, cover one eye, and read the smallest line he can. Record the smallest line in which he can read at least one-half the letters as a fraction. 20/70 means that a normal eye could read the line from 70 feet away, but your patient could read it only from 20 feet. (PCPP 2–60 EPC 636)

53.

D. Shining a light into one eye and observing its reaction to light is checking its direct response. Observing the other eye is checking its consensual response. Both eyes should constrict simultaneously in response to the light. (PCPP 2–64 EPC 637)

Matching (PCPP 2–64 EPC 640)

54. D Unilateral sluggish pupil
55. C Bilateral sluggishness
56. B Constricted pupil
57. A Fixed and dilated pupil

A. Brain death
B. Opiate poisoning
C. Global hypoxia
D. Increased intracranial pressure

58.

A. As you focus on an object right in front of you, your pupils should constrict. This is known as the near response and is an effective way to evaluate pupil response outside on a sunny day. (PCPP 2–64 EPC 640)

59.

C. In the "H" test, have your patient follow your finger as you move it in an "H" pattern in front of him. This tests the integrity of the extraoccular muscles and cranial nerves III (occulomotor), IV (trochlear), and VI (abducens). Normal eye movements should be conjugate (together). (PCPP 2–64 EPC 640)

60.

B. To assess for papilledema and retinal hemorrhaging, you will need an ophthalmoscope. Examining the eye's interior is a detailed process that is very difficult to master, requiring skill and practice. (PCPP 2–65 EPC 640)

61.

D. An inner or middle ear infection (otitis) will cause tenderness to the tragus and warrant inspection of the tympanic membrane and ear canal with an otoscope. (PCPP 2–66 EPC 640)

62.

D. Watery, clear rhinitis and "cobblestoning" usually suggest allergies. If the rhinitis or conjunctival discharge appears thick and yellow, suspect an infection. (PCPP 2–70 EPC 642)

63.

D. To palpate the maxillary sinuses, press upward just underneath the zygomatic arches and look for tenderness. You can also tap on the area, as you would percuss the chest. Swelling or tenderness suggests a sinus infection or obstruction. (PCPP 2–70 EPC 642)

64.

A. Make sure to inspect the sides and bottom of the tongue in patients who smoke, chew, and drink because this is where malignancies are likely to appear. Simply hold the tongue and manipulate it with a 2×2 gauze pad. (PCPP 2–72 EPC 645)

65.

C. To examine the thyroid, stand behind your patient and palpate the gland with two fingers of each hand on each side of the trachea. Now ask him to swallow and feel for the gland moving under your touch. It should be smooth, small, and nodule-free. (PCPP 2–75 EPC 645)

Matching (PCPP 2–75 EPC 647)

66. I Posterior auricular
67. B Preauricular
68. F Occipital
69. C Supraclavicular
70. G Posterior cervical
71. D Anterior cervical
72. H Deep cervical
73. A Submental
74. E Submandibular

A. Under the chin
B. Anterior to the tragus
C. Just above the clavicle
D. Anterior to the sternocleidomastoid
E. Under the lateral jaw
F. At the base of the skull
G. Posterior to the sternocleidomastoid
H. Deep into the sternocleidomastoid
I. Behind the ear

75.

D. Common chest abnormalities include funnel chest (pectus excavatum), pigeon chest (pectus carinatum), and barrel chest. (PCPP 2–78 EPC 648)

76.

D. Perform tactile fremitus when you wish to evaluate the consistency of lung tissue. If you detect increased fremitus (vibration) in a particular area, this suggests consolidation of lung tissue as in pneumonia, tumor, or pulmonary fibrosis. (PCPP 2–79   EPC 648)

77.

C. Hyperresonance suggests an area abnormally filled with air. In a unilateral lung, you would suspect pneumothorax. Bilaterally you would suspect diseases such as asthma or emphysema, which trap air in the distal alveoli. (PCPP 2–79   EPC 650)

78.

C. The phrenic nerve (left and right) leaves the spinal cord at C3, C4, C5 (remember: C3,4,5 keeps us alive) and innervates the diaphragm bilaterally. If one of the branches is paralyzed, the result is loss of function on that side and asymmetrical movement. (PCPP 2–79   EPC 650)

79.

D. Wheezes are caused by bronchiole constriction. These tiny airways collapse when the positive pressure exerted on them from the outside is greater than the pressure available on the inside to keep them patent. This happens first at the end of exhalation, and as your patient's condition worsens, it occurs earlier in the cycle. (PCPP 2–81   EPC 651)

80.

D. Any patient whom you suspect has a lower airway infection or who has abnormal breath sounds should receive the following tests to identify abnormally transmitted voice sounds, which suggest areas of consolidated tissue: whispered pectoriloquoy (have him whisper "99"), egophony (have him say "e"), and bronchophony (have him say "99") while you auscultate. (PCPP 2–82   EPC 651)

81.

A. If, when palpating the carotid arteries you note a thrill, or humming vibration, immediately auscultate the artery for bruits, the sound of rushing blood around an obstructed artery. Avoid deep manipulative palpation, which could loosen the obstruction (plaque) and cause a cerebral embolism (stroke). (PCPP 2–86   EPC 653)

82.

B. The point of maximum impulse (PMI) signifies the apex of the heart. Here you can find the apical pulse. This point is usually found at the fifth intercostal space, just medial to the midclavicular line. Lateral displacement suggests right ventricle enlargement from systemic hypertension. (PCPP 2–88   EPC 655)

83.

C. With the diaphragm of your stethoscope, listen for the high-pitched sounds of S_1 at the fifth intercostal space, left sternal border (tricuspid valve) and at the PMI (mitral valve). (PCPP 2–88   EPC 655)

84.

B. With the diaphragm of your stethoscope, listen for the high-pitched sounds of S_2 at the second intercostal space, right sternal border (aortic valve) and left sternal border (pulmonic valve). (PCPP 2–88 EPC 655)

85.

C. A relaxed patient is the key to an effective abdominal exam. Have him lay supine with a pillow underneath his head and his knees to relax the abdominal muscles. Have him place his arms at his sides and make sure his bladder is empty prior to the exam if possible. (PCPP 2–93   EPC 656)

86.

B. Discoloration over the umbilicus (Cullen's sign) or over the flanks (Grey-Turner's sign) is a classic late sign of intra-abdominal hemorrhage. (PCPP 2–94 EPC 656)

87.

D. A bulge just above the pubic bone suggests a pregnant uterus or a distended bladder. A bulge in the inguinal or femoral area suggests a hernia. (PCPP 2–94   EPC 656)

88.

C. Proximal to an intestinal obstruction where the bowels are trying to force debris through the obstruction, you will hear the increased sounds of hyperperistalsis. (PCPP 2–94   EPC 656)

89.

C. An inflamed peritoneum will be very irritable. Even the slightest movement causes severe pain. To test for rebound tenderness, press down gently but firmly on an area away from the patient's complaint, and then release your hand quickly. The sudden jarring will cause pain if the peritoneum is irritated. (PCPP 2–95   EPC 657)

90.

A. Ascites is the collection of fluid in the abdominal cavity and flanks caused by congestive heart failure. Test for ascites by causing a fluid wave across your patient's abdomen. (PCPP 2–95   EPC 657)

91.

B. A yellow, green, or gray discharge with a fishy or foul odor suggests a bacterial infection, such as gonorrhea or Gardnarella. If the discharge is white or curd-like and odorless, suspect a fungal infection, such as candidiasis. (PCPP 2–98   EPC 660)

Matching (PCPP 2–104–127   EPC 662–673)

92.	A	DIP, PIP, MCP
93.	A, G	Wrist
94.	A, C	Elbow
95.	A, B, D	Shoulder
96.	A, H	Ankle
97.	A, D	Knee
98.	A, B, D	Hip
99.	A, D, E, F	Spine

A. Flexion/extension
B. Abduction/adduction
C. Supination/pronation
D. Internal/external rotation
E. Lateral bending
F. Rotation
G. Deviation
H. Inversion/eversion

100.

B. Redness, swelling, and warmth suggest increased circulation to the area. Difficulty with both active and passive range of motion tests suggests a nontraumatic joint inflammation, such as arthritis, gout, or rheumatic fever. (PCPP 2–103   EPC 661)

101.

C. Carpal tunnel syndrome is caused by inflammation of the median nerve, which runs through the middle groove at the inside of the wrist. During acute flexion of the wrist, your patient will complain of numbness of the palmar surface of the thumb, the

index finger, the middle finger, and part of his ring finger. (PCPP 2–106   EPC 662)

102.

A. Nontraumatic inflammation of the lateral epicondyles (tennis elbow) or medial epicondyles (golfer's elbow) suggests tendonitis at those muscle insertion sites. (PCPP 2–107   EPC 662)

103.

C. Lateral ankle sprains are common. Your patient will present with pain, tenderness, and swelling to the outside of the ankle. During inversion and plantar flexion tests, expect him to complain of severe pain. In these cases, do not continue the exam. (PCPP 2–116   EPC 665)

104.

D. The drawer test evaluates the stability of the anterior and posterior cruciate ligaments. Simply try to move the knee joint anterior and posterior like opening and closing a drawer. There should be little movement, if any, if the ligaments are intact. (PCPP 2–118   EPC 668)

105.

C. Inspect your patient's spine and note any irregularities. The spine should be straight and plumb from the neck to the buttocks. Abnormal lateral curvature is known as scoliosis. Observe the spine from the side. An exaggerated lumbar concavity is known as lordosis or swayback. An exaggerated thoracic convexity is known as kyphosis or hunchback. (PCPP 2–126   EPC 668)

106.

C. Pulse quality is quantified according to the following scale:

0   Absent
1+ Weak and thready
2+ Normal
3+ Bounding

(PCPP 2–131   EPC 673

107.

B. When assessing the extremities, unilateral coldness suggests an arterial occlusion. Bilateral coldness suggests an environmental problem, bilateral occlusion, or global circulatory collapse (shock). (PCPP 2–131   EPC 673)

108.

D. Assess pitting edema by pressing on the top of the foot or over the shins and note the depression. Then grade it according to the following scale:

1+ One-quarter inch or less
2+ One-quarter inch to one-half inch
3+ One-half to one inch
4+ One inch or more

(PCPP 2–133   EPC 675)

109.

A. Classic signs of a deep vein thrombosis (DVT) include a swollen, painful lower leg; visible venous distention; femoral vein tenderness; and a tender calf. A DVT can become a pulmonary embolism if it breaks away from the vein wall. (PCPP 2–133 EPC 675)

110.

D. Manic behavior is characterized by a general state of overexuberance and expansive movements. Manic patients may have bipolar disease. In this case, they alternate between manic behavior and depression. (PCPP 2–135   EPC 676)

111.

C. Speech pattern abnormalities can be the result of dysarthria (from a motor deficit), dysphonia (from vocal cord damage), or aphasia (from neurological damage to the brain). (PCPP 2–136   EPC 676)

Matching (PCPP 2–136   EPC 677)

112. **C** Loose associations
113. **F** Flight of ideas
114. **J** Incoherence
115. **A** Confabulation
116. **I** Compulsion
117. **D** Obsession
118. **G** Feelings of unreality
119. **H** Delusions
120. **E** Illusions
121. **B** Hallucinations

A. Makes up facts and events
B. Sees things that are not real
C. Often shifts to unrelated topics
D. Has recurrent, uncontrollable feeling of doom
E. Misinterprets what is real
F. Rambles in related areas with no real conclusion
G. Senses things in environment are strange
H. Has false personal beliefs not shared by group
I. Is driven to prevent some unrealistic future event
J. Rambles on with unrelated, illogical thoughts

122.

B. Hallucinations can be caused by post-traumatic stress disorders and organic brain syndrome. Auditory hallucinations (hearing things) are commonly caused by psychedelic drug ingestion, while tactile hallucinations (feeling things) suggest alcohol withdrawal. (PCPP 2–137   EPC 677)

123.

B. Repeating a series of numbers (digit span), counting from 100 backward by sevens (serial sevens), and spelling a common 5 letter word backward all test your patient's ability to concentrate. (PCPP 2–137   EPC 677)

124.

C. Memory is divided into three grades. Immediate memory is the ability to recall the names of several unrelated objects and is similar to digit span. Recent memory is the ability to recall something that happened earlier that day. Remote memory is the ability to recall events from the past. (PCPP 2–137 EPC 678)

125.

A. When you test for pupillary response with a penlight, you are evaluating the integrity of two cranial nerves. The optic nerve (CN-II) senses the light, and the occulomotor nerve (CN–III) responds by constricting the pupil. (PCPP 2–141   EPC 678)

126.

D. When you conduct the "H" test to evaluate the function of the extraoccular muscles, you are assessing the integrity of the occulomotor (CN-III), trochlear (CN-IV), and abducens (CN-VI) nerves. (PCPP 2–141   EPC 679)

127.

C. The motor portion of the trigeminal nerve (CN-V) innervates the temporal muscles (at the temples) and the masseter muscles (between the cheek and jaw). The sensory portion innervates the forehead (ophthalmic branch), the cheeks (maxillary branch), and the chin (mandibular branch). (PCPP 2–144   EPC 681)

128.

A. The facial nerve (CN-VII) innervates the muscles of facial expression. To evaluate this nerve, ask your patient to make a variety of facial expressions for you, such as smiling and frowning. (PCPP 2–145 EPC 681)

129.

D. The acoustic nerve (CN-VIII), also known as the vestibulocochlear nerve, innervates the structures of the inner ear and is responsible for both hearing and balance. A great way to test for both aspects is, after he closes his eyes, to tell him to open them up again. If he does, his gross hearing is also intact. (PCPP 2–145 EPC 681)

130.

A. The glossopharyngeal (CN-IX) and vagus (CN-X) nerves are responsible for the gag reflex. (PCPP 2–145 EPC 681)

131.

D. When your patient says "aaaahhhhh," his soft palate (and uvula) will rise symmetrically if the vagus nerve is intact. A lesion to the vagus nerve will cause the uvula to deviate to the side of the lesion. (PCPP 2–145 EPC 681)

132.

C. The hypoglossal (CN-XII) nerve innervates the tongue. A lesion to this nerve will cause the tongue to deviate to the opposite side of the lesion, hence the "Q" sign. (PCPP 2–145 EPC 681)

133.

D. Postural tremors occur only when the patient tries to perform a task such as lifting a spoon or handwriting. Tremors at rest, which may disappear with voluntary movement, suggest Parkinson's disease. (PCPP 2–148 EPC 682)

134.

C. Cog-wheel rigidity is a common finding in a patient who is either faking his symptoms or resisting the exam. True rigidity, known as lead-pipe rigidity, will be constant throughout the range of motion. Rigidity at the extreme limits of movement is known as spasticity. (PCPP 2–148 EPC 682)

135.

B. When assessing muscle strength, put the muscle and the related joint through a range of motion exam and grade according to the following scale:

0 No visible muscle contraction, flaccid
1 Barely palpable muscle contraction with no movement
2 Active movement with gravity eliminated
3 Active movement against gravity
4 Active movement against some resistance and gravity
5 Active movement against full resistance with no fatigue (PCPP 2–151 EPC 683)

136.

D. Cerebellar function is assessed by the Romberg, pronator drift, rapid alternating movements, point-to-point, and heel-to-shin tests. Any abnormalities in these exams suggest cerebellar or extrapyramidal tract dysfunction. (PCPP 2–151 EPC 683)

137.

B. You can assess your patient's sensory system by assessing for pain, light touch, temperature, position, vibration, and discrimination. Discrimination is the ability to identify an object by touch. (PCPP 2–153 EPC 685)

138.

B. Assess your patient's deep tendon reflexes and grade them according to the following scale:

0   No response
+   Diminished, below normal
++   Average, normal
+++   Brisker than normal
++++   Hyperactive, associated with clonus (PCPP 2–154 EPC 687)

139.

A. To test the deep tendon reflex of the biceps, place the arm in a slightly flexed position, put your thumb directly over the tendon, strike your thumb with the point of the hammer, and observe the briskness of the response (elbow flexion). (PCPP 2–153 EPC 687)

16

Patient Assessment in the Field

DIRECTIONS Each of the questions or incomplete statements below is followed by suggested answers or completions. Select the **one answer** that is best in each case.

1. Which of the following is NOT a component of an assessment conducted on a responsive medical patient?
   A. Initial assessment
   B. Rapid medical assessment
   C. Focused history and physical exam
   D. Ongoing assessment

2. Which of the following is NOT a component of the scene size-up?
   A. Body substance isolation
   B. Mechanism of injury
   C. Initial assessment
   D. Location of all patients

3. The HEPA mask is designed to protect you from
   A. tuberculosis
   B. AIDS
   C. hepatitis
   D. meningitis

4. The top priority in any emergency situation is
   A. patient assessment
   B. bystander cooperation
   C. customer service
   D. your personal safety

5. As you approach a scene, something just does not seem right. It is not anything you can put your finger on, just a sense that something is wrong or is about to happen. What should you do about it?
   A. Wait until law enforcement arrives before entering
   B. Ignore your feelings and enter the scene
   C. Enter the scene with something with which to protect yourself
   D. Call out for the patient to come outside

6. You are responding to a shooting at a well-known bar. How should you approach the scene?
   A. Stage outside the bar until the police arrive
   B. Wait for another ambulance or rescue crew before entering
   C. Just enter the scene
   D. Stage your ambulance a few blocks away until law enforcement arrives

7. You arrive on the scene and see that a power line lies close to your pediatric patient. You are fairly sure the line is live and decide to move it with a dry piece of equipment. Which of the following should you use?
   A. A wooden-handled ax
   B. A fallen tree branch
   C. A nylon rope
   D. None of the above

8. When you and your partner arrive at a multiple-patient incident, you should
   A. begin assessing and treating the first patient you encounter
   B. establish command and begin triage
   C. provide intensive emergency care to the most critical patient
   D. start at opposite ends and begin assessing patients

9. Of the following components of the initial assessment, which should you perform first?
   A. Airway
   B. Priority determination
   C. Circulation
   D. Mental status

10. To maintain proper alignment of a child's head and neck, you should place a folded towel under his
   A. head
   B. neck
   C. shoulders
   D. none of the above

11. Your patient presents with his eyes open, and he responds to you when you speak to him. He answers your questions but is obviously disoriented as to time and place. You grade him _____ on the AVPU scale.
   A. A
   B. V
   C. P
   D. U

12. Your patient fails to respond to your shouting commands. When you pinch his fingernails and rub his sternum, he exhibits decorticate posturing. He receives a/an _____ on the AVPU scale.
   A. A
   B. V
   C. P
   D. U

Match the following upper airway obstruction situations with their respective treatments:

13. ____ Snoring
14. ____ Gurgling
15. ____ Foreign body
16. ____ Burns
17. ____ Anaphylaxis
18. ____ Epiglottitis

   A. Vasoconstrictor medications
   B. Orotracheal suctioning
   C. Blow-by oxygen and a quiet ride
   D. Immediate endotracheal intubation
   E. Heimlich/Magill forceps
   F. Head-tilt/chin-lift

19. Which of the following is NOT a possible diagnosis for a patient with diffuse expiratory wheezing?
   A. Epiglottitis
   B. Bronchitis
   C. Asthma
   D. Bronchiolitis

20. When performing positive pressure ventilation on a nonbreathing patient, provide _____ breaths per minute for adults and _____ breaths per minute for children.
   A. 20, 30
   B. 25, 50
   C. 12, 20
   D. 12, 15

21. Your patient presents unconscious, without a gag reflex, and with a decreased minute volume. You should do all of the following EXCEPT
   A. intubate the patient
   B. perform bag-valve-mask ventilation
   C. administer 100% oxygen
   D. complete the initial assessment before treating

22. Your patient presents with warm, pink skin; a radial pulse rate of 80/minute; and a capillary refill time of :02 second. From this information, what can you conclude about her circulatory condition?
   A. It is normal
   B. It shows signs of early circulatory compromise
   C. It shows signs of severe circulatory collapse
   D. None of the above

23. Which of the following patients should be prioritized for rapid transport?
   A. Cardiac arrest

B. Isolated femur fracture

C. Altered mental status

D. All of the above

24. Which of the following mechanisms is NOT considered a predictor of serious internal injury for an adult?

   A. Fall from higher than 10 feet

   B. Ejection from vehicle

   C. Vehicle rollover

   D. Motorcycle crash

25. You arrive on the scene of a head-on motor vehicle crash and notice that the airbag on the driver's side has been deployed. When you lift the bag, you also notice that the steering wheel is deformed. What is the most likely reason for this finding?

   A. The airbag malfunctioned

   B. The seat belt was not fastened

   C. The crash was not of high speed

   D. The steering wheel was bent before the crash

26. The rapid trauma assessment is designed to

   A. provide a detailed physical exam

   B. identify life-threatening injuries not found in the initial assessment

   C. find and treat minor injuries

   D. rule out the need for rapid transport

27. Which of the following is NOT a component of the DCAP–BTLS mnemonic?

   A. Lacerations

   B. Contusions

   C. Deformities

   D. Broken bones

28. Your patient presents with a major jugular vein laceration. You must immediately

   A. stop the bleeding with a gauze pressure dressing

   B. clamp the vessel with a hemostat

C. tie the vessel off with a surgical string

D. apply an occlusive dressing

29. Your major trauma patient presents with jugular vein distention while sitting up. Which of the following conditions may be the cause?

   A. Pericardial tamponade

   B. Massive hemothorax

   C. Flail chest

   D. Diaphragmatic hernia

30. Your patient's trachea tugs to the left side each time he breathes. The most likely cause for this is

   A. tension pneumothorax

   B. tracheal tear

   C. pneumothorax on the left

   D. pneumothorax on the right

31. Infants and small children _____ to maintain back pressure to keep the airways open.

   A. use accessory muscles

   B. use retractions

   C. grunt

   D. flare their nares

32. Which bone fractures more easily and more often than any other in the body?

   A. Clavicle

   B. Radius

   C. Tibia

   D. Cranium

33. If your patient presents with fractures of the first three ribs, you should suspect

   A. no major systemic complications

   B. pericardial tamponade

   C. major underlying damage

   D. esophageal damage

34. Paradoxical chest wall movement is a classic sign of
    A. pneumothorax
    B. diaphragmatic hernia
    C. tracheo-bronchial tear
    D. flail chest

35. Your patient presents with jugular vein distention, absent breath sounds on the left side, diminished breath sounds on the right side, tachycardia, and profound hypotension. You should
    A. monitor and transport the patient to the trauma center
    B. decompress the left chest immediately
    C. place your patient on his right side
    D. perform pericardiocentesis

36. Which of the following is **NOT** a component of a SAMPLE history?
    A. Past medical history
    B. Medications
    C. Signs
    D. Allergies

37. Which of the following do you **NOT** use to evaluate a basketball player who has twisted his knee?
    A. Milking the joint
    B. Drawer test
    C. Side-to-side test
    D. Full range of motion, regardless of the pain

38. The "H" test evaluates the integrity of
    A. the optic nerve
    B. cranial nerves III, IV, and V
    C. the extraoccular muscles
    D. all of the above

39. Your patient complains of chest pain. You should include an examination of the mouth to assess
    A. central oxygenation
    B. presence of fluids
    C. buccal pallor
    D. all of the above

40. Your cardiac patient presents with jugular vein distention while sitting up. This could suggest
    A. right heart failure
    B. left heart failure
    C. simple pneumothorax
    D. systemic hypertension

41. A localized wheeze could be the result of
    A. asthma
    B. pneumonia
    C. acute pulmonary edema
    D. COPD

42. Your patient presents with unequal femoral pulses and a cool, ashen left leg. This could be the result of a/an
    A. thoracic aneurysm
    B. abdominal aneurysm
    C. pulsus paradoxus
    D. deep vein thrombosis

43. Your patient presents with pinpoint pupils, a classic finding in
    A. shock
    B. anticholinergic poisoning
    C. brain anoxia
    D. narcotic overdose

44. At the far extremes of your "H" test, you note that your patient's eyes begin fine, jerking movements. This is known as
    A. doll's eyes
    B. nystagmus
    C. decortication
    D. hyphema

45. Which of the following patients should receive a "rapid alternating movements" exam?
    A. The acute abdomen
    B. The acute myocardial infarction
    C. The stroke
    D. The arm injury

46. Voluntary abdominal rigidity and guarding suggest
    A. peritoneal irritation
    B. intra-abdominal hemorrhage
    C. massive infection
    D. an anxious patient

47. Which of the following statements best describes the detailed physical exam?
    A. It is a luxury, designed for use en route to the hospital
    B. It follows the primary survey prior to transport
    C. It is an abbreviated version of the comprehensive physical exam
    D. None of the above

48. The ongoing assessment is designed to
    A. reevaluate the effectiveness of your interventions
    B. detect trends
    C. review the ABCs every 5 minutes for critical patients
    D. all of the above

49. You are transporting a patient with a chest injury following a motor vehicle crash. Your partner has intubated the patient and is performing bag-valve ventilation. He suddenly complains that the bag is becoming increasingly more difficult to squeeze. You reassess your patient and note pronounced JVD, tachycardia, and hypotension. The most likely cause for this sudden change in condition is
    A. pericardial tamponade
    B. tension pneumothorax
    C. massive hemothorax
    D. diaphragmatic hernia

50. A narrowing pulse pressure, along with JVD and muffled heart sounds, suggests
    A. tension pneumothorax
    B. cardiac tamponade
    C. hypovolemic shock
    D. massive hemothorax

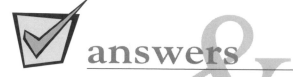

answers & rationales

1.

B. For the responsive patient who can answer your questions, you conduct an initial assessment, a focused history and physical exam, and an ongoing assessment en route to the hospital. (PCPP 2–173 EPC 700)

2.

C. Scene size-up is the essential first step at any emergency. A proper scene size-up includes body substance isolation, scene safety, location of patients, mechanism of injury, and nature of illness. (PCPP 2–175 EPC 701)

3.

A. The high-efficiency particulate air (HEPA) mask is designed to filter out the tuberculosis bacillus. Always wear the mask when performing high-risk procedures, such as endotracheal intubation, or suctioning on patients suspected of having tuberculosis. (PCPP 2–176 EPC 703)

4.

D. Never forget this! Your personal safety is jeopardized every time you answer an alarm. The safety of you and your crew is the top priority at any emergency scene. (PCPP 2–176 EPC 704)

5.

A. Your instincts are the subconscious sum of your experiences. Listen to them. They are probably correct. (PCPP 2–177 EPC 705)

6.

D. Entering an unstable or dangerous environment without law enforcement is the foolish behavior of inexperienced emergency personnel. Better to stage your ambulance a few blocks away from the scene, so as not to rile the bystanders, and wait for the police to secure the scene. (PCPP 2–179 EPC 705)

7.

D. Another example of foolish behavior by inexperienced emergency personnel is to try to move a live wire with ANY piece of equipment. No matter how dry you believe the wooden handles are, they contain moisture and will conduct electricity. Leave it for the professionals with equipment tested to do the job safely. A foolish hero is not a hero. (PCPP 2–179 EPC 705)

8.

B. The first crew on the scene of a multiple-patient incident must avoid the urge to begin treating patients. It is more important to establish a command center, assess your needs, call for help, and begin triage. These steps are patient care. (PCPP 2–183 EPC 709)

9.

D. The initial assessment consists of the following steps: forming a general impression, stabilizing the cervical spine as needed, assessing a baseline mental status, assessing the airway, assessing breathing, assessing circulation, and determining priority. (PCPP 2–186 EPC 712)

10.

C. A child's occiput is very large. To compensate for this, place a folded towel under his shoulders to maintain proper alignment of his head and neck. (PCPP 2–187 EPC 713)

11.

A. An alert patient is awake, as evidenced by open eyes, even though he is disoriented. (PCPP 2–188 EPC 714)

12.

C. If your patient responds to your painful stimulus by abnormal posturing, he receives a P on the AVPU scale. (PCPP 2–188 EPC 714)

Matching (PCPP 2–191   EPC 715)

13. **F** Snoring
14. **B** Gurgling
15. **E** Foreign body
16. **D** Burns
17. **A** Anaphylaxis
18. **C** Epiglottitis

A. Vasoconstrictor medications
B. Orotracheal suctioning
C. Blow-by oxygen and a quiet ride
D. Immediate endotracheal intubation
E. Heimlich/Magill forceps
F. Head-tilt/chin-lift

19.

A. Expiratory wheezing is usually the result of lower airway spasm or obstruction. This can be the result of diseases such as asthma, bronchiolitis, emphysema, and bronchitis. Epiglottitis is an upper airway problem that causes stridor. (PCPP 2–191 EPC 716)

20.

C. According to the American Heart Association, when performing positive pressure ventilation on a nonbreathing patient, provide 12 breaths per minute for adults and 20 breaths per minute for children. (PCPP 2–191   EPC 716)

21.

D. If your patient presents unconscious, without a gag reflex, and with a decreased minute volume, you should first perform bag-valve-mask ventilation with 100% oxygen and plan to intubate the patient. Most important, you should do these things before completing the rest of the initial assessment. (PCPP 2–185   EPC 717)

22.

A. Normal circulatory status in the healthy adult is evidenced by warm, dry skin; the presence of a radial pulse at a rate of 60–100 per minute; and a capillary refill time of less than 2 seconds. (PCPP 2–198 EPC 717)

23.

C. Top priority and rapid transport are reserved for patients with significant airway, breathing, or circulation problems and those with an uncorrectable altered mental status. Cardiac arrest patients can be managed effectively and more efficiently on the scene. (PCPP 2–199   EPC 721)

24.

A. Predictors of serious internal injury for an adult patient include ejection from the vehicle, fall from higher than 20 feet, vehicle rollover, high-speed collision, motorcycle crash, and penetration of the trunk or head. (PCPP 2–200   EPC 722)

25.

B. Within seconds after inflation, an airbag deflates so as not to suffocate the patient. Unfortunately, if your patient does not have his seat belt fastened, he could be propelled into the steering wheel and sustain life-threatening injuries. (PCPP 2–201   EPC 723)

26.

B. The rapid trauma assessment is conducted on trauma patients with a significant mechanism of injury or an altered mental status. It is designed to identify life-threatening injuries not found in the initial assessment. (PCPP 2–202   EPC 724)

27.

D. When performing a rapid trauma assessment, use the mnemonic DCAP–BTLS. It stands for **D**eformities, **C**ontusions, **A**brasions, **P**enetrations, **B**urns, **T**enderness, **L**acerations, and **S**welling. (PCPP 2–203   EPC 725)

28.

D. Aside from major blood loss, consider the possibility of an air embolism because of the negative pressure generated each time your patient inhales. The negative pressure in the chest may draw air into an exposed jugular vein. An occlusive dressing will prevent this. (PCPP 2–203   EPC 725)

29.

A. Jugular vein distention following chest trauma is usually caused by either pericardial tamponade or tension pneumothorax, in which blood is inhibited from returning to the heart. To differentiate, listen for lung sounds. They will be clear bilaterally in pericardial tamponade and absent in tension pneumothorax. (PCPP 2–203   EPC 725)

30.

C. If the trachea tugs to one side during inspiration, the probable cause is a simple pneumothorax on that side. (PCPP 2–203   EPC 725)

31.

C. Grunting is a sign of serious respiratory distress in infants and children. They grunt to create back pressure to keep their lower airways open in such diseases as asthma and bronchiolitis. If your patient is grunting, it is serious. (PCPP 2–204   EPC 726)

32.

A. The clavicles, being so thin and so unprotected and vulnerable, fracture more easily and more often than any other bones in the body. (PCPP 2–204 EPC 726)

33.

C. The first three ribs are well-supported and well-protected. It takes a tremendous force to cause a fracture. Thus, you should expect major damage to organs lying underneath these ribs, especially vascular structures. (PCPP 2–204   EPC 726)

34.

D. A flail chest is defined as two or more rib fractures in two or more places, causing a floating segment. The floating segment moves in opposition to the rest of the chest wall in a paradoxical fashion. (PCPP 2–204   EPC 726)

35.

B. Jugular vein distention, absent breath sounds on one side and diminished breath sounds on the other, tachycardia, and hypotension paint the classic picture of a left-sided tension pneumothorax. You would immediately decompress the left chest with a large-bore angiocatheter. (PCPP 2–205 EPC 727)

36.

C. The SAMPLE history is comprised of the following components: **S**ymptoms, **A**llergies, **M**edications, **P**ast history, **L**ast eaten, and **E**vents preceding the incident. It is used to elicit a quick history from a trauma patient. (PCPP 2–211   EPC 733)

37.

D. For a person with an isolated injury, such as a twisted knee, you inspect and palpate the joint for any irregularities, which includes "milking the joint" for a fluid wave. You then conduct the side-to-side test to evaluate the stability of the medial and lateral collateral ligaments. You use the drawer test to assess the stability of the anterior and posterior cruciate ligaments. Finally, you put the knee through its passive range of motion unless this causes pain. (PCPP 2–212   EPC 734)

38.

C. Anybody with an eye injury should receive a full eye exam. This includes inspection and palpation of the external eye for discoloration, deformity, tenderness, and hyphema; a visual acuity test; direct and consensual response to light; the near-far reflex; accommodation; and the "H" test. The "H" test evaluates the integrity of the cranial nerves and the extraoccular muscles they innervate: CN-III (occulomotor) superior rectus, inferior rectus, inferior oblique; CN-IV (trochlear) superior oblique; and CN-VI (abducens) lateral rectus. An easy way to remember this is SO4–LR6–AR3. In other words, **S**uperior **O**blique is CN-IV, **L**ateral **R**ectus is CN-VI, and **A**ll the **R**est are CN-III. (PCPP 2–212   EPC 734)

39.

D. Examining the mouth of a chest pain patient may reveal important clues as to the seriousness of his condition. Examine the buccal mucosa for signs of central hypoxemia (cyanosis) and circulatory collapse (pallor). Also observe for any fluids, such as pink frothy sputum, which could indicate acute pulmonary edema. (PCPP 2–215   EPC 737)

40.

A. Jugular vein distention (JVD) indicates that blood return to the heart is inhibited. Some common causes for JVD include tension pneumothorax, cardiac tamponade, massive pulmonary embolism, and right heart failure. (PCPP 2–215   EPC 737)

41.

B. Localized wheezing is the result of a lower airway obstruction in one area of the lung from conditions such as an infection (pneumonia), a pulmonary embolism, or foreign body aspiration. Diffuse, or global, wheezing is the result of conditions that affect the entire lung, such as asthma, COPD, and acute pulmonary edema. (PCPP 2–215   EPC 737)

42.

B. An abdominal aneurysm usually blocks the blood flow path to one or the other leg. This results in a weaker femoral pulse on the affected side, absent pulses in the foot, and cool, ashen skin. (PCPP 2–216   EPC 738)

43.

D. Pinpoint pupils, along with unconsciousness and depressed respirations, are a classic sign of narcotic drug overdose. They also can suggest a pontine (from the pons) hemorrhage. (PCPP 2–217 EPC 738)

44.

B. A nystagmus is a fine, jerking movement of the eyes during an extraocular muscle exam. If it occurs at the far extremes of the test, it is normal. If it occurs during the entire range of motion, it is considered pathological. (PCPP 2–217   EPC 739)

45.

C. The "rapid alternating movements" test is used to evaluate the integrity of the cerebellum and the pyramidal system. Any patient with neurological deficits should receive a complete cerebellar exam, which also includes point-to-point and heel-to-shin tests. (PCPP 2–217   EPC 739)

46.

D. If you detect abdominal rigidity or guarding, you must determine whether it is voluntary, because your patient is anxious or resisting your exam, or involuntary, suggesting peritoneal irritation. (PCPP 2–218   EPC 740)

47.

A. The detailed physical is a careful, thorough history and physical exam designed to be conducted en route to the hospital if time and conditions allow. It is a luxury because seldom is there enough time to perform a complete one. (PCPP 2–222   EPC 744)

48.

D. The ongoing assessment is designed to reevaluate the ABCs to detect trends in vital signs and to record the effectiveness of your interventions. (PCPP 2–229   EPC 751)

49.

B. A bag that becomes increasingly more difficult to squeeze is cause for great concern because something is inhibiting lung inflation. This is a classic description of a tension pneumothorax. If you assess lung sounds, you will note absence on the affected side and diminished on the other side. In this case, immediately decompress the chest with a large-bore catheter on the affected side. (PCPP 2–229   EPC 751)

50.

B. Cardiac tamponade is characterized by a narrowing pulse pressure, JVD, and muffled heart sounds—known as Beck's triad. (PCPP 2–231   EPC 753)

17

Clinical Decision Making

DIRECTIONS Each of the questions or incomplete statements below is followed by suggested answers or completions. Select the **one answer** that is best in each case.

1. Another word that describes your patient's severity is
   A. nulliparity
   B. acuity
   C. tonicity
   D. accommodation

2. Which patient acuity level poses the greatest challenge to the paramedic?
   A. Obvious critical life threat
   B. Potential life threat
   C. Non-life-threatening
   D. None of the above

3. A schematic flowchart that outlines patient care procedures is known as a/an
   A. protocol
   B. standing order
   C. algorithm
   D. advanced directive

4. You are authorized to administer an albuterol treatment to patients with diffuse wheezing. This is an example of a/an
   A. protocol
   B. algorithm
   C. mandate
   D. standing order

5. The major disadvantage to using protocols is that they
   A. apply only to atypical patients
   B. apply only to patients with vague presentations
   C. do not allow the paramedic the flexibility to adapt to an atypical patient with an unusual presentation
   D. all of the above

6. The style that requires you to focus on the most important aspect of a critical situation is known as
   A. anticipatory
   B. reflective
   C. divergent
   D. convergent

7. The style that requires you to respond instinctively to a situation rather than thinking about it is known as
   A. impulsive
   B. reflective
   C. divergent
   D. anticipatory

8. To raise your skill level to the pseudo-instinctive level means to be able to
   A. describe each step in detail
   B. do it without thinking about it
   C. consider all the possibilities before attempting a skill
   D. perform the skill while blocking out all other thoughts

9. Place the following steps of the decision-making process in chronological order:
   A. Maintain control
   B. Stop and think
   C. Reevaluate
   D. Scan the situation
   E. Decide and act

10. Which of the following is **NOT** a part of the critical decision process?
   A. Forming a concept
   B. Evaluating
   C. Reflecting
   D. Researching

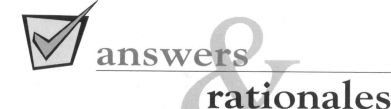

answers & rationales

1.

B. Acuity is a term that describes the severity or acuteness of your patient's condition. There are three general classes of patient acuity: obvious critical life threats, potential life threats, and non-life-threatening presentations. (PCPP 2–237   EPC 758)

2.

B. Patients who fall between minor and life-threatening on the acuity scale pose the greatest challenge to the paramedic because, while stable, they may become unstable at any time. These patients require extreme vigilance and ongoing assessments. (PCPP 2–238   EPC 759)

3.

C. An algorithm is a schematic outline of patient care procedures for specific signs and symptoms. An example is the algorithm recommended by the American Heart Association for managing a patient in recurrent ventricular fibrillation. (PCPP 2–238   EPC 759)

4.

D. Standing orders are treatments you can perform before contacting the medical direction physician for permission. (PCPP 2–238   EPC 759)

5.

C. Protocols are standard guidelines for managing certain patient conditions. Unfortunately they address only typical patients with classic presentations and rarely allow the paramedic to adapt to the atypical patient with an unusual presentation or with multiple symptoms. (PCPP 2–238   EPC 759)

6.

D. The convergent approach to decision making requires you to focus on the most important aspect of your patient's situation and not be distracted by other stimuli. (PCPP 2–243   EPC 763)

7.

A. There is a time to think and a time to act. When confronted with a patient with a sucking chest wound, an uncontrollable hemorrhage, or a complete airway obstruction, paramedics need to react impulsively and fix the situation (seal the wound, stop the bleeding, perform the Heimlich). (PCPP 2–242   EPC 763)

8.

B. As a paramedic, you must raise your technical skill level to the pseudo-instinctive level. This means that you have developed such muscle memory that you can perform the skill while you think about something else, such as managing the scene and carrying out the treatment plan. You should be able to start an IV the same way you tie your shoes—without thinking about each step. (PCPP 2–243 EPC 763)

9.

D, B, E, A, C. First, scan the situation (take a look around), stop and think (don't just jump in), decide and act (do something; even a bad plan is better than no plan), maintain control (control yourself first, then others), and finally reevaluate (if things are going badly, change your plan). (PCPP 2–244 EPC 764)

10.

D. The critical decision process includes forming a concept (field diagnosis), interpreting the data (patient assessment), applying the principles (treatment plan), evaluating (ongoing assessment), and reflecting (post-call critique). (PCPP 2–245   EPC 765)

18 Communications

DIRECTIONS Each of the questions or incomplete statements below is followed by suggested answers or completions. Select the **one answer** that is best in each case.

1. A device that receives a transmission from a low-power source on one frequency and re-transmits it at a higher power on another frequency is a/an
   A. mobile transmitter
   B. repeater
   C. encoder
   D. decoder

2. A group of radio frequencies that are close together is called a
   A. band
   B. spectrum
   C. multiplex
   D. UHF configuration

3. Which of the following radio bands is best suited for cities?
   A. VHF lo
   B. VHF hi
   C. UHF
   D. AM

4. Which of the following radio bands is best suited for large rural areas?
   A. VHF lo
   B. VHF hi
   C. UHF
   D. FM

5. Which of the following is NOT a feature of an enhanced 911 system?
   A. Caller telephone number
   B. Caller location
   C. Instant call-back
   D. Best route of travel

6. Which of the following is a component of a priority dispatch system?
   A. Medically approved caller interrogation

B. Predetermined response configurations
C. Pre-arrival instructions
D. All of the above

7. In which type of communications system do transmission and reception occur on the same frequency?
   A. Simplex
   B. Duplex
   C. Multiplex
   D. Biotelemetry

8. In which type of communications system can transmission and reception occur simultaneously?
   A. Simplex
   B. Duplex
   C. Multiplex
   D. Biotelemetry

9. In which type of communications system can biotelemetry information be transmitted during conversation on the same frequency?
   A. Simplex
   B. Duplex
   C. Multiplex
   D. Biotelemetry

10. Trunking is a communications term that describes
    A. computerized frequency allocation
    B. hardwiring for ambulance radios
    C. base station radio procedures
    D. multiple-antenna installation

11. Which of the following statements is true regarding digital technology?
    A. It is much faster and more accurate than analog
    B. It causes frequency overcrowding

C. Digital communications are monitored by scanners

D. None of the above

12. Which of the following is an advantage of using cellular communications?

A. Twelve-lead EKGs can be transmitted

B. Fax and computer messages can be transmitted

C. Dedicated paramedic lines can be established

D. All of the above

13. Place the following information into the proper order for a radio report:

A. SAMPLE

B. ETA

C. unit and provider ID

D. patient age, sex, weight

E. treatment prior to calling

F. OPQRST

G. scene description

H. chief complaint

I. request for orders

J. physical exam

14. The echo procedure refers to

A. repeating a transmission for clarification

B. writing down the address as dispatched

C. using the siren as you pass underneath a bridge

D. pushing the microphone button and waiting for a few seconds before speaking

15. The government agency that regulates all radio communications is the

A. Department of Transportation

B. Department of Communications

C. Federal Communications Commission

D. National Association of Broadcasting

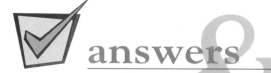

1.

B. A repeater is a device that receives a transmission from a low-power portable or a mobile radio on one frequency and retransmits it at a higher power on another frequency. Repeaters are important in large geographical areas because portable and mobile radios may not have enough range to communicate with each other, with medical control, or with the dispatcher. (PCPP 2–255   EPC 773)

2.

A. A group of radio frequencies that are close together on the electromagnetic spectrum is called a band. Some examples of radio bands are AM, FM, citizen band, shortwave, UHF, and VHF. (PCPP 2–255 EPC 774)

3.

C. Ultrahigh frequency (UHF; 300–3000 MHz) penetrates concrete and steel well and is less susceptible to interference, making it an excellent radio band for cities. (PCPP 2–255   EPC 774)

4.

A. Very high frequency (VHF) lo (150–170 MHz) follows the curvature of the earth and is best suited for large areas with varied geographical terrain. (PCPP 2–255   EPC 774)

5.

D. With an enhanced 911 system, you receive the caller's location and telephone number and instant call-back capability. (PCPP 2–257   EPC 775)

6.

D. A priority dispatch system includes medically approved caller interrogation, predetermined response configurations, and pre-arrival instructions. This system, developed by Dr. Jeff Clawson for the Salt Lake City Fire Department, is used throughout the country. (PCPP 2–258   EPC 776)

7.

A. In a simplex system, transmission and reception cannot occur at the same time because they both occur on the same frequency. A person must transmit a message, release the button, and wait for a response. (PCPP 2–261   EPC 779)

8.

B. In a duplex system, two frequencies are used much like telephone communications. This means that transmission and reception can occur at the same time. (PCPP 2–261   EPC 780)

9.

C. In a multiplex system, radio communications and other data, such as EKG, can be transmitted simultaneously, using multiple frequencies. (PCPP 2–262   EPC 780)

10.

A. In a trunked system, all frequencies are pooled. A computer routes a radio transmission to the first available frequency. All subsequent transmissions are routed in the same manner. This eliminates the need to search for unused frequencies. (PCPP 2–262   EPC 780)

11.

A. Digital technology is the wave of the present and is here to stay. It translates sound into digital code for transmission. It is much faster, more accurate, and more secure than analog communications. You cannot monitor digital transmissions without a decoder, and this technology eases the overcrowding of emergency frequencies. (PCPP 2–262   EPC 781)

12.

D. Many EMS systems are using cellular communications. Advantages include the ability to transmit 12-lead EKGs, as well as fax and computer messages, and the ability to establish dedicated paramedic lines into the base station hospital. (PCPP 2–263   EPC 781)

13.

C, G, D, H, F, A, J, E, I, B. (PCPP 2–265   EPC 783)

14.

A. The echo procedure refers to repeating back a transmission for clarification. It is a major component of the feedback loop and essential in emergency communications. The best example is verifying a medication order with the physician prior to administering it. (PCPP 2–266   EPC 785)

15.

C. The Federal Communications Commission is the government agency responsible for assigning frequencies, regulating all radios, and controlling all radio communications in the United States. (PCPP 2–268   EPC 786)

19 Documentation

DIRECTIONS Each of the questions or incomplete statements below is followed by suggested answers or completions. Select the **one answer** that is best in each case.

1. The prehospital care report is likely to be reviewed by which of the following?
   A. Surgical team
   B. Insurance providers
   C. Emergency department staff
   D. All of the above

2. Which of the following is NOT a time commonly recorded on the PCR?
   A. Call received
   B. Unit alerted
   C. Arrival at patient side
   D. Departure from scene

3. When is the ideal time to complete your PCR?
   A. En route to the hospital
   B. Immediately after the call
   C. At the station
   D. At the end of the shift

4. If you misspell a word or check the wrong box on your PCR, you should
   A. scribble the correction over the mistake
   B. draw one line through it and initial
   C. blacken out the entire mistake
   D. place parentheses around the mistake

5. If you detect an error after you have submitted your PCR to the hospital, you should
   A. write an addendum
   B. call the hospital and have the clerk make the correction
   C. do nothing
   D. none of the above

6. Which of the following statements could place you in danger of being sued for libel?
   A. "The patient smelled of alcohol."
   B. "The patient walked with a staggering gait."
   C. "The patient used abusive language."
   D. "The patient was an obnoxious drunk."

7. Which of the following is included in the subjective narrative?
   A. History of present illness
   B. Vital signs
   C. HEENT exam
   D. Labs and ECG

8. SOAP stands for
   A. Scene—Objective—Assessment—Post call
   B. Subjective—Objective—Assessment—Plan
   C. Systems—Observation—Anterior—Posterior
   D. Status—Ongoing—Arrival—Past history

9. In general, a patient who refuses your care demonstrates mental competence by
   A. understanding the circumstances
   B. understanding the risks associated with refusing care
   C. accepting the risks and responsibility
   D. all of the above

10. If you are canceled as you arrive on an emergency call, you should
    A. return to the station or post
    B. document "canceled en route" on your PCR
    C. document the canceling authority
    D. get the patient's name and vital signs

Provide the abbreviation for each of the following medical terms:

11. Coronary artery bypass graft _____
12. Atherosclerotic heart disease _____

13. Against medical advice _____

14. Blood sugar _____

15. Body surface area _____

16. Bag-valve-mask _____

17. Birth control pills _____

18. Cubic centimeter _____

19. Chief complaint _____

20. Centimeter _____

21. Congestive heart failure _____

22. Complains of _____

23. Carbon monoxide _____

24. Carbon dioxide _____

25. Chronic obstructive pulmonary disease _____

26. Chest pain _____

27. Cerebrospinal fluid _____

28. Carotid sinus massage _____

29. Cerebrovascular accident _____

30. Discontinue _____

31. Dyspnea on exertion _____

32. Deep vein thrombosis _____

33. Estimated date of confinement _____

34. Alcohol (ethanol) _____

35. Occasional _____

36. Fracture _____

37. Gastrointestinal _____

38. Gunshot wound _____

39. Hour _____

40. Headache _____

41. History _____

42. Intramuscular _____

43. Intraosseous _____

44. Jugular venous distention _____

45. Potassium _____

46. Kilogram _____

47. Keep vein open _____

48. Deciliter _____

49. Laceration _____

50. Lactated Ringer's _____

51. Moves all extremities well _____

52. Microgram _____

53. Milliequivalent _____

54. Milligram _____

55. Milliliter _____

56. Morphine sulfate _____

57. Sodium _____

58. Sodium chloride _____

59. No known allergies _____

60. Nitroglycerine _____

61. Nausea/vomiting _____

62. Organic brain syndrome _____

63. Penicillin _____

64. Hydrogen ion concentration _____

65. Pelvic inflammatory disease _____

66. As needed _____

67. Patient _____

68. Every _____

69. Rule out _____

70. Range of motion _____

71. Positive-end expiratory pressure _____

72. Signs/symptoms _____

73. Subcutaneous _____

74. Sublingual _____

75. Within normal limits _____

76. Translate the following medical report into everyday English:

Pt is a 45 y.o. male, AO × 4, c/o sudden onset CP and SOB × 2h. Pt also c/o DOE, N/V, and weakness. Pt has Hx of ASHD and AMI × 2 with CHF, and TIA × 1. He takes NTG 0.4 mg SL PRN for CP. NKA. VS as follows: BP 170/80, pulse 80, respirations 28, BS clear bilaterally, skin WNL. ECG shows NSR with PVC's. BS is 120. R/O AMI. Plan—O_2 − 10 LPM, NTG 0.4 mg SL q5 minutes PRN, MS 2 mg IV repeat PRN.

answers & rationales

1.

D. The prehospital care report (PCR) is likely to be reviewed by the emergency department staff, surgical staff, floor or intensive care unit personnel, EMS administrators, billing department, researchers, insurance providers, and lawyers. Your PCR is a direct reflection of your care. (PCPP 2–273   EPC 790)

2.

C. The times commonly recorded on the PCR include call received, crew alerted, en route to scene, arrival at scene, departure from scene, arrival at hospital, in service, and in quarters. One major omission is the actual time of arrival at the patient's side, which gives a false impression of the true response time. (PCPP 2–285   EPC 790)

3.

B. The best time to complete your PCR is at the hospital immediately following the call, when the information is fresh in your mind. En route to the hospital, generally you should be attending to your patient, not filling out your PCR. (PCPP 2–289   EPC 801)

4.

B. If you make a mistake, and you will, simply place a line through the mistake, initial it, and make the correction. Never try to cover up a mistake. If you are early in the report, simply start over. (PCPP 2–289   EPC 801)

5.

A. If you detect a mistake, or receive additional information, after you have submitted your PCR to the hospital, you should write an addendum, noting the reason, the date and time, and the pertinent information. (PCPP 2–289   EPC 801)

6.

D. Always be objective and describe your patient's behavior. Avoid subjective opinions and comments that may damage your patient's character. Even if accurate, a comment such as "The patient was an obnoxious drunk" is still just your opinion and is a potentially libelous statement. (PCPP 2–290 EPC 802)

7.

A. The subjective narrative includes all the information elicited during the history: the chief complaint, history of present illness, past history, current health status, and review of systems. (PCPP 2–290 EPC 802)

8.

B. SOAP stands for **S**ubjective (the history)—**O**bjective (the physical exam) —**A**ssessment (your field diagnosis)—**P**lan (treatment). This mnemonic is commonly used to document your patient assessment. (PCPP 2–293   EPC 803)

9.

D. A patient who refuses care and transportation must demonstrate competence by understanding the circumstances and the risks of refusing care and by accepting the risks of and responsibility for his actions. (PCPP 2–296   EPC 808)

10.

C. Sometimes your services are not needed, and you will be canceled by the on-scene command officer. In this case, document the name of the person and agency canceling your services, and document that you never made patient contact. (PCPP 2–297 EPC 810)

Fill-ins (PCPP 2c–277–2-284   EPC 794–797)

11.	Coronary artery bypass graft	CABG
12.	Atherosclerotic heart disease	ASHD
13.	Against medical advice	AMA
14.	Blood sugar	BS
15.	Body surface area	BSA
16.	Bag-valve-mask	BVM
17.	Birth control pills	BCP
18.	Cubic centimeter	cc
19.	Chief complaint	CC
20.	Centimeter	cm
21.	Congestive heart failure	CHF
22.	Complains of	c/o
23.	Carbon monoxide	CO
24.	Carbon dioxide	CO_2
25.	Chronic obstructive pulmonary disease	COPD
26.	Chest pain	CP
27.	Cerebrospinal fluid	CSF
28.	Carotid sinus massage	CSM
29.	Cerebrovascular accident	CVA
30.	Discontinue	D/C
31.	Dyspnea on exertion	DOE
32.	Deep vein thrombosis	DVT
33.	Estimated date of confinement	EDC
34.	Alcohol (ethanol)	ETOH
35.	Occasional	occ
36.	Fracture	Fx
37.	Gastrointestinal	GI
38.	Gunshot wound	GSW
39.	Hour	h
40.	Headache	H/A
41.	History	Hx
42.	Intramuscular	IM
43.	Intraosseous	IO
44.	Jugular venous distention	JVD
45.	Potassium	K^+
46.	Kilogram	kg
47.	Keep vein open	KVO
48.	Deciliter	dL
49.	Laceration	lac
50.	Lactated Ringer's	LR
51.	Moves all extremities well	MAEW
52.	Microgram	mcg

53.	Milliequivalent	mEq
54.	Milligram	mg
55.	Milliliter	ml
56.	Morphine sulfate	MS
57.	Sodium	Na^+
58.	Sodium chloride	NaCl
59.	No known allergies	NKA
60.	Nitroglycerine	NTG
61.	Nausea/vomiting	N/V
62.	Organic brain syndrome	OBS
63.	Penicillin	PCN
64.	Hydrogen ion concentration	pH
65.	Pelvic inflammatory disease	PID
66.	As needed	prn
67.	Patient	Pt
68.	Every	q
69.	Rule out	R/O
70.	Range of motion	ROM
71.	Positive-end expiratory pressure	PEEP
72.	Signs/symptoms	S/S
73.	Subcutaneous	SC, SQ
74.	Sublingual	SL
75.	Within normal limits	wnl

76.

The patient is a 45-year-old male, alert and oriented to person, place, and time, who complains of a sudden onset of chest pain and shortness of breath that began 2 hours ago. The patient also complains of dyspnea upon exertion, nausea, vomiting, and weakness. The patient has a history of atherosclerotic heart disease and has had two heart attacks with congestive heart failure, and one transient ischemic attack. He takes nitroglycerine 0.4 milligrams sublingually as needed for chest pain. He has no known allergies. His vital signs are as follows: blood pressure 170/80, pulse 80, respirations 28, breath sounds clear bilaterally, skin within normal limits. His electrocardiogram shows normal sinus rhythm with premature ventricular contractions. Blood sugar is 120. Rule out acute myocardial infarction. Plan—oxygen at 10 liters/minute; nitroglycerine 0.4 milligrams sublingually every 5 minutes as needed; morphine sulfate 2 milligrams intravenously, repeat as needed.

20

Pulmonology

DIRECTIONS Each of the questions or incomplete statements below is followed by suggested answers or completions. Select the **one answer** that is best in each case.

1. The term that means "difficulty in breathing" is
   A. orthopnea
   B. apnea
   C. hypopnea
   D. dyspnea

2. A patient who presents with orthopnea
   A. has difficulty in breathing when sitting straight up
   B. has difficulty in breathing when lying flat
   C. uses only the diaphragm
   D. depends on hypoxic drive to breathe

3. Coughing up blood from the respiratory tree is called
   A. hematemesis
   B. hematoma
   C. hemoptysis
   D. hymenoptera

4. Pulsus paradoxus occurs when
   A. the pulse increases during inspiration
   B. the systolic blood pressure decreases 10 torr while breathing
   C. the pulse rises and blood pressure drops when the patient sits up
   D. none of the above

5. Vibratory tremors felt through the chest by palpation are called
   A. percussive tremors
   B. tactile fremitus
   C. bronchophony
   D. pectoriloquy

6. If your patient presents with carpopedal spasms, this is most likely the result of
   A. hyperventilation
   B. severe respiratory acidosis
   C. metabolic alkalosis
   D. congestive heart failure

7. Which of the following measures the maximum amount of air in liters/minute that your patient can expire?
   A. Pulse oximeter
   B. Wright spirometer
   C. Capnograph
   D. Colormetric capnometer

8. A form of noncardiogenic pulmonary edema that is caused by fluid accumulation in the interstitial space within the lungs is known as
   A. cor pulmonale
   B. polycythemia
   C. ARDS
   D. status edematous

9. Management of a patient with ARDS includes
   A. positive-end expiratory pressure
   B. fluid challenge
   C. diuretics, such as furosemide
   D. IV nitroglycerine

SCENARIO

Questions 10–14 refer to the following scenario.

Your patient is a 59-year-old male who presents sitting at the kitchen table in moderate respiratory distress. His elbows are on the table in a tripod position, and he appears to be really working at breathing. Although this problem came on gradually today, his family states that he has had lung disease for a long time. He is a lifetime smoker and is on home oxygen at 2 liters/minute via nasal cannula. He takes Atrovent® (ipratropium bromide) inhaler, Theolair® (theophylline), and Proventil® (albuterol) inhaler. He appears very thin and barrel chested with a pink complexion. You immediately notice the pronounced accessory muscles in his neck and chest along with retractions. He labors to breathe, pursing his lips during exhalation. His vital signs are pulse 90, BP 140/80, respiratory rate 40, skin warm and pink, diffuse expiratory wheezes, and O_2 saturation 90%.

10. Your prehospital diagnosis is
    A. asthma
    B. congestive heart failure
    C. chronic bronchitis
    D. emphysema

11. This disease is characterized by
    A. alveolar wall destruction
    B. hypermucous secretion
    C. decreased left ventricular function
    D. allergic reaction

12. His pink complexion is caused by
    A. decreased carbon dioxide levels
    B. increased oxygen levels
    C. increased red blood cell production
    D. decreased tidal volume

13. Ipratropium bromide is a drug in which class?
    A. Sympathomimetic
    B. Corticosteroid
    C. Bronchodilator
    D. Mast cell stabilizer

14. Immediate management of this patient includes
    A. continued oxygen at 2 liters/minute via nasal cannula
    B. bronchodilation
    C. IV fluid replacement with normal saline
    D. all of the above

SCENARIO

Questions 15–21 refer to the following scenario.

Your patient is a 24-year-old male who presents in severe respiratory distress. His wife states that he has had increasing difficulty in breathing all morning but now is much worse. He has a history of asthma and takes two oral medications: Theo-Dur® (theophylline) and prednisone. He also takes two metered-dose inhalers: Ventolin® (albuterol) and Beclovent® (beclomethasone). Upon examination, you find an otherwise healthy person who speaks in words only. His vital signs are pulse 120 and strong, BP 140/80, respirations 40 and very labored, and skin pale. You auscultate inspiratory and expiratory wheezes and rhonchi bilaterally. He is hyperressonant to percussion.

15. Asthma is a disease characterized by
    A. airway edema
    B. bronchospasm
    C. hypermucous secretion
    D. all of the above

16. The above reactions are caused by the
    A. sympathetic nervous system response
    B. release of norepinephrine
    C. release of histamine
    D. blockage of parasympathetic action

17. Prednisone and beclomethasone are drugs that
    A. dilate the bronchioles directly
    B. decrease inflammation
    C. stimulate the respiratory center
    D. block the allergic response

18. Albuterol and theophylline are prescribed to
    A. dilate the bronchioles directly
    B. decrease inflammation
    C. inhibit the respiratory center
    D. block the allergic response

19. The hyperresonance is due to
    A. collapsed alveoli
    B. associated pneumothorax
    C. air trapped in the alveoli
    D. decreased duration of the expiratory phase

20. The Wright's meter measures
    A. peak expiratory flow
    B. residual volume
    C. oxygen saturation
    D. total lung capacity

21. Prehospital management of this patient includes
    A. 100% oxygen
    B. Proventil/Atrovent combination
    C. IV access
    D. all of the above

22. A patient who presents with shortness of breath, chest pain, fever, chills, general malaise, a productive yellow sputum streaked with blood, and rales and wheezes in the lower-right lobe probably has
    A. congestive heart failure
    B. emphysema
    C. an acute asthma attack
    D. pneumonia

23. The problem described in the previous question is a respiratory infection caused by a
    A. virus
    B. bacteria
    C. fungus
    D. all of the above

24. Patients with lung cancer will often have _____ as a coexisting disease.
    A. CHF
    B. COPD
    C. ARDS
    D. URI

25. Your first concern in dealing with any patient with a suspected toxic inhalation injury is
    A. managing the airway
    B. administering 100% oxygen
    C. maintaining your own personal safety
    D. removing the patient from the course

SCENARIO

Questions 26–28 refer to the following scenario.

Your patient is a firefighter who took off his self-contained breathing apparatus (SCBA) while performing overhaul procedures in a house fire. He presents with a headache, irritability, loss of coordination, and confusion.

26. This patient is probably suffering from
    A. acute myocardial infarction
    B. carbon monoxide poisoning

    C. transient ischemic attack
    D. stroke

27. The pathophysiology of this problem includes
    A. CO binding on hemoglobin
    B. cellular hypoxia
    C. metabolic acidosis
    D. all of the above

28. Management of this situation includes
    A. airway management
    B. 100% oxygenation
    C. transportation to a hyperbaric chamber
    D. all of the above

SCENARIO

Questions 29–31 refer to the following scenario.

Your patient is a 45-year-old man who complains of sudden onset of upper right-sided stabbing chest pain and shortness of breath. He has no other medical history except for being hospitalized with pneumonia two weeks ago and sent home to recuperate. Earlier this week he had experienced some lower calf pain. He presents in moderate distress with the following vital signs: pulse 100, BP 140/80, respirations 28, skin warm and dry, and some expiratory wheezing in the area of chest pain.

29. Your prehospital diagnosis is
    A. acute asthma attack
    B. acute myocardial infarction
    C. acute pulmonary embolism
    D. spontaneous pneumothorax

30. This problem is characterized by
    A. an allergic reaction
    B. coronary artery ischemia
    C. a moving blood clot
    D. a ruptured lung

31. A predisposing factor of this condition is
    A. prolonged immobilization
    B. atherosclerosis

C. a congenital defect

D. hyperreactive airways

32. Your patient is a tall, thin male in his late twenties who presents with sudden onset of sharp pain in the upper right chest and mild shortness of breath. He has no history and takes no medications but has smoked for 10 years. He has decreased lung sounds in the upper right apex and some subcutaneous emphysema in the same area. He is tachycardic, diaphoretic, and pale. Your field diagnosis is

A. spontaneous pneumothorax

B. traumatic asphyxia

C. ruptured aortic aneurysm

D. aortic valve stenosis

SCENARIO

Questions 33–39 refer to the following scenario.

Your patient is a 79-year-old female who presents in moderate respiratory distress. She sits upright and can answer your questions only with short phrases. She describes having a recent cold and this worsening shortness of breath and cough. She denies any chest pain. She has a long history of breathing problems. She claims that she gets this every year at this time and it lasts about 2 months. She also admits to smoking 2 packs of cigarettes each day for the past 50 years. Her vital signs are pulse 100 and regular, BP 150/80, respiratory rate 36 and labored, and skin cyanotic. You auscultate diffuse expiratory wheezes. She has a very productive cough, with her sputum being yellowish-brown and sticky. She has pitting pedal edema and ascites.

33. Your prehospital diagnosis should be

A. acute asthma

B. emphysema

C. chronic bronchitis

D. acute pulmonary embolism

34. The cause of this disease is

A. allergies

B. venous stasis

C. years of toxic inhalation

D. none of the above

35. The pathophysiology of this disease involves

A. the destruction of alveolar walls

B. increased mucus production

C. a traveling blood clot

D. hyperreactive airways

36. This patient's smoking history is described as

A. 50 pack/years

B. 2 pack/years

C. 100 pack/years

D. none of the above

37. Her sputum indicates

A. respiratory infection

B. pulmonary edema

C. hematemesis

D. hemoptysis

38. Her pedal edema is probably caused by

A. left heart failure

B. acute pulmonary edema

C. peripheral vasoconstriction

D. cor pulmonale

39. Her cyanosis is caused by

A. hypocarbia

B. hypoxia

C. pulmonary hypertension

D. increased residual volume

40. The base station physician orders you to administer albuterol via nebulizer in an attempt to

A. decrease pulmonary edema

B. stop the allergic reaction

C. dilate the airways

D. increase cardiac contractions

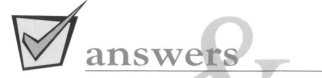

answers & rationales

1.

D. The term "dyspnea" means "shortness of breath." It describes the patient's subjective sensation of not being able to breathe. (PCPP 3–24   EPC 1164)

2.

B. Orthopnea is the patient's sensation of difficulty in breathing while lying flat. It is a common complaint in patients with congestive heart failure. (PCPP 3–25   EPC 1165)

3.

C. Hemoptysis is the coughing up of blood from the respiratory tree. Hemoptysis can be caused by tumors, pulmonary emboli, and many forms of blunt or penetrating chest trauma. (PCPP 3–25 EPC 1165)

4.

B. Pulsus paradoxus occurs when there is a drop in the systolic blood pressure of 10 torr or more with each respiratory cycle. It is associated with chronic obstructive pulmonary disease and cardiac tamponade. As a rule, in the field, you should not take the time to look for pulsus paradoxus. (PCPP 3–31 EPC 1169)

5.

B. In some patients, it may be appropriate to assess for tactile fremitus. This is a vibration felt in the chest during speaking. When evaluating tactile fremitus, compare one side of the chest with the other. This sign is common in pneumonia, where the sound vibrations travel farther through areas of lung consolidation. (PCPP 3–28   EPC 1167)

6.

A. A patient with carpopedal spasms presents with his fingers and toes in flexion. This is the result of transient shifts in blood calcium caused by changes in the serum CO_2 and pH levels from hyperventilating. Your main job in these cases is to find out **WHY** your patient was or is still hyperventilating. (PCPP 3–30   EPC 1168)

7.

B. A Wright spirometer measures your patient's peak flow in liters/minute. It is useful in determining the degree of lower airway resistance and measuring the efficacy of treatments. For example, if before treatment your asthmatic patient can blow only 45% of normal, and after an albuterol treatment he can blow 75%, you can assume your treatments are working. (PCPP 3–33 EPC 1171)

8.

C. Adult respiratory distress syndrome (ARDS) is a noncardiogenic pulmonary edema caused by fluid accumulation in the interstitial space within the lungs. ARDS is usually the result of increased capillary permeability and decreased venous drainage from the lung. Mortality for patients who develop ARDS approaches 70%. (PCPP 3–36 EPC 1174)

9.

A. Management of the patient with ARDS includes oxygen administration with a bag-valve-mask and positive-end expiratory pressure (PEEP), IV lifeline, and ECG monitoring. Customary medications such as nitroglycerine and furosemide are not helpful because this is not a preload or fluid overload problem. (PCPP 3–38   EPC 1176)

10.

D. The prehospital diagnosis of this patient should be emphysema. (PCPP 3–39   EPC 1177)

11.

A. Emphysema results from destruction of the alveolar walls distal to the terminal bronchioles. This disease is caused by exposure to noxious substances, such as cigarette smoke, and results in the gradual destruction of the walls of the alveoli, decreasing the alveolar membrane surface area and lessening the area available for gas exchange. (PCPP 3–41   EPC 1177)

12.

C. Patients with emphysema tend to be pink in color due to polycythemia and are referred to as "pink puffers." The polycythemia occurs as an excess of red blood cells is produced. (PCPP 3–42   EPC 1178)

13.

C. Ipratropium bromide is a bronchodilating drug in the anticholinergic class. This class of drugs blocks the effects of acetylcholine. Acetylcholine causes bronchoconstriction. Blocking this action allows for relaxation of the smooth muscle in the airways. (PCPP 3–43   EPC 1183)

14.

B. Immediate management of this patient includes administering 100% oxygen via a non-rebreather mask and attempting to dilate the lower airways with albuterol, ipratropium, or a combination of both. (PCPP 3–43   EPC 1183)

15.

D. Asthma is a disease characterized by lower airway edema, bronchospasm, and hypermucous secretion. This is the classic pathophysiological triad of asthma. (PCPP 3–43   EPC 1181)

16.

C. The first phase of asthma is characterized by the release of chemical mediators, such as histamine. These mediators cause contraction of the bronchial smooth muscle and leakage of fluid from the capillaries. This results in both bronchoconstriction and bronchial edema. (PCPP 3–43   EPC 1181)

17.

B. Prednisone and beclomethasone are drugs that decrease inflammation. These belong to a class known as corticosteroids. (PCPP 3–44   EPC 1182)

18.

A. Albuterol (beta agonist) and theophylline (xanthine) are prescribed to directly dilate the bronchioles. (PCPP 3–44   EPC 1182)

19.

C. The asthma patient may exhibit hyperresonance upon percussion. This hyperresonance is due to the collapse of the bronchioles upon exhalation, trapping air in the distal airways and alveoli. (PCPP 3–45   EPC 1182)

20.

A. The Wright's meter measures the peak expiratory flow rate. This flow rate occurs during a maximum exhalation and is a reliable indicator of air flow. It is used to measure asthma severity and to monitor the patient's response to therapy. (PCPP 3–45   EPC 1183)

21.

D. Prehospital management of this patient includes 100% oxygen, Proventil/Atrovent combination via nebulizer, IV access, ECG monitoring, and reassessment for deterioration or signs of status asthmaticus. (PCPP 3–45   EPC 1183)

22.

D. A patient who presents with shortness of breath, chest pain, fever, chills, general malaise, a productive yellow sputum streaked with blood, and rales and wheezing in the lower-right lobe probably has pneumonia. Other clues include pleuritic chest pain, dull to percussion, and egophony. Pneumonia is an infection of the lungs and a common medical problem. (PCPP 3–50   EPC 1185)

23.

D. Pneumonia is a common respiratory disease caused when an infectious agent invades the lungs. Pneumonia can be bacterial, viral, or fungal. It may involve part or all of the lung. (PCPP 3–50   EPC 1185)

24.

B. Patients with lung cancer often have COPD as a co-existing disease from years of inhaling toxic substances, such as cigarette smoke. (PCPP 3–50   EPC 1187)

25.

C. The paramedic's first concern in any toxic inhalation situation is his own personal safety. (PCPP 3–53   EPC 1189)

26.

B. A particular hazard for firefighters and rescue personnel is carbon monoxide poisoning, particularly during overhaul operations when some smoldering still occurs. A smoldering fire yields much carbon monoxide. (PCPP 3–53   EPC 1189)

27.

D. Carbon monoxide is an odorless, tasteless, and colorless gas produced from the incomplete burning of fossil fuels. Carbon monoxide easily binds to the hemoglobin molecule. Once bound, receptor sites on the hemoglobin can no longer transport oxygen to the peripheral tissues. The result is hypoxia at the cellular level and ultimately metabolic acidosis. (PCPP 3–53   EPC 1189)

28.

D. Management of any patient suspected of having carbon monoxide poisoning includes ensuring a patent airway, providing 100% oxygen, and transporting the patient rapidly to a hyperbaric chamber. Hyperbaric oxygen increases PaO_2 and promotes oxygen uptake on hemoglobin molecules not yet bound by carbon monoxide. (PCPP 3–54   EPC 1190)

29.

C. This patient, who complains of sudden onset of upper right-sided stabbing chest pain and shortness of breath following hospitalization and confinement to bed for a couple of weeks and of lower leg pain, probably has suffered an acute pulmonary embolism. (PCPP 3–54   EPC 1190)

30.

C. Pulmonary embolism is a blood clot or some other particle that lodges in a pulmonary artery. The condition is potentially life-threatening because it can significantly decrease pulmonary blood flow, thus leading to hypoxemia. The problem occurs when a blood clot travels up the venous circulatory system and lodges in a pulmonary artery. (PCPP 3–55 EPC 1190)

31.

A. Factors predisposing a patient to blood clots include prolonged immobilization, thrombophlebitis, the use of certain medications, and atrial fibrillation. (PCPP 3–55   EPC 1190)

32.

A. A spontaneous pneumothorax occurs in the absence of trauma usually in tall, thin males between 20 and 40 years old. Risk factors include cigarette smoking. As with a pneumothorax, it is important to ensure adequate ventilation of the lungs while you monitor for a developing tension pneumothorax. (PCPP 3–56   EPC 1192)

33.

C. Your patient presents with the classic signs and symptoms of chronic bronchitis. (PCPP 3–41 EPC 1179)

34.

C. Following prolonged exposure to cigarette smoke, the number of mucus-secreting cells in the respiratory tree increases, producing a large quantity of sputum. (PCPP 3–42   EPC 1180)

35.

B. The pathophysiology of chronic bronchitis involves increased mucus production. This increased mucus becomes a place for bacteria to grow, making the patient susceptible to frequent respiratory tract infections. (PCPP 3–42   EPC 1180)

36.

C. Every patient suspected of having lung disease should be questioned about cigarette and tobacco use. This is generally reported in pack/years. Multiply the number of cigarette packs smoked per day by the number of years smoked. This patient smoked 2 packs per day for 50 years, making her a 100 pack/years smoker (and a member of the Century Club). (PCPP 3–42   EPC 1180)

37.

A. Yellow sputum indicates a lower respiratory infection typical of patients with exacerbations of chronic bronchitis. (PCPP 3–42   EPC 1180)

38.

D. Patients with chronic obstructive pulmonary disease maintain chronic high levels of carbon dioxide. Carbon dioxide is a potent pulmonary vasoconstrictor, resulting in pulmonary hypertension. This condition may lead to right heart failure or cor pulmonale. (PCPP 3–42   EPC 1180)

39.

B. Patients with chronic bronchitis tend to be overweight and cyanotic. Because of this, they are referred to as "blue bloaters." This is due to the chronic hypoxia. (PCPP 3–42   EPC 1180)

40.

C. Common first-line treatment for chronic bronchitis is to administer a sympathomimetic bronchodilator via nebulizer in an attempt to dilate the lower airways. These inhaled beta agonists include albuterol, metaproterenol, and isoetharine. Inhaled anticholinergics, such as ipratropium bromide, are also indicated. (PCPP 3–43   EPC 1180)

21 Cardiovascular Emergencies

DIRECTIONS Each of the questions or incomplete statements below is followed by suggested answers or completions. Select the **one answer** that is best in each case.

1. The great vessels enter the heart through its
   A. base
   B. apex
   C. midline
   D. ventricles

2. The innermost layer of the heart, which lines the chambers, is the
   A. myocardium
   B. endocardium
   C. epicardium
   D. pericardium

3. The muscular layer of the heart is the
   A. myocardium
   B. endocardium
   C. epicardium
   D. pericardium

4. The visceral pericardium is contiguous with the
   A. myocardium
   B. endocardium
   C. epicardium
   D. pleura

5. The protective sac surrounding the heart is the
   A. myocardium
   B. endocardium
   C. epicardium
   D. pericardium

6. The inferior chambers are the
   A. atria
   B. auricles
   C. ventricles
   D. vesicles

7. The only arteries that carry oxygen-poor blood are the
   Λ. coronary arteries

B. carotid arteries
   C. mesenteric arteries
   D. pulmonary arteries

8. The only veins that carry oxygen-rich blood are the
   A. vena cava
   B. pulmonary veins
   C. coronary veins
   D. jugular veins

9. The greatest muscle mass is found in the
   A. right atrium
   B. right ventricle
   C. left atrium
   D. left ventricle

10. Which valves are open during systole?
    A. Mitral and tricuspid valves
    B. Aortic and pulmonic valves
    C. AV valves
    D. None of the above

11. Which valves are open during diastole?
    A. Mitral and tricuspid valves
    B. Aortic and pulmonic valves
    C. Semilunar valves
    D. None of the above

12. The heart muscle is perfused by the
    A. coronary arteries
    B. cerebral arteries
    C. inferior vena cava
    D. subclavian arteries

13. The development of collateral circulation is possible by the presence of
    A. the coronary sinus
    B. the aorta

C. anastomoses

D. automaticity

14. Blood from the coronary veins empties into the
    A. right atrium
    B. left atrium
    C. right ventricle
    D. left ventricle

15. The innermost lining of the peripheral blood vessels is the
    A. tunica intima
    B. tunica media
    C. tunica adventitia
    D. none of the above

16. The muscular layer of the peripheral blood vessels is the
    A. tunica intima
    B. tunica media
    C. tunica adventitia
    D. none of the above

17. Poiseuille's law states that blood flow through a vessel is most dependent on the
    A. pump force
    B. fluid viscosity
    C. vessel length
    D. vessel diameter

18. Gas exchange and cellular respiration occur at what level of the circulation system?
    A. Arterioles
    B. Venules
    C. Arteries
    D. Capillaries

19. Which of the following does not occur during diastole?
    A. Ventricular filling
    B. Coronary artery perfusion
    C. AV valve closure
    D. Atrial contraction

20. The amount of blood ejected by the heart in one contraction is called
    A. preload
    B. cardiac output
    C. blood pressure
    D. stroke volume

21. Which of the following does not directly affect stroke volume?
    A. Preload
    B. Afterload
    C. Heart rate
    D. Contractile force

22. Up to a point, the greater the preload, the greater the
    A. contractile force
    B. heart rate
    C. afterload
    D. blood pressure

23. The resistance against which the heart must pump is called
    A. preload
    B. afterload
    C. Starling's affect
    D. end-diastolic volume

24. Another name for preload is
    A. afterload
    B. end-diastolic volume
    C. blood pressure
    D. stroke volume

25. A person with a stroke volume of 70 ml and a heart rate of 80 has a cardiac output of
    A. 5600 ml
    B. 1500 ml
    C. 560 ml
    D. 150 ml

26. Preload is dependent on
    A. arteriole vasoconstriction
    B. venous return

C. stroke volume

D. ventricular strength

27. The sympathetic nervous system innervates the heart via which receptors?
    A. Beta 1
    B. Beta 2
    C. Alpha 1
    D. Dopaminergic

28. The primary parasympathetic nerve that innervates the heart is the _____ nerve.
    A. phrenic
    B. cardiac
    C. vagus
    D. acetylcholine

29. Which of the following could produce a parasympathetic response?
    A. Pressure on the epiglottis
    B. Pressure on the carotid sinus
    C. Bladder distention
    D. All of the above

30. A positive inotropic drug increases
    A. heart rate
    B. conduction velocity
    C. contractile force
    D. refractoriness

31. A negative chronotropic drug decreases
    A. heart rate
    B. conduction velocity
    C. contractile force
    D. refractoriness

32. Specialized structures designed to speed conduction from one muscle fiber to the next are the
    A. syncytial tissues
    B. inotropic fibers
    C. intercalated discs
    D. autonomic cells

33. The ventricular syncytium occurs in an inferior to superior direction in order to
    A. direct blood to the aorta and pulmonary artery
    B. direct conduction through the AV node
    C. enhance conduction velocity toward the atria
    D. avoid the vagus nerve

34. Which of the following is true regarding the resting potential?
    A. Sodium is pumped into the cell
    B. Potassium is pumped out of the cell
    C. The inside of the cell is more negative than the outside
    D. The inside of the cell is more positive than the outside

35. Which of the following best characterizes the action potential?
    A. Potassium is actively pumped into the cell
    B. Sodium rapidly diffuses into the cell
    C. The inside of the cell becomes more negative
    D. The outside of the cell becomes more positive

36. The cells of the cardiac conductive system have
    A. automaticity
    B. excitability
    C. conductivity
    D. all of the above

37. The normal intrinsic firing rate of the SA node is
    A. 20–40 beats per minute
    B. 40–60 beats per minute
    C. 60–100 beats per minute
    D. none of the above

38. The normal intrinsic firing rate of the AV junction is
    A. 20–40 beats per minute
    B. 40–60 beats per minute

C. 60–100 beats per minute

D. none of the above

39. The normal intrinsic firing rate of the Purkinje system is

A. 20–40 beats per minute

B. 40–60 beats per minute

C. 60–100 beats per minute

D. none of the above

40. According to Einthoven's triangle, lead 2 is characterized by

A. right leg negative, left arm positive

B. left leg positive, right arm negative

C. right leg positive, left arm negative

D. left leg negative, right arm positive

41. Which of the following can be obtained from a single-lead ECG reading?

A. The presence of an infarct

B. Cardiac output

C. Chamber enlargement

D. Heart rate

42. On the vertical axis of a standard ECG graph paper, a deflection of two large boxes signifies

A. 1 mV of amplitude

B. 10 mV of amplitude

C. 0.4 second duration

D. 2.0 seconds duration

43. On the horizontal axis of a standard ECG graph paper, a deflection of one large box signifies

A. 1 mV of amplitude

B. 10 mV of amplitude

C. 0.2 second duration

D. 0.04 second duration

44. The P wave represents

A. atrial depolarization

B. ventricular depolarization

C. delay at the AV node

D. ventricular repolarization

45. The T wave represents

A. atrial depolarization

B. ventricular depolarization

C. delay at the AV node

D. ventricular repolarization

46. The QRS complex represents

A. atrial depolarization

B. ventricular depolarization

C. delay at the AV node

D. ventricular repolarization

47. The P–R interval represents

A. atrial depolarization

B. ventricular depolarization

C. delay at the AV node

D. ventricular repolarization

48. Which of the following is true regarding the absolute refractory period?

A. The heart may depolarize

B. The heart cannot depolarize

C. It is represented by the T wave

D. It is the most vulnerable part of the cardiac cycle

49. Which of the following may produce artifact on the ECG?

A. Muscle tremors

B. Loose electrodes

C. 60 Hz interference

D. All of the above

50. Using the "triplicate method," what will the heart rate be if the R–R interval is three large boxes?

A. 60 beats per minute

B. 100 beats per minute

C. 150 beats per minute

D. 75 beats per minute

51. In normal sinus rhythm, the P waves should be

A. present

B. upright

C. alike

D. all of the above

52. The normal P–R interval is
   A. <0.12 second
   B. 0.12–0.20 second
   C. 0.04–0.1 second
   D. none of the above

53. The normal QRS complex is
   A. <0.04 second
   B. 0.12–0.20 second
   C. 0.04–0.12 second
   D. none of the above

54. Which of the following could cause a cardiac dysrhythmia?
   A. Lateral wall myocardial infarction
   B. Hyperkalemia
   C. Hypoxia and acidosis
   D. All of the above

55. Cardiac depolarization resulting from a focus other than a normal pacemaker cell is called
   A. antegrade
   B. retrograde
   C. ectopic
   D. reentry

SCENARIO

Questions 56–58 refer to the following scenario.

Your patient is a 45-year-old male who experienced some chest discomfort while jogging. The pain is substantial and does not radiate. He has no previous medical history and takes no medications. The pain is somewhat relieved by rest. His BP is 150/88, pulse 96 and regular, respirations 18, and skin warm and pink. His lungs are clear bilaterally, and he has no other remarkable signs or symptoms. His ECG strip is shown in Figure 21–1.

56. This patient's probable diagnosis is
   A. stable angina
   B. unstable angina
   C. pre-infarction angina
   D. Prinzmetal's angina

57. His ECG strip is
   A. sinus tachycardia
   B. wandering atrial pacemaker
   C. premature atrial contractions
   D. normal sinus rhythm

58. Initial prehospital management of this patient should include oxygen and
   A. morphine IV
   B. nitroglycerine SL
   C. epinephrine SC
   D. atropine IV

SCENARIO

Questions 59–62 refer to the following scenario.

Your patient is a 56-year-old female who complains of sudden onset of substernal chest pressure with no radiation while watching television. She denies any shortness of breath or nausea. She has a history of atherosclerotic heart disease and takes diltiazem. Her BP is 160/90, pulse 110, respirations 16, skin warm and dry, and lungs clear

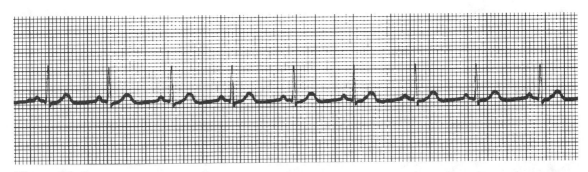

Figure 21–1

bilaterally. She has no other remarkable physical findings. Her ECG is shown in Figure 21–2.

59. This patient is probably suffering from
    A. stable angina
    B. unstable angina
    C. cardiogenic shock
    D. Ludwig's angina

60. Her ECG strip is
    A. normal sinus rhythm
    B. premature atrial contraction
    C. wandering atrial pacemaker
    D. sinus dysrhythmia

61. The process by which fatty deposits collect within arterial walls is known as
    A. arteriosclerosis
    B. atherosclerosis
    C. arteriosclerotitis
    D. atheritis

62. Diltiazem is a drug in which class?
    A. Nitrate
    B. Beta blocker
    C. Calcium channel blocker
    D. Diuretic

SCENARIO

Questions 63–66 refer to the following scenario.

Your patient is a 65-year-old man who complains of sudden onset of substernal chest pain radiating to the neck and left shoulder. It began while eating 1 hour ago and has not subsided. He also complains of some shortness of breath, nausea, and dizziness. He has a history of coronary artery disease and hypertension. He takes Procardia XL once a day. His BP is 180/80, pulse 80 and irregular, respirations 26, lungs clear, and skin warm and dry. His ECG strip is shown in Figure 21–3.

63. This patient is probably suffering from
    A. stable angina
    B. unstable angina
    C. acute myocardial infarction
    D. cardiogenic shock

64. His ECG strip is
    A. normal sinus rhythm
    B. premature atrial contraction

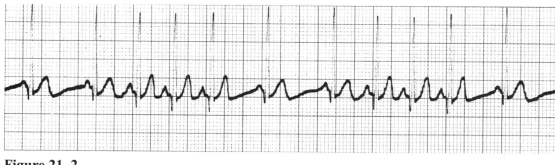

Figure 21–2

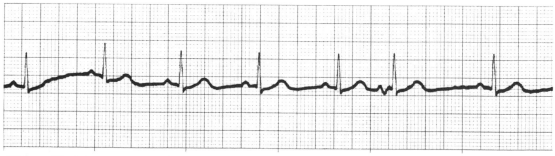

Figure 21–3

C. wandering atrial pacemaker

D. sinus dysrhythmia

65. Procardia XL is a drug in which class?

A. Nitrate

B. Beta blocker

C. Calcium channel blocker

D. Diuretic

66. Prehospital management of this patient includes

A. high-flow oxygen

B. pain management

C. reassurance

D. all of the above

SCENARIO

Questions 67–70 refer to the following scenario.

Your patient is a 45-year-old female who complains of mild-to-moderate shortness of breath and some chest discomfort. She has a long history of cardiac problems and takes digoxin, Lasix, and Slow-K. Her BP is 180/80, pulse 94 and very irregular, respirations 20, and skin cool and pink. She has bilateral crackles (rales) in the lower lobes. She has no peripheral edema or JVD. Her ECG is shown in Figure 21–4.

67. Your diagnosis of this patient is

A. right heart failure

B. left heart failure

C. cardiogenic shock

D. acute pulmonary edema

68. Her medications suggest she has

A. abnormal cardiac dysrhythmias

B. aortic valve problems

C. cor pulmonale

D. congestive heart failure

69. Her ECG is

A. wandering atrial pacemaker

B. atrial flutter

C. atrial fibrillation

D. junctional rhythm

70. Prehospital pharmacological management of this patient should include oxygen and

A. nitroglycerine, furosemide, morphine

B. furosemide, albuterol, lidocaine

C. morphine, naloxone, furosemide

D. potassium, furosemide, morphine

SCENARIO

Questions 71–74 refer to the following scenario.

Your patient is an 80-year-old male who presents in severe respiratory distress, sitting bolt upright, and gasping for each breath. He has a history of high blood pressure and breathing problems. He takes Inderal each day. His BP is 170/70, pulse 72 and irregular, respirations 40 and extremely labored, and skin warm and diaphoretic. Upon auscultation, you hear diffuse bilateral crackles and wheezing. He coughs up blood-tinged sputum. His ECG is shown in Figure 21–5.

71. This patient is suffering from

A. acute pulmonary edema

B. cor pulmonale

C. cardiogenic shock

D. aortic aneurysm

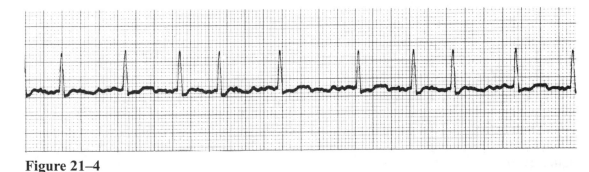

Figure 21–4

72. His ECG is
    A. wandering atrial pacemaker
    B. atrial flutter
    C. atrial fibrillation
    D. junctional rhythm

73. Inderal is a drug in which class?
    A. Beta blocker
    B. Nitrate
    C. Calcium channel blocker
    D. Cardiac glycoside

74. Which of the following is not a prehospital management goal for this patient?
    A. Oxygenation
    B. Preload increase
    C. Diuresis
    D. Coronary artery dilation

SCENARIO

Questions 75–79 refer to the following scenario.

Your patient is a 57-year-old woman who lies unconscious on her living room floor. Her husband claims she "just collapsed after clutching her chest." She has a previous medical history and takes Cardizem. Her BP is 70 palpated; pulse 140; respirations rate 20 and shallow; skin cool, pale, and clammy; lungs congested; and chemstrip 130. Her ECG strip is shown in Figure 21–6.

75. This patient is suffering from
    A. cardiogenic shock
    B. acute pulmonary edema
    C. right heart failure
    D. left heart failure

76. Her ECG is
    A. atrial fibrillation
    B. paroxysmal supraventricular tachycardia
    C. sinus tachycardia
    D. atrial flutter

77. The primary cause for this dysrhythmia is
    A. ectopic focus
    B. reentry focus
    C. compensatory mechanism
    D. parasympathetic stimulation

78. Cardizem is a drug in which class?
    A. Nitrate
    B. Cardiac glycoside

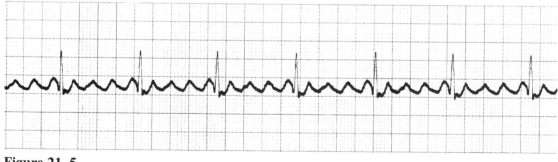

Figure 21–5

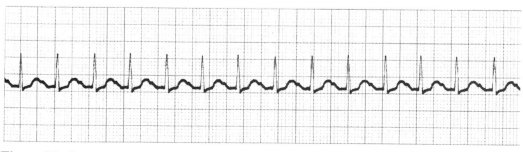

Figure 21–6

C. Beta blocker

D. Calcium channel blocker

79. Prehospital management of this patient includes all of the following except
   A. dopamine IV
   B. oxygen
   C. IV fluid challenge
   D. positive pressure ventilation

SCENARIO

Questions 80–82 refer to the following scenario.

Your patient is a 78-year-old male who collapsed in the bathroom while moving his bowels. He sits slumped on the toilet, moaning, pale, and extremely diaphoretic. He has no history of cardiac problems and takes no medications. His BP is 70 palpated, pulse 36, respirations 28 and shallow, lungs clear, and chemstrip 120. His ECG is shown in Figure 21–7.

80. The most likely cause of this man's symptoms is
   A. hypoglycemia
   B. decreased cardiac output
   C. narcotic overdose
   D. sympathetic overstimulation

81. His ECG strip is
   A. junctional rhythm
   B. sinus arrhythmia
   C. sinus bradycardia
   D. idioventricular rhythm

82. The first prehospital treatment after oxygen is
   A. transcutaneous cardiac pacing
   B. adenosine IV
   C. epinephrine IV
   D. atropine IV

SCENARIO

Questions 83–85 refer to the following scenario.

Your patient is a 35-year-old female who developed heart palpitations while exercising. She complains of lightheadedness and some dizziness. She denies any chest pain. She has a history of Wolff-Parkinson-White syndrome and takes Pronestyl. Her BP is 140/70, pulse 190, respirations 18, skin warm and dry, and lungs clear bilaterally. Her ECG is shown in Figure 21–8.

83. This patient's rhythm is
   A. sinus tachycardia
   B. ventricular tachycardia
   C. supraventricular tachycardia
   D. atrial flutter

84. The probable cause of this dysrhythmia is
   A. ectopic focus in the ventricle
   B. reentry focus in the atria
   C. compensatory mechanism
   D. sympathetic stimulation

85. The initial treatment of this patient includes oxygen and
   A. immediate cardioversion
   B. immediate defibrillation

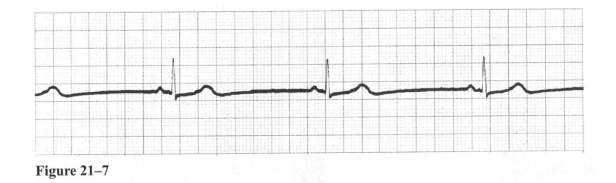

Figure 21–7

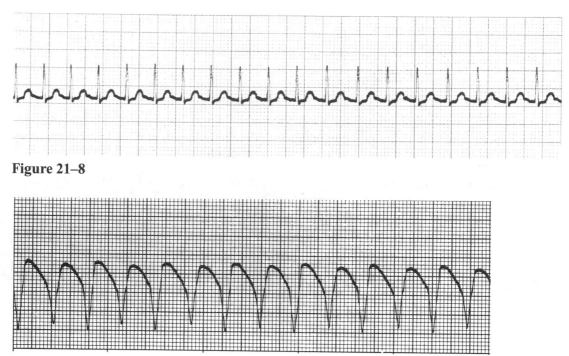

Figure 21–8

Figure 21–9

C. vagal maneuvers

D. verapamil IV

SCENARIO

Questions 86–88 refer to the following scenario.

Your patient is a 67-year-old man who collapsed in the kitchen while cooking dinner. He presents on the floor, pale, clammy, and moaning, with vomit around his mouth. His wife states he has no history and takes no medications. His BP is 70/30, pulse 170 and weak, respirations 28 and shallow, lungs clear bilaterally, and chemstrip 120. His ECG is shown in Figure 21–9.

86. His ECG is
    A. ventricular tachycardia
    B. SVT with aberrancy
    C. ventricular fibrillation
    D. idioventricular rhythm

87. Initial management of this patient includes
    A. immediate synchronized cardioversion
    B. aggressive airway management
    C. diazepam IV
    D. all of the above

88. Which of the following drugs may be ordered for this patient?
    A. Atropine and epinephrine
    B. Adenosine and verapamil
    C. Naloxone and 50% dextrose
    D. Lidocaine and procainamide

SCENARIO

Questions 89–92 refer to the following scenario.

Your patient is a 45-year-old male who complains of chest pain and shortness of breath. During your workup, he suddenly loses consciousness and slumps over. His ECG changes are shown in Figure 21–10.

89. This patient's new ECG is
    A. ventricular fibrillation
    B. ventricular tachycardia
    C. asystole
    D. idioventricular rhythm

90. Your first move is to
    A. defibrillate at 200 joules
    B. deliver a precordial thump

C. begin CPR

D. check your patient

91. All of the following will decrease intra-thoracic resistance during defibrillation **EXCEPT**

   A. using electrode jelly

   B. using proper paddle pressure

   C. using proper paddle positioning

   D. waiting 3–5 minutes between defibrillation attempts

92. Pharmacological management of this patient includes which of the following drugs?

   A. Oxygen, epinephrine, atropine

   B. Oxygen, epinephrine, lidocaine, amiodarone

   C. Oxygen, adenosine, verapamil, lidocaine

   D. Oxygen, epinephrine, isoproterenol, lidocaine

SCENARIO

Questions 93–96 refer to the following scenario.

Your patient is a 99-year-old male found in cardiac arrest by his family. CPR was begun immediately and is ongoing upon your arrival. After a quick look, your patient is in the following rhythm (see figure 21–11). He is pulseless, apneic, and unconscious.

93. This patient's rhythm is

   A. supraventricular tachycardia

   B. idioventricular rhythm

   C. ventricular tachycardia

   D. none of the above

94. This patient's condition is described as

   A. AV dissociation

   B. pulseless electrical activity

   C. complete heart block

   D. none of the above

95. Management of this patient includes all of the following **EXCEPT**

   A. CPR and intubation

   B. epinephrine and atropine IV

   C. defibrillation and amiodarone

   D. IV fluids

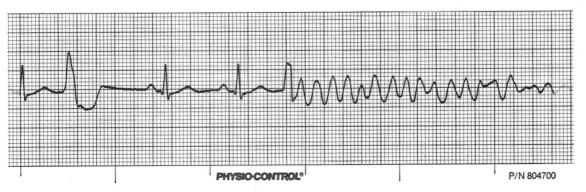

Figure 21–10

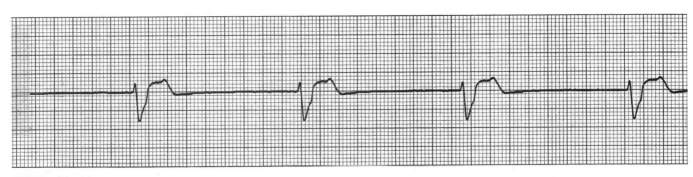

Figure 21–11

96. Causes for this condition include
    A. hypovolemia
    B. pericardial tamponade
    C. hypoxia and acidosis
    D. all of the above

SCENARIO

Questions 97–98 refer to the following scenario.

Your patient is a 65-year-old male complaining of malaise. He has no medical history and takes no medications. His BP is 120/70, pulse 60 and irregular, respirations 20, lungs clear, and skin warm and dry. His ECG is shown in Figure 21–12.

97. This patient's rhythm is
    A. second-degree AV block type 2
    B. second-degree AV block type 1
    C. third-degree AV block
    D. first-degree AV block

98. Prehospital management of this patient includes
    A. oxygen and monitoring only
    B. oxygen, atropine IV
    C. oxygen, transcutaneous pacing
    D. oxygen, atropine, transcutaneous pacing

SCENARIO

Questions 99–100 refer to the following scenario.

Your patient is an 89-year-old female who collapsed while shopping. No one is available to give you a history, and she responds to deep pain only. Her BP is 70/30, pulse 36, respirations 30 and shallow, skin pale and clammy, lungs clear bilaterally, and chemstrip 100. Her ECG is shown in Figure 21–13.

99. Her ECG is
    A. second-degree AV block type 2
    B. junctional escape rhythm
    C. third-degree AV block
    D. ventricular escape rhythm

100. Prehospital management of this patient includes
    A. CPR and intubation
    B. atropine and transcutaneous pacing
    C. lidocaine and bretylium
    D. adenosine and verapamil

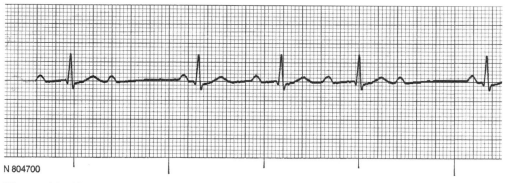

N 804700

Figure 21–12

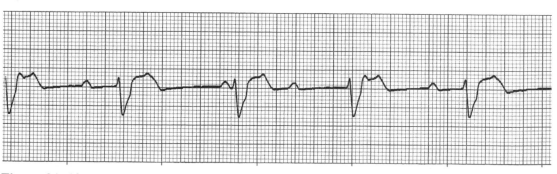

Figure 21–13

answers & rationales

1.

A. The great vessels enter the heart through its base. The base is the top portion of the heart, located at the level of the second rib. The great vessels include the inferior and superior vena cava, aorta, pulmonary arteries, and veins. (PCPP 3–74   EPC 207)

2.

B. The innermost layer of the heart, which lines the chambers, is the endocardium. It is the smoothest surface known to man. (PCPP 3–71   EPC 207)

3.

A. The thick middle layer of the heart wall, containing the bulk of the muscle mass, is the myocardium. The myocardium muscle cells are unique in that they physically resemble skeletal muscles, but they have electrical properties like smooth muscle. (PCPP 3–71   EPC 207)

4.

C. The visceral pericardium is the layer in contact with the heart muscle itself. The outermost lining of the heart, the epicardium, is contiguous with the visceral pericardium. (PCPP 3–71   EPC 207)

5.

D. Surrounding the heart is a protective sac, the pericardium. The pericardium consists of two layers, the visceral pericardium and the parietal pericardium. Situated between the two layers is pericardial fluid, which acts as a lubricant during cardiac contraction. (PCPP 3–71   EPC 207)

6.

C. The heart contains four chambers. The two superior chambers, which receive incoming blood, are called atria. The larger inferior chambers are called ventricles. (PCPP 3–71   EPC 208)

7.

D. The only arteries in the body that carry oxygen-poor blood are the pulmonary arteries. These arteries carry blood from the right ventricle to the lungs for oxygenation. (PCPP 3–74   EPC 210)

8.

B. The only veins in the body that carry oxygen-rich blood are the pulmonary veins. These veins carry blood from the lungs back to the left atrium. (PCPP 3–74   EPC 210)

9.

D. The greatest muscle mass is found in the left ventricle. The left ventricle receives blood from the left atrium and pumps it out of heart into the aorta. The left side of the heart is the high-pressure side of the pump because of the high level of resistance present in the peripheral circulation. (PCPP 3–74   EPC 207)

10.

B. During systole, the aortic and pulmonic valves are open, allowing the heart to eject blood into the aorta and the pulmonary artery. (PCPP 3–73   EPC 209)

11.

A. During diastole, the mitral and tricuspid valves open to allow the atria to dump blood into the ventricles. (PCPP 3–73   EPC 209)

12.

A. The heart muscle itself is perfused by the coronary arteries. These vessels originate in the aorta just above the leaflets of the aortic valve and lie on the surface of the heart. (PCPP 3–75   EPC 211)

13.

C. Anastomoses between various branches of the coronary arteries allow for the development of collateral circulation. This is a protective mechanism that allows for an alternate path of blood flow in the event of vascular occlusion. (PCPP 3–75   EPC 211)

14.

A. Deoxygenated blood is removed from the heart through the coronary veins. The coronary veins roughly correspond to the coronary arteries and drain into the right atrium. (PCPP 3–75   EPC 211)

15.

A. The innermost lining of the blood vessels, the tunic intima, is a single layer thick. This layer allows for rapid diffusion of blood gases to and from the tissues. (PCPP 3–76   EPC 218)

16.

B. The muscular layer of the peripheral blood vessels is the tunica media, consisting of elastic fibers and muscle. This layer gives blood vessels the strength and recoil that result from the difference in pressure inside and outside the cell. (PCPP 3–76   EPC 218)

17.

D. Poiseuille's law states that blood flow through a vessel is directly proportional to the fourth power of the vessel's diameter. This means that an increase or decrease in a blood vessel's size greatly influences the amount of blood flow through that vessel. (PCPP 3–76   EPC 218)

18.

D. Gas exchange and cellular respiration occur at the capillary level. The walls of the capillaries are a single cell layer thick, which allows for the exchange of gases, fluids, and nutrients between the vascular system and the tissues. (PCPP 3–76   EPC 211)

19.

C. During diastole, the ventricles fill with blood, the coronary arteries are perfused, and the artia contract, sending blood down to the ventricles. The AV valves are open, allowing this flow of blood. (PCPP 3–77   EPC 211)

20.

D. Stroke volume is the amount of blood ejected by the heart in one contraction. Stroke volume is measured in milliliters. The average stroke volume is 60–100 milliliters, although this capacity can in-

crease significantly in a healthy heart. (PCPP 3–78 EPC 1203)

21.

C. Stroke volume is a reflection of three factors: preload, cardiac contractility, and afterload. (PCPP 3–78   EPC 1203)

22.

A. The pressure in the ventricle at the end of diastole is referred to as preload. Preload influences the force of the next contraction. This is based on Starling's law of the heart, which states that the more the myocardial muscle is stretched, up to a limit, the greater its force of contraction will be. (PCPP 3–78   EPC 1203)

23.

B. The resistance against which the heart must pump is called afterload. In general, the greater the resistance or afterload, the less the stroke volume. An increase in peripheral vascular resistance will decrease stroke volume. Conversely, a decrease in peripheral vascular resistance, up to a point, will increase stroke volume. (PCPP 3–78   EPC 1204)

24.

B. Another name for preload is end-diastolic volume. (PCPP 3–78   EPC 1203)

25.

A. Cardiac output is defined as the volume of blood pumped by the heart in 1 minute. It is a calculation of stroke volume times heart rate. A person with a stroke volume of 70 milliliters and heart rate of 80 beats per minute has a cardiac output of 5600 milliliters. (PCPP 3–78   EPC 1204)

26.

B. Preload represents the amount of blood or pressure in the ventricles prior to contraction. It is dependent on venous return from the body. (PCPP 3–78 EPC 1203)

27.

A. The sympathetic nervous system innervates the heart via the beta 1 receptors. When these receptors are stimulated, they cause the heart to increase its rate, force of contractions, and conductivity. (PCPP 3–80 EPC 212)

28.

C. The primary parasympathetic nerve that innervates the heart is the vagus nerve. The vagus nerve, also called cranial nerve X, arises from the base of the brain. It is responsible for regulating the heart's resting rate. (PCPP 3–80   EPC 214)

29.

D. The parasympathetic response can be produced by pressure on the epiglottis, by pressure on the carotid sinus, or by bladder distention. (PCPP 3–80   EPC 214)

30.

C. The term "inotropy" refers to the strength of a muscular contraction of the heart. Therefore, a positive inotropic agent is one that increases the strength of a cardiac contraction. (PCPP 3–80   EPC 214)

31.

A. The term "chronotrope" refers to heart rate. A drug that is a negative chronotropic agent is one that suppresses the heart rate. (PCPP 3–80   EPC 214)

32.

C. Within the cardiac muscle fibers are special structures called intercalated discs. These discs connect cardiac muscle fibers and conduct electrical impulses quickly from one muscle fiber to the next. (PCPP 3–80   EPC 214)

33.

A. A syncytium is a group of cardiac muscle cells that physiologically functions as a unit. The ventricular syncytium occurs in an inferior to superior direction in order to direct blood flow to the aorta and the pulmonary artery. (PCPP 3–80   EPC 214)

34.

C. The resting potential is the normal electrical state of cardiac cells. During this phase, a pump actively pumps sodium out of the cell membrane. This causes more negatively charged ions to remain inside the cell than positively charged ions, which results in a difference of voltage across the cell membrane. Therefore, the inside of the cell is more negatively charged than the outside. (PCPP 3–81   EPC 215)

35.

B. During the action potential, the membrane surrounding the cell changes instantaneously to allow sodium ions to rush into the cell, bringing their positive charge. (PCPP 3–82   EPC 215)

36.

D. The cells of the cardiac conductive system have several important properties. First, they have excitability. They can respond to electrical stimulus. Second, they have conductivity. They can conduct an electrical impulse from one cell to another. Third, they have automaticity, the ability to self-depolarize without an impulse from an outside source. (PCPP 3–83   EPC 1205)

37.

C. The normal intrinsic firing rate of the SA node is 60–100 beats per minute. (PCPP 3–84   EPC 1205)

38.

B. The normal intrinsic firing rate of the AV junction is 40–60 beats per minute. (PCPP 3–84   EPC 1205)

39.

A. The normal intrinsic firing rate of the Purkinje system is 20–40 beats per minute. (PCPP 3–84   EPC 1205)

40.

B. According to Einthoven's triangle, lead 2 is characterized by left leg positive, right arm negative. (PCPP 3–85   EPC 1207)

41.

D. Only a very limited amount of information can be obtained from a single-lead ECG reading. You can tell how fast the heart is beating, how regular the heart beat is, and how long it takes to conduct the impulse through various parts of the heart. You cannot tell the presence or location of an infarct or a chamber enlargement or the quality or presence of pumping action. (PCPP 3–84   EPC 1206)

42.

A. On the vertical axis of the standard ECG graph paper, a deflection of two large boxes signifies 1 millivolt of amplitude. (PCPP 3–87   EPC 1209)

43.

C. On the horizontal axis of the standard ECG graph paper, a deflection of one large box signifies 0.2 second duration. (PCPP 3–87   EPC 1209)

44.

A. The P wave represents each atrial depolarization. (PCPP 3–88   EPC 1210)

45.

D. The T wave represents ventricular repolarization. (PCPP 3–89   EPC 1211)

46.

B. The QRS complex represents ventricular depolarization. (PCPP 3–88   EPC 1210)

47.

C. The P–R interval represents delay at the AV node. The normal P–R interval is 0.12–0.20 second. (PCPP 3–93   EPC 1215)

48.

B. The absolute refractory period represents the period of the cardiac cycle when stimulation will not produce any depolarization whatsoever. This usually lasts from the beginning of the QRS complex to the tip of the T wave. (PCPP 3–94   EPC 1216)

49.

D. Artifacts are deflections produced by factors other than the heart's electrical activity. Common causes of artifacts include muscle tremors, shivering, patient movement, loose electrodes, 60 Hz interference, and machine malfunction. (PCPP 3–84   EPC 1206)

50.

B. Using the triplicate method, if the R–R interval is three large boxes, the rate will be 100. First, locate an R wave that falls on a dark line bordering a large box on the graph paper; then assign numbers corresponding to the heart rate to the next six dark lines to the right. The order is 300, 150, 100, 75, 60, and 50. The number corresponding to the dark line closest to the peak of the next R wave is a rough estimate of the heart rate. (PCPP 3–96   EPC 1218)

51.

D. In normal sinus rhythm, the P waves should be present and upright in lead 2; all P waves should look alike. (PCPP 3–97   EPC 1219)

52.

B. The normal P–R interval is 0.12 to 0.20 second. (PCPP 3–93   EPC 1219)

53.

C. The normal QRS complex is 0.04 to 0.12 second. (PCPP 3–93   EPC 1219)

54.

D. Dysrhythmias are deviations from the normal electrical rhythm of the heart and can be caused by a number of situations: myocardial ischemia and infarction; electrolyte imbalances, such as hyperkalemia; and blood gas abnormalities, including hypoxia and an abnormal pH. (PCPP 3–97 EPC 1219)

55.

C. Cardiac depolarization, resulting from depolarization from cells in the heart that are not a part of the heart's normal pacemaker system, is known as ectopic beats. (PCPP 3–98   EPC 1220)

56.

A. Stable angina occurs during activity when the oxygen demands of the heart are increased. Angina can be of relatively short duration (3–5 minutes) or prolonged (lasting 15 minutes or more). The pain is often relieved by rest, nitroglycerine, or oxygen. (PCPP 3–191   EPC 1307)

57.

D. Sinus rhythm is the standard heartbeat. It is distinguished by the following features: rate is 60–100 beats per minute; P–P and R–R rhythms are regular; P waves are normal in shape, are upright, and appear only before each QRS complex. The P–R interval lasts 0.12 to 0.20 second and is constant. The QRS complex looks normal and has a duration of less than 0.12 second. (PCPP 3–97 EPC 1219)

58.

B. Initial prehospital management of this patient should include oxygen and nitroglycerine sublingually. Nitroglycerine decreases myocardial work and dilates the coronary arteries. (PCPP 3–195 EPC 1311)

59.

B. Unstable angina occurs at rest. Because this condition often indicates severe atherosclerotic heart disease, it is also called pre-infarction angina. (PCPP 3–191   EPC 1307)

60.

D. Sinus dysrhythmia is often a normal finding and is sometimes related to the respiratory cycle and changes in intrathoracic pressure. It can also be caused by enhanced vagal tone. The identifying feature of sinus dysrhythmia is an irregular rhythm. In all other ways, it is identical to normal sinus rhythm. (PCPP 3–104 EPC 1227)

61.

B. The major underlying factor in many cardiovascular emergencies is atherosclerosis. Atherosclerosis is a progressive, degenerative disease of the medium and large arteries. It results from the deposition of fats under the tunica intima layer of the involved vessels. (PCPP 3–196 EPC 1307)

62.

C. Diltiazem (Cardizem) is a calcium channel blocker used increasingly for angina pectoris, dysrhythmias, hypertension, and other cardiovascular problems. It works by inhibiting calcium from entering the cells. (PCPP 3–180 EPC 1311)

63.

C. Acute myocardial infarction is the death of a portion of the heart muscle from prolonged deprivation of arterial blood supply. It can also occur when the oxygen demand of the heart exceeds its supply for an extended period of time. It is most often associated with atherosclerotic heart disease. (PCPP 3–196 EPC 1312)

64.

B. Premature atrial contractions (PACs) result from a single electrical impulse originating in the atria outside the SA node, which, in turn, causes a premature depolarization of the heart before the next expected sinus beat. Identifying features of a PAC include an early beat with a normal-looking P wave and normal-looking QRS. (PCPP 3–112 EPC 1235)

65.

C. Nifedipine (Procardia XL) is a calcium channel blocker. (PCPP 3–180 EPC 1311)

66.

D. Prehospital management of a patient with acute myocardial infarction includes preventing pain and apprehension by reassuring the patient, administering high-flow oxygen, managing pain with nitroglycerine and morphine, and screening for the use of thrombolytics or angioplasty. (PCPP 3–199 EPC 1315)

67.

B. Left ventricular failure occurs when the left ventricle fails as an effective forward pump, causing back pressure of blood into the pump pulmonary circulation and often resulting in pulmonary edema. The patient with left heart failure usually presents with bilateral rales in the lower lobes and shortness of breath. (PCPP 3–202 EPC 1318)

68.

D. A patient with a history of congestive heart failure may take digoxin to increase cardiac output by increasing the force of contraction of the left ventricle. He may take a diuretic to decrease venous return and stimulate the kidneys to produce more urine and a potassium supplement, such as Slow-K, to replenish potassium lost through excessive diuresis. (PCPP 3–204 EPC 1319)

69.

C. Atrial fibrillation is a dysrhythmia that results from multiple areas of reentry within the atria or from multiple ectopic foci bombarding an AV node. Identifying features of atrial fibrillation include a grossly irregular rhythm and no discernible P waves. (PCPP 3–120 EPC 1243)

70.

A. The goals of prehospital management of a patient in left ventricular failure include decreasing venous return to the heart, decreasing myocardial oxygen demands, and improving ventilation and oxygenation. Pharmacologically we do this by administering nitroglycerine, furosemide, and morphine. (PCPP 3–205 EPC 1320)

71.

A. Acute pulmonary edema is the most serious complication of left ventricular failure when the lungs are literally bombarded with fluid. The fluid leaks out of the capillary beds into the interstitial spaces. (PCPP 3–205 EPC 1320)

72.

B. Atrial flutter results from a rapid atrial reentry circuit and an AV node that cannot handle all impulses through to the ventricles. Identifying features of atrial flutter include the absence of P waves and the presence of flutter waves at a rate of 250–350 per minute. The flutter waves resemble a sawtooth or picket fence pattern. (PCPP 3–118 EPC 1241)

73.

A. Beta blockers are frequently used to control dysrhythmias, high blood pressure, and angina. Many beta blockers, such as propranolol (Inderal), are nonselective, while others are selective for beta 1 or beta 2 receptors. (PCPP 3–180 EPC 1311)

74.

B. Prehospital management of a patient in acute pulmonary edema includes decreasing the venous return of the heart, decreasing myocardial oxygen demands, and improving ventilation and oxygenation. (PCPP 3– 205 EPC 1320)

75.

A. Cardiogenic shock is the most severe form of pump failure. It occurs when left ventricular function is so compromised that the heart cannot meet the metabolic demands of the body and compensatory mechanisms are exhausted. (PCPP 3–209 EPC 1324)

76.

C. Sinus tachycardia results from an increase in the rate of SA node discharge. Tachycardia is identical to normal sinus rhythm except that the rate is greater than 100. (PCPP 3–102 EPC 1225)

77.

C. Sinus tachycardia is often a benign process. In some cases, it is a compensatory mechanism for decreased stroke volume. (PCPP 3–103 EPC 1225)

78.

D. Diltiazem (Cardizem) is a calcium channel blocker. Calcium channel blockers are used increasingly for angina, dysrhythmias, hypertension, and other cardiovascular problems. (PCPP 3–180 EPC 1311)

79.

C. Prehospital management of the patient in cardiogenic shock is difficult. Even when the best technology is available, mortality rates approach 80–90%. Prehospital management should include rapid transport, high-flow oxygen, and a dopamine drip. (PCPP 3–210 EPC 1325)

80.

B. The most common cause of this man's symptoms is decreased cardiac output from a decreased heart rate. Remember that cardiac output is rate times stroke volume. A decrease or increase in either component without compensation directly affects the cardiac output. (PCPP 3–99 EPC 1223)

81.

C. Sinus bradycardia results from the slowing of the SA node. It can result from increased parasympathetic tone, SA node disease, or drug effects. (PCPP 3–101 EPC 1223)

82.

D. Treatment of sinus bradycardia is unnecessary unless hypotension or ventricular irritability is present. If treatment is required, administer 0.5 mg bolus of atropine sulfate. This can be repeated every 3–5 minutes until a satisfactory rate has been obtained or 0.04 mg/kg of the drug has been given. (PCPP 3–101 EPC 1223)

83.

C. Supraventricular tachycardia occurs when rapid atrial depolarization overrides the SA node. It often occurs with a sudden onset and may last minutes to hours. (PCPP 3–115 EPC 1237)

84.

B. Supraventricular tachycardia may be caused by increased automaticity of a single atrial focus or by reentry phenomena at the AV node. (PCPP 3–115 EPC 1237)

85.

C. Initial treatment of a patient in supraventricular tachycardia with stable vital signs includes administering oxygen and performing vagal maneuvers, such as Valsalva or carotid sinus massage. (PCPP 3–116 EPC 1237)

86.

A. Ventricular tachycardia is a rhythm that consists of three or more ventricular complexes in succession at a rate of 100 beats per minute or more. This rhythm overrides the normal pacemaker of the heart. (PCPP 3–144 EPC 1266)

87.

A. Initial management of this patient includes immediate synchronized cardioversion. (PCPP 3–145 EPC 1267)

88.

D. Pharmacological management of this patient may include lidocaine, procainamide, or amiodarone. (PCPP 3–145 EPC 1267)

89.

A. Ventricular fibrillation is a chaotic ventricular rhythm usually resulting from the presence of many reentry circuits within the ventricles. There is no ventricular depolarization or contraction. (PCPP 3–148 EPC 1271)

90.

D. The initial management of this patient is to check him clinically. Always correlate your patient's pulse with what you see on the ECG. In this case, a disconnected lead or faulty monitor could produce this ECG pattern. If you cannot detect a pulse, consider the rhythm ventricular fibrillation. (PCPP 3–149 EPC 1271)

91.

D. Reducing intrathoracic resistance is an important factor in a successful defibrillation. Using electrode jelly, using proper paddle positioning and pressure, and delivering successive countershocks as quickly as possible will all decrease intrathoracic resistance. (PCPP 3–181 EPC 1297)

92.

B. Pharmacological management of the patient with ventricular fibrillation includes oxygen, epinephrine, amiodarone, and lidocaine. (PCPP 3–149 EPC 1271)

93.

B. Ventricular escape rhythm or idioventricular rhythm results when either impulses from the higher pacemakers fail to reach the ventricles or the rate of discharge of the higher pacemakers becomes less than that of the ventricles, normally 15–45 beats per minute. (PCPP 3–140 EPC 1263)

94.

B. When a patient with a rhythm has no associated pulse, this is known as pulseless electrical activity. (PCPP 3–154 EPC 1276)

95.

C. Management of a patient in idioventricular rhythm with pulseless electrical activity includes CPR; airway management and oxygenation, including intubation; epinephrine and atropine IV; and rapid IV fluid administration. (PCPP 3–155 EPC 1276)

96.

D. Common causes for pulseless electrical activity include hypovolemia, hypoxia, acidosis, and cardiac tamponade. (PCPP 3–155 EPC 1276)

97.

B. Second-degree AV block type 1 (Wenkebach phenomenon) is an intermittent block at the level of the AV node. It produces a characteristic cyclic pattern in which the P–R intervals become progressively longer until an impulse is blocked or not conducted through the AV node. This cycle is repetitive. An identifying feature of second-degree AV block type 1 is a P–R interval that progressively lengthens until a QRS complex is dropped. (PCPP 3–126 EPC 1249)

98.

A. There is generally no treatment other than observation for patients in second-degree AV block type 1 with stable vital signs. (PCPP 3–127 EPC 1249)

99.

C. Third-degree block, or complete heart block, is the absence of conduction between the atria and the ventricles, resulting from complete electrical block at or below the AV node. The atria and ventricles subsequently pace the heart independent of each other. (PCPP 3–130 EPC 1253)

100.

B. Third-degree heart block can severely compromise cardiac output because of decreased heart rate and the loss of coordinated atrial kick. The prehospital management of this patient would include parasympathetic blockers, such as atropine, and transcutaneous external pacing. (PCPP 3–131 EPC 1253)

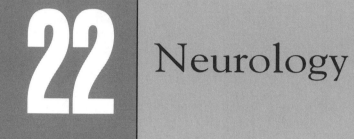

22 Neurology

DIRECTIONS
Each of the questions or incomplete statements below is followed by suggested answers or completions. Select the **one answer** that is best in each case.

1. The central nervous system consists of the
   A. sympathetic and parasympathetic branches
   B. cranial nerves and peripheral nerves
   C. axial and appendicular skeleton
   D. brain and spinal cord

2. Which of the following is NOT a component of a neuron?
   A. Cell body
   B. Synapse
   C. Axon
   D. Dendrite

3. During the resting state, the inside of the neuron is _____.
   A. negatively charged
   B. positively charged
   C. neutral
   D. none of the above

4. During the action potential, the inside of the nerve cell becomes
   A. negative
   B. positive
   C. neutral
   D. none of the above

5. Neurons connect with other neurons at junctions called
   A. neurojunctions
   B. synapses
   C. axons
   D. dendrites

6. The primary neurotransmitter(s) for the autonomic nervous system is/are
   A. epinephrine
   B. norepinephrine
   C. acetylcholine
   D. B and C

7. The outermost meningeal layer is the
   A. pia mater
   B. arachnoid
   C. subdura
   D. dura mater

Match the six main divisions of the brain with their respective definitions:

8. ____ Cerebrum
9. ____ Diencephalon
10. ____ Mesencephalon
11. ____ Pons
12. ____ Medulla
13. ____ Cerebellum

A. The midbrain
B. Contains the higher centers
C. Coordinates motor control and balance
D. Contains the thalamus, hypothalamus, and limbic system
E. Contains the respiratory and vasomotor centers
F. Lies between the midbrain and the medulla

14. The right and left hemispheres of the cerebrum are connected by the
    A. medulla oblongata
    B. midbrain
    C. circle of Willis
    D. corpus callosum

Match the five areas of specialization of the brain with their respective lobes:

15. ____ Temporal
16. ____ Occipital

17. ____ Frontal
18. ____ Cerebellum
19. ____ Parietal

  A. Personality, motor skills
  B. Sensory
  C. Speech center
  D. Coordination and balance
  E. Vision

20. The circle of Willis joins the
  A. carotid and vertebrobasilar circulatory systems
  B. midbrain and brain stem
  C. right and left brain
  D. venous sinuses and jugular veins

21. Nerve fibers that transmit impulses from the brain to the body are called
  A. afferent fibers
  B. efferent fibers
  C. dermatomes
  D. neurotransmitters

22. Each nerve route has a corresponding area of the body to which it supplies sensation. These areas are called
  A. afferent areas
  B. efferent areas
  C. dermatomes
  D. neurotransmitters

23. The pupils are controlled by which cranial nerve?
  A. I
  B. III
  C. V
  D. X

24. Which of the following is an early sign of increased intracranial pressure?
  A. Dilated, nonreactive pupils
  B. Dilated, reactive pupils

  C. Unilaterally dilated pupil
  D. None of the above

Match the following respiratory patterns with their respective descriptions:

25. ____ Cheyne-Stokes
26. ____ Central neurogenic
27. ____ Ataxic
28. ____ Apneustic
29. ____ Diaphragmatic

  A. Prolonged inspiration
  B. No intercostal movement
  C. Increase/decrease/apnea
  D. Rapid, deep breathing; hyperventilation
  E. Ineffective muscular coordination

30. Which of the following is true?
  A. Carbon dioxide is a potent vasodilator
  B. Hyperventilation can decrease intracranial pressure
  C. At a $PaCO_2$ of approximately 25 mm/Hg, the cerebral blood vessels constrict
  D. All of the above

31. A patient who responds to questions but is disoriented is categorized
  A. A
  B. V
  C. P
  D. U

32. Decorticate posturing is characterized by
  A. arms extended, legs extended
  B. arms flexed, legs extended
  C. arms extended, legs flexed
  D. arms flexed, legs flexed

33. A common mnemonic for remembering the causes for coma is
  A. PQRST
  B. AEIOU–TIPS

C. SLUDGE

D. ABCDE

34. Inadequate thiamine intake may result in all of the following **EXCEPT**

A. Wernicke's syndrome

B. Kernig's sign

C. Korsakoff's psychosis

D. encephalopathy

SCENARIO

Questions 35–39 refer to the following scenario.

Your patient is a 75-year-old female who presents at home slumped to one side of the couch. She appears awake but disoriented. Per her family, she has a long history of hypertension and one stroke. Her respiratory rate is 18, pulse 90 and regular, BP 170/90, and pupils equal and reactive. Her left side is obviously weakened, she slurs her speech, and she has facial drooping. According to her family, these signs are all new.

35. Strokes are caused by

A. hemorrhage of cerebral blood vessels

B. thrombus formation

C. embolism

D. all of the above

36. Transient ischemic attacks are defined as

A. minor strokes

B. temporary strokes

C. strokes caused by hypoxia

D. none of the above

37. Patients with strokes commonly present with

A. bilateral paralysis or paresthesia

B. polyuria, polydipsia, polyphagia

C. hemiparesis or hemiplegia

D. all of the above

38. Hemiplegia means

A. weakness to the legs

B. inability to speak

C. unilateral paralysis

D. numbness

39. Management of this patient should include

A. blood glucose determination

B. 100% oxygen administration

C. cardiac monitoring

D. all of the above

SCENARIO

Questions 40–47 refer to the following scenario.

Your patient is a 56-year-old homeless man who, per bystanders, suffered a seizure. He presents to you on the street, comatose, and smelling of alcohol and urine, with vomit and blood around his mouth. Further examination finds him responsive to deep pain with purposeful movement, breathing at 20/minute, heart rate 90 and regular, BP 140/70, and pupils equal but sluggish to react. As you prepare to examine him further, he seizes once again, full grand mal.

40. The most common cause of seizures is

A. hypoglycemia

B. hypoxia

C. drug overdose

D. epilepsy

Match the following types of seizures with their respective descriptions:

41. ____ Grand mal

42. ____ Petit mal

43. ____ Jacksonian

44. ____ Psychomotor

45. ____ Pseudoseizure

A. Brief loss of consciousness

B. Dysfunction to one area of body

C. Tonic/clonic extremity movement

D. Involves temporal lobe with aura

E. Can be interrupted, no postictal period

46. Status epilepticus is defined as

A. a seizure due to epilepsy

B. a seizure that does not stop following diazepam therapy

C. two or more seizures without a lucid interval

D. all of the above

47. Which of the following is **NOT** recommended in the management of this patient?
    A. IV D_5W
    B. Blood glucose determination
    C. Diazepam IV push
    D. 100% oxygen administration

48. Your patient suffered a sudden loss of consciousness and was unresponsive for approximately 5 minutes. Your differential field diagnosis includes all of the following **EXCEPT**
    A. syncope
    B. seizure
    C. TIA
    D. cardiac dysrhythmia

49. Which of the following is a cause of syncope?
    A. Idiopathic reasons
    B. Cardiovascular conditions
    C. Hypoglycemia
    D. All of the above

50. Your patient is a 30-year-old woman who complains of recurring right-sided headaches. She describes them as intense and throbbing. She also complains of photophobia, nausea, and vomiting. She claims she can feel it coming on through some auditory signals. Her neck is supple. Your probable field diagnosis is
    A. cluster headache
    B. migraine headache
    C. tension headache
    D. organic headache

51. Which of the following statements is true regarding brain tumors?
    A. Most originate in the brain itself
    B. Only malignant tumors are harmful
    C. Breast cancer often metastasizes to the brain
    D. All of the above

52. A degenerative brain disorder that is the most common cause of dementia in the elderly is
    A. multiple sclerosis
    B. Parkinson's
    C. muscular dystrophy
    D. Alzheimer's

53. A group of genetic diseases characterized by progressive muscle weakness and degeneration of skeletal or voluntary muscle fibers is
    A. multiple sclerosis
    B. Parkinson's
    C. muscular dystrophy
    D. Alzheimer's

54. A disease that involves inflammation of certain nerve cells followed by demyelination is
    A. multiple sclerosis
    B. Parkinson's
    C. muscular dystrophy
    D. Alzheimer's

55. A chronic and progressive motor system disorder that appears to be caused by a decrease in dopamine in the brain is
    A. multiple sclerosis
    B. Parkinson's
    C. muscular dystrophy
    D. Alzheimer's

56. Which of the following is **NOT** a characteristic of Parkinson's disease?
    A. Tremors
    B. Flaccidity
    C. Bradykinesia
    D. Postural instability

57. Your patient presents unable to close his left eye, tearing, drooling, and hypersensitive to sound, with some taste impairment. The entire left side of his face and forehead seems to droop.

He has no other neurological deficits. Your field diagnosis is

A. stroke

B. Bell's palsy

C. myoclonus

D. central pain syndrome

58. Which of the following neurological diseases is caused by a virus?

A. Amyotrophic lateral sclerosis

B. Spina bifida

C. Myoclonus

D. Polio

59. Which of the following statements is true regarding back pain?

A. Fifteen percent of lower back pain is due to sciatica

B. The cause of most lower back pain is unknown

C. Sciatica never causes motor or sensory deficits

D. Men report 50% more lower back pain than women

60. Which is the most common cause of a herniated disc?

A. Degeneration

B. Trauma

C. Improper lifting

D. None of the above

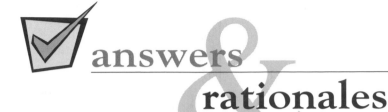

answers & rationales

1.

D. The central nervous system consists of the brain and spinal cord. (PCPP 3–263   EPC 177)

2.

B. The fundamental unit of the nervous system is the nerve cell, or neuron. The neuron consists of the cell body containing the nucleus; the dendrites, which carry nervous impulses to the cell body; and the axons, which transmit nervous impulses away from the cell body. (PCPP 3–264   EPC 177)

3.

A. The transmission of nervous impulses in the nervous system resembles the conduction of electrical impulses through the heart. In its resting state, the neuron is positively charged on the outside and negatively charged on the inside. (PCPP 3–264 EPC 177)

4.

B. When stimulated, sodium rapidly enters the cell and potassium rapidly leaves it, producing a positive charge at the entry site. (PCPP 3–264   EPC 177)

5.

B. The neuron joins with other neurons at junctions called synapses. The neurons do not come into contact with each other at these synapses. Upon reaching the synapse, the axon releases a chemical neurotransmitter, which crosses the synapse and stimulates the connecting nerve. (PCPP 3–264 EPC 177)

6.

D. The primary postsynaptic neurotransmitter for the sympathetic nervous system is norepinephrine. The transmitter for the parasympathetic nervous system is acetylcholine. (PCPP 3–264   EPC 179)

7.

D. The outermost layer of the meninges is the dura mater. An easy way to recall the meningeal layers is to remember that they provide a PAD for the brain (**P**ia—**A**rachnoid—**D**ura). (PCPP 3–265   EPC 179)

Matching (PCPP 3–268   EPC 182)

8. B Cerebrum
9. D Diencephalon
10. A Mesencephalon
11. F Pons
12. E Medulla
13. C Cerebellum

A. The midbrain
B. Contains the higher centers
C. Coordinates motor control and balance
D. Contains the thalamus, hypothalamus, and limbic system
E. Contains the respiratory and vasomotor centers
F. Lies between the midbrain and the medulla

14.

D. The right and left hemispheres of the cerebrum are connected by the corpus collosum. (PCPP 3–268 EPC 182)

Matching (PCPP 3–269   EPC 182)

15. C Temporal
16. E Occipital
17. A Frontal
18. D Cerebellum
19. B Parietal

A. Personality, motor skills
B. Sensory
C. Speech center
D. Coordination and balance
E. Vision

20.

A. Blood flow to the brain is provided by two systems. The carotid system is anterior, while the vertebrobasilar system is posterior. Both join at the circle of Willis before entering the substance of the brain. (PCPP 3–269   EPC 182)

21.

B. Nerve fibers that transmit motor impulses from the brain to the body are called efferent fibers. Those that transmit sensory impulses from the body to the brain are called afferent fibers. (PCPP 3–271   EPC 185)

22.

C. Each nerve route has a corresponding area of the body, called the dermatome, to which it supplies sensation. (PCPP 3–271   EPC 187)

23.

B. The pupils are controlled by the third cranial nerve (CN-III), also called the occulomotor nerve. This nerve follows a long course through the skull and is easily compressed by brain swelling. Thus, it can be an early indicator of increasing intracranial pressure. (PCPP 3–274   EPC 679)

24.

C. A unilaterally dilated pupil that remains reactive to light may be the earliest sign of increasing intracranial pressure. The patient who presents with or develops the unilaterally dilated pupil is in the immediate transport category. (PCPP 3–280   EPC 1347)

Matching (PCPP 3–281   EPC 1348)

25. C   Cheyne-Stokes
26. D   Central neurogenic
27. E   Ataxic
28. A   Apneustic
29. B   Diaphragmatic

A. Prolonged inspiration
B. No intercostal movement
C. Increase/decrease/apnea
D. Rapid, deep breathing; hyperventilation
E. Ineffective muscular coordination

30.

D. The blood level of carbon dioxide has a critical effect on cerebral blood vessels. The normal blood $PaCO_2$ is 40 mm/Hg. Increasing the $PaCO_2$ causes cerebral vasodilation, while decreasing it results in cerebral vasoconstriction. If the patient is poorly ventilated, the $PaCO_2$ will increase, causing even further vasodilation with a subsequent increase in intracranial pressure. Hyperventilation can decrease the $PaCO_2$ to nearly 25 mm/Hg, effectively causing vasoconstriction of the cerebral vessels. This will help minimize brain swelling. Therefore, hyperventilate any patient suspected of having increased intracranial pressure at a rate of 24 breaths per minute or more. (PCPP 3–282   EPC 1349)

31.

A. A patient who responds to questions but is disoriented is categorized A for alert. He is alert but disoriented. To be oriented, he must know who he is, where he is, and the approximate time. (PCPP 3–278   EPC 1345)

32.

B. Decorticate posturing is characterized by flexion of the arms and extension of the legs. Decerebrate posturing is characterized by arm and leg extension. Both signify deep cerebral or brain stem injury. (PCPP 3–283   EPC 1350)

33.

B. Unconsciousness or coma is a state in which the patient cannot be aroused even by powerful external stimuli. There generally are only two mechanisms capable of producing alterations in mental status: structural lesions and toxic-metabolic states. Within these two general categories, there are many causes of altered mental status. The mnemonic AEIOU–TIPS is an easy way to remember some of them. (PCPP 3–287 EPC 1354)

A—acidosis, alcohol
E—epilepsy
I—infection
O—overdose
U—uremia (kidney failure)
T—trauma, tumor, toxin
I—insulin
P—psychosis, poison
S—stroke, seizure

34.

B. Thiamine deficiency may cause Wernicke's syndrome (an acute and reversible encephalopathy) or Korsakoff's psychosis. (PCPP 3–289   EPC 1356)

35.

D. A stroke or CVA is a term that describes injury or death of brain tissue, usually due to interruption of cerebral blood flow from either ischemic or hemorrhagic lesions. This may be caused by hemorrhage in the brain tissue, an embolus in the cerebral blood vessels, or thrombus formation that occludes arterial supply to the brain. (PCPP 3–289   EPC 1356)

36.

B. Transient ischemic attacks or TIAs are temporary strokes. These are usually caused by emboli that temporarily interfere with the blood supply to the brain, producing symptoms of neurologic deficit. These symptoms may last for only a few minutes or for several hours. (PCPP 3–292   EPC 1359)

37.

C. Patients with strokes commonly present with hemiplegia or hemiparesis, unilateral facial droop, speech disturbances, confusion and agitation, eating disturbances, uncoordinated fine motor movements, vision problems, inappropriate behavior with excessive laughing or crying, or coma. (PCPP 3–292 EPC 1359)

38.

C. Hemiplegia means paralysis of one side of the body. (PCPP 3–292   EPC 1359)

39.

D. Management of a patient with stroke symptoms should include blood glucose determination and administration of 50% dextrose if the patient is hypoglycemic, administration of 100% oxygen, and cardiac monitoring. Of utmost importance are ascertaining the time of onset of symptoms and rapidly transporting the patient to a stroke center if still within the 3-hour window for administering fibrinolytic therapy. (PCPP 3–293   EPC 1360)

40.

D. A seizure is a temporary alteration in behavior due to massive electrical discharge of one or more groups of neurons in the brain. The most common cause is idiopathic epilepsy. (PCPP 3–295   EPC 1361)

Matching (PCPP 3–295   EPC 1362)

41. C   Grand mal
42. A   Petit mal
43. B   Jacksonian
44. D   Psychomotor
45. E   Pseudoseizure

A. Brief loss of consciousness
B. Dysfunction to one area of body
C. Tonic/clonic extremity movement
D. Involves temporal lobe with aura
E. Can be interrupted, no postictal period

46.

C. Status epilepticus is a series of two or more generalized motor seizures without an intervening return of consciousness. The most common cause in adults is failure to take prescribed anticonvulsive medications. (PCPP 3–298   EPC 1365)

47.

A. Managing the patient in status epilepticus includes aggressive airway management, oxygenation, IV access with normal saline or lactated Ringer's, determination of blood glucose level and administration of 50% dextrose if the patient is hypoglycemic, and administration of a diazepam IV push. (PCPP 3–298   EPC 1365)

48.

A. Syncope is, by definition, a transient loss of consciousness due to inadequate blood flow to the brain. Syncope involves rapid recovery of consciousness. If your patient does not regain consciousness within a few moments, it is not syncope but something more serious. (PCPP 3–299   EPC 1366)

49.

D. Syncope can be caused by cardiovascular conditions, such as dysrhythmias (e.g., bradycardia, tachycardia) or mechanical problems; noncardiovascular disease, such as metabolic (e.g., hypoglycemia), neurological (e.g., transient ischemic attack), or psychiatric (e.g., anxiety) conditions; or idiopathic (unknown) reasons. (PCPP 3–299   EPC 1366)

50.

B. Migraine headaches afflict approximately 17 million people. They are characterized by an intense, throbbing, unilateral headache, accompanied by photophobia, nausea, and vomiting. Often patients experience a visual or auditory aura just prior to the headache. (PCPP 3–300   EPC 1367)

51.

C. Most brain tumors are metastases from cancer that started somewhere else in the body, such as in the breast. While malignant tumors are always more dangerous, even a benign tumor within the confines of the skull can be life-threatening if it jeopardizes vital functions. (PCPP 3–302   EPC 1369)

52.

D. A degenerative brain disorder that is the most common cause of dementia in the elderly is Alzheimer's disease. It results from the death and disappearance of nerve cells in the cerebral cortex and causes marked atrophy of the brain. (PCPP 3–304   EPC 1371)

53.

C. A group of genetic diseases characterized by progressive muscle weakness and degeneration of skeletal or voluntary muscle fibers is muscular dystrophy (MD). The prognosis of MD varies, depending on the type and progression of the disorder. (PCPP 3–304   EPC 1371)

54.

A. A disease that involves inflammation of certain nerve cells followed by demyelination, or destruction of the myelin sheath, which is the fatty insulation surrounding nerve fibers of the brain and spinal cord, is multiple sclerosis. Severe cases can be debilitating, rendering a patient unable to care for himself. (PCPP 3–304   EPC 1371)

55.

B. A chronic and progressive motor system disorder that appears to be caused by a decrease in dopamine in the brain is Parkinson's. First described in the

nineteenth century, 50,000 new cases are reported each year. (PCPP 3–305   EPC 1372)

56.

B. The four main characteristics of Parkinson's disease are tremor (pill rolling), rigidity (resistance to movement), bradykinesia (slowed autonomic movement), and postural instability (impaired balance and coordination). (PCPP 3–305   EPC 1372)

57.

B. Bell's palsy is paralysis of the facial muscles due to inflammation of the facial nerve (CN-VII). Patients present with unilateral facial paralysis, inability to close one eye, taste impairment, pain, tearing, and drooling. Emergency management is aimed at protecting the eye. Steroids are prescribed, and most patients recover within 3 months. (PCPP 3–306   EPC 1373)

58.

D. Poliomyelitis (polio) is an infectious, inflammatory viral disease of the central nervous system that sometimes results in permanent paralysis. The Salk vaccine in the 1950s all but eradicated the disease, but thousands of prevaccine survivors are alive today. (PCPP 3–306   EPC 1373)

59.

B. Most back pain is idiopathic. That is, the cause may be difficult or impossible to diagnose. This makes the treatment of many cases of lower back pain frustrating and sometimes unsuccessful. (PCPP 3–308 EPC 1374)

60.

C. This is probably the most important question and answer in this book for a paramedic. Improper lifting is the most common cause of disc herniation. Through adequate exercise and proper mechanics, you can avoid this career-ending injury. (PCPP 3–308   EPC 1375)

23 Endocrinology

DIRECTIONS Each of the questions or incomplete statements below is followed by suggested answers or completions. Select the **one answer** that is best in each case.

1. Chemical substances released by a gland that control or affect other glands or body systems are called
   A. endocrines
   B. hormones
   C. polypeptides
   D. ketones

2. The _____ is the junction between the central nervous system and the endocrine system.
   A. pituitary gland
   B. pineal
   C. hypophysis
   D. hypothalamus

3. The master gland whose function is to control the other endocrine glands is the _____ gland.
   A. pituitary
   B. thyroid
   C. adrenal
   D. endocrine

4. The hormone(s) produced by the posterior pituitary gland that help(s) control fluid regulation is/are
   A. antidiuretic hormone
   B. vasopressin
   C. prolactin
   D. A and B

5. Oxytocin, when released, causes
   A. uterine contractions
   B. egg implantation in the uterus
   C. feminization
   D. maturation of the egg

6. You can suppress preterm labor by administering a fluid bolus because
   A. the mother is usually dehydrated
   B. oxytocin release is inhibited

C. the fluid increase fools the thyroid gland
D. less ACTH is secreted

7. Graves' disease, characterized by insomnia, tachycardia, hypertension, and fatigue, is the result of
   A. hyponatremia
   B. hyperadrenalism
   C. hyperthyroidism
   D. hypocalcemia

8. Myxcdema, characterized by facial bloating, weakness, altered mental status, and oily skin is caused by
   A. hypothyroidism
   B. hyperadrenalism
   C. hypernatremia
   D. hypocalcemia

9. The parathyroid glands are responsible for regulating the blood level of
   A. glucose
   B. calcium
   C. insulin
   D. ADH

10. Which of the following hormones stimulates the liver to transform its glycogen stores into glucose for immediate use?
    A. Prolactin
    B. Glucagon
    C. Insulin
    D. Somatostatin

11. Which of the following hormones is **NOT** produced by the islets of Langerhans?
    A. Glucagon
    B. Somatostatin
    C. Prolactin
    D. Insulin

12. Insulin is necessary to
    A. facilitate transport of glucose into the cells
    B. produce glucose from muscle tissue
    C. enhance glycogen formation in the liver
    D. promote gluconeogenesis

13. Catecholamines are released by the
    A. adrenal medulla
    B. adrenal cortex
    C. islets of Langerhans
    D. pancreas

14. The adrenal cortex releases
    A. corticosteroids
    B. anti-inflammatory agents
    C. mineralocorticoids
    D. all of the above

15. Oversecretion by the adrenal cortex results in a condition known as
    A. Graves' disease
    B. myxedema
    C. diabetes mellitus
    D. Cushing's disease

16. The ovaries are responsible for all of the following EXCEPT
    A. manufacturing estrogen and progesterone
    B. preparing the uterus for egg implantation
    C. secreting testosterone
    D. aiding female sexual development

17. The testes are controlled by the hormone(s)
    A. estrogen and progesterone
    B. FSH and LH
    C. TSH and GH
    D. prolactin

18. Which of the following is NOT a characteristic of diabetes mellitus?
    A. Ketone production
    B. Excessive insulin production
    C. Osmotic diuresis
    D. Associated heart and kidney disease

19. Diabetic ketoacidosis is a direct result of
    A. the cells burning inefficient fuels
    B. the pancreas secreting excessive insulin
    C. the kidneys reabsorbing glucose
    D. rapid, deep respirations

20. Insulin shock is a direct result of
    A. insufficient insulin levels
    B. insufficient blood glucose levels
    C. hyperglycemia
    D. not taking enough insulin

21. Nonketotic hyperosmolar coma differs from DKA in that
    A. the pancreas produces some insulin
    B. ketones are eliminated by the kidneys
    C. osmotic diuresis does not occur
    D. blood glucose levels do not rise greatly

SCENARIO

Questions 22–30 refer to the following scenario.

Your patient is a 45-year-old male who lies unconscious in bed. His daughter states that he has a long history of diabetes and takes insulin daily. He lives alone and had not been seen for a few days. He has no other history. His heart rate is 100, BP 90/60, respirations 40 and deep with a fruity odor, lungs clear, skin warm and dry, chemstrip 380. He had vomited twice prior to your arrival.

22. This patient is most likely suffering from
    A. hypoglycemia
    B. insulin shock
    C. hyperglycemia
    D. nonketotic hyperosmolar coma

23. His problem probably resulted from
    A. taking his insulin and not eating enough
    B. not taking his insulin
    C. taking his insulin and overeating
    D. recent illness

24. His hypotension and dehydrated look result from
    A. osmotic diuresis
    B. overproduction of ketones

C. increased insulin levels

D. increased ADH release

25. His respiratory pattern is known as
    A. Cheyne-Stokes
    B. Kussmaul's
    C. Graves'
    D. Biot's

26. This respiratory pattern occurs as the body attempts to
    A. increase insulin production
    B. correct metabolic acidosis
    C. decrease hypoxia from insulin shock
    D. produce more ketonic acids

27. The fruity breath results from _____ in the expired air.
    A. glucose
    B. insulin
    C. ketones
    D. glucagon

28. His chemstrip reads 380 because
    A. he cannot transport glucose into his cells
    B. he cannot transform glycogen into glucose
    C. he is hypoglycemic
    D. he is in insulin shock

29. Classic early signs of this disease include all of the following EXCEPT
    A. polydipsia
    B. polyuria
    C. polyphagia
    D. polyphasia

30. Emergency prehospital treatment for this patient includes
    A. crystalloid fluid infusion
    B. 50% dextrose IV
    C. glucagon IM
    D. naloxone IV

SCENARIO

Questions 31–35 refer to the following scenario.

Your patient is a 39-year-old female who collapsed in a supermarket and lies unconscious on the floor. She is alone, and no one is available to provide you with a history. She has no medications in her purse, except for some Glucotabs. She is wearing a bracelet that states she is diabetic. Her heart rate is 110, BP 100/70, respirations 28 and shallow, skin cool and clammy, lungs clear, and chemstrip 40.

31. This patient is most likely suffering from
    A. hypoglycemia
    B. insulin shock
    C. hyperglycemia
    D. A and B

32. This patient's condition could have resulted from any of the following EXCEPT
    A. taking her insulin and not eating enough
    B. not taking her insulin
    C. too much exercise/activity
    D. recent illness

33. Her unconsciousness is due to
    A. cerebral hypoxia
    B. cerebral hypoglycemia
    C. ketoacidosis
    D. osmotic diuresis

34. Prehospital management of this patient includes
    A. insulin SC
    B. 250 ml of lactated Ringer's
    C. 50% dextrose IV
    D. all of the above

35. If an accurate chemstrip cannot be obtained, management should include all of the following EXCEPT
    A. thiamine IV
    B. 50% dextrose IV
    C. insulin SC
    D. oral glucose

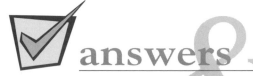

answers & rationales

1.

B. Hormones are chemical substances released by glands that control or affect other glands or body systems. Endocrine glands secrete hormones directly into the bloodstream. Exocrine glands transport their hormones to target tissues via ducts. Emergencies are usually caused by the underproduction or overproduction of hormones. (PCPP 3–315   EPC 1379)

2.

D. The hypothalamus is the junction between the central nervous system and the endocrine system. Its cells act as both nerve cells and gland cells. It receives messages from the nervous system and translates them into a glandular response. (PCPP 3–317 EPC 200)

3.

A. The pituitary gland is known as the "master gland." Its primary function is to regulate the other endocrine glands. It is located at the base of the brain and is very well protected. (PCPP 3–320   EPC 201)

4.

D. The posterior pituitary gland produces two hormones: oxytocin and antidiuretic hormone (ADH). ADH, also called vasopressin, stimulates the kidneys to retain water by reabsorbing sodium to compensate for fluid volume losses. After fluid levels stabilize, the pituitary gland inhibits ADH secretion. (PCPP 3–320   EPC 201)

5.

A. Oxytocin stimulates contraction of the uterine musculature and milk "let down" from the breast. Oxytocin is the naturally occurring form of the drug pitocin. In the hospital, it is used to induce labor by contracting the uterus. In the field, paramedics administer oxytocin to control postpartum hemorrhage. (PCPP 3–320   EPC 201)

6.

B. Oxytocin and ADH have an interesting relationship. They are both secreted by the posterior pituitary gland. Preterm labor, also called Braxton-Hicks labor, is caused by premature uterine contractions. By administering a fluid bolus, intravascular fluid volume is increased, signaling the brain to stop secreting ADH. Since oxytocin is secreted by the same area of the pituitary, its release is also inhibited. By stopping oxytocin release, the uterine contractions subside, and the labor pains stop. (PCPP 3–321 EPC 201)

7.

C. The thyroid gland controls the rate of metabolism. Overproduction of thyroid hormones causes Graves' disease. It is characterized by insomnia, fatigue, tachycardia, hypertension, heat intolerance, and weight loss. In severe cases, thyrotoxicosis may occur—a medical emergency. (PCPP 3–322   EPC 1388)

8.

A. Inadequate levels of thyroid hormones result in myxedema. Characteristics of this disorder include facial bloating, weakness, cold intolerance, oily skin and hair, altered mental status, and a 50% mortality rate. People with hypothyroidism take a synthetic thyroid hormone. (PCPP 3–338   EPC 1390)

9.

B. The parathyroid glands produce a hormone called parathyroid hormone, which increases the blood level of calcium. These glands are located in the neck near the thyroid. (PCPP 3–322   EPC 203)

10.

B. Glucagon stimulates the liver to transform its glycogen stores into glucose for immediate use. It also stimulates the liver to manufacture glucose from other substances in a process called gluconeogenesis. Glucagon raises the blood level of glucose. (PCPP 3–323   EPC 204)

11.

C. The islets of Langerhans are specialized tissues within the pancreas that contain three types of hormone-secreting cells: alpha cells, beta cells, and delta cells. Alpha cells secrete glucagon; beta cells secrete insulin; delta cells secrete somatostatin. (PCPP 3–322   EPC 203)

12.

A. Insulin is a hormone secreted by the beta cells of the islets of Langerhans. It is antagonistic to glucagon and causes the blood level of glucose to decrease. It combines with insulin receptors on the cell membrane and allows glucose to enter the cell. It is an absolute necessity for survival. (PCPP 3–323   EPC 204)

13.

A. The catecholamines, epinephrine and norepinephrine, are secreted by the adrenal glands, specifically the adrenal medulla. These hormones stimulate the sympathetic nervous system to prepare the body for extreme stressors. (PCPP 3–324   EPC 205)

14.

D. The adrenal cortex secretes three classes of hormones: glucocorticoids, mineralocorticoids, and androgenic hormones. Like the catecholamines, these steroidal hormones respond to body stressors by raising the blood glucose level and performing anti-inflammatory and immune suppression duties. (PCPP 3–324   EPC 205)

15.

D. Prolonged secretion of adrenal cortex hormones may result in Cushing's disease. This disease is characterized by increased blood sugar levels, unusual body fat distribution, and rapid mood swings. If electrolyte imbalances occur as a result of this disease, serious complications may arise, including cardiac dysrhythmias, coma, and death. This condition is usually caused by a tumor. (PCPP 3–340   EPC 1391)

16.

C. The ovaries are the female sex glands, located adjacent to the uterus. They produce eggs for reproduction and manufacture estrogen and progesterone, which aid in sexual development and in preparation of the uterus for egg implantation. The ovaries are controlled by the anterior pituitary hormones FSH (follicle stimulating hormone) and LH (luteinizing hormone). (PCPP 3–325   EPC 205)

17.

B. The testes are the male sex glands, located in the scrotum. They produce sperm for reproduction and manufacture testosterone, which promotes male growth and masculinization. The testes are also controlled by the anterior pituitary hormones FSH (follicle stimulating hormone) and LH (luteinizing hormone). (PCPP 3–325   EPC 206)

18.

B. Diabetes mellitus is a disease characterized by decreased insulin production by the beta cells of the islets of Langerhans of the pancreas. Insulin facilitates glucose transport into the cells. As the body cells become starved for glucose, they use other sources of energy, resulting in ketone production. Increased blood glucose levels cause an osmotic gradient, resulting in a water shift into the vascular compartment. This, in turn, causes glucose to be spilled into the urine, taking water with it. The diabetic is at risk for heart disease, kidney failure, and blindness. (PCPP 3–326   EPC 1380)

19.

A. Diabetic ketoacidosis is a direct result of the cells using other sources of energy, such as fats. This inefficient fuel produces many by-products, such as ketones and other organic acids. If enough ketones are produced, metabolic acidosis and coma may ensue. (PCPP 3–330   EPC 1384)

20.

B. Insulin shock (hypoglycemia) is a result of insufficient glucose to meet tissue demands. Usually this occurs as a result of taking injected insulin and not eating enough to feed the tissues. The insulin transports all available glucose into the cells, leaving very low blood levels. Untreated, the patient may sustain brain injury, since the brain receives its energy from glucose metabolism. Hypoglycemia is a true emergency. (PCPP 3–333   EPC 1387)

21.

A. Nonketotic hyperosmolar coma differs from diabetic coma. Patients suffering the former produced enough insulin to feed the cells but not enough to maintain normal blood glucose levels. Their glucose can reach extremely high levels, causing a tremendous osmotic gradient and dehydration. Ketones are not produced because glucose is burned as fuel in the cells. (PCPP 3–332   EPC 1386)

22.

C. This patient is most likely suffering from diabetic ketoacidosis (DKA) or hyperglycemia. The history (positive for diabetes), onset (slow), chemstrip (high), respirations (rapid and deep), and skin condition (warm and dry) are all classic signs. (PCPP 3–331   EPC 1385)

23.

B. Hyperglycemia most often results from not taking sufficient amounts of prescribed insulin. Without this messenger, glucose cannot enter the cells. (PCPP 3–330   EPC 1383)

24.

A. Increased blood glucose levels cause an osmotic gradient. This gradient draws interstitial water into the intravascular compartment, resulting in glucose spillage into the urine. As water follows glucose, patients become dehydrated. If enough fluid is lost, hypotension and tachycardia follow. (PCPP 3–331 EPC 1383)

25.

B. Kussmaul's respirations, characterized by rapid, deep breathing, represent the body's attempt to increase minute volume. (PCPP 3–331   EPC 1385)

26.

B. Kussmaul's respirations are the body's attempt to compensate for the metabolic acidosis caused by excessive ketone production. As the buffer system changes metabolic acids (ketones) to respiratory acids (carbon dioxide), the respiratory system eliminates the excess by increasing minute volume ventilation. Minute volume is increased by breathing faster and deeper than normal. (PCPP 3–331   EPC 1385)

27.

C. When ketones are eliminated through the respiratory tract, the patient will exhibit a fruity, or acetone, breath odor. (PCPP 3–331   EPC 1385)

28.

A. Because this patient cannot transport glucose into his cells, blood levels rise dramatically. (PCPP 3–328   EPC 1382)

29.

D. The early signs of diabetes include polyuria (frequent urination from osmotic diuresis), polydipsia (excessive thirst from the dehydration), and polyphagia (excessive hunger from the cells being starved of glucose). (PCPP 3–329   EPC 1383)

30.

A. If blood glucose levels can be accurately determined to be high and the patient exhibits the signs and symptoms of DKA, a crystalloid infusion should be administered to reverse the dehydration and hypotension. A red top can be drawn to obtain baseline blood glucose levels. If allowed, insulin may be administered in the field. (PCPP 3–332 EPC 1386)

31.

D. Your patient is most likely suffering from insulin shock (hypoglycemia). Her history (Medic-Alert bracelet and Glucotabs), level of consciousness (altered), and chemstrip (low) all strongly suggest hypoglycemia. An altered level of consciousness, low chemstrip, and improvement following dextrose therapy are known as Whipple's triad. (PCPP 3–333   EPC 1387)

32.

B. Hypoglycemia may result from taking too much insulin, not eating enough, excessive exercise, or illness. (PCPP 3–333   EPC 1387)

33.

B. This patient has no available glucose for brain metabolism. The brain is a very greedy organ, demanding a constant supply of oxygen and glucose. Withhold either from the brain for an extended period of time and death may result. (PCPP 3–333 EPC 1387)

34.

C. Prehospital treatment of this patient includes a rapid bolus of 25 grams of 50% dextrose IV. A red top can be drawn to determine baseline blood glucose levels. (PCPP 3–336   EPC 1388)

35.

C. If blood glucose levels cannot be determined, a rapid bolus of 25 grams of 50% dextrose IV followed by 100 mg of thiamine IV should be administered. (PCPP 3–336   EPC 1388)

24

Allergies and Anaphylaxis

DIRECTIONS Each of the questions or incomplete statements below is followed by suggested answers or completions. Select the **one answer** that is best in each case.

1. Anaphylaxis is defined as
   A. an acute, generalized, violent reaction
   B. an antigen/antibody process
   C. a life-threatening emergency
   D. all of the above

2. Any substance capable of producing an immune system response is a/an
   A. antibody
   B. antigen
   C. receptor
   D. idiosyncrasy

3. The type of immune response that involves a chemical attack on the foreign substance by antibodies is known as _____ immunity.
   A. cellular
   B. anaphylactoid
   C. humoral
   D. anaphylactic

4. Antibodies are produced by specialized cells of the immune system called _____ cells.
   A. B
   B. G
   C. T
   D. E

5. During the primary response, _____ is/are released.
   A. IgA
   B. IgG
   C. IgM
   D. B and C

6. Which of the following types of immunity develops through vaccination?
   A. Acquired
   B. Natural
   C. Naturally acquired
   D. Induced active

7. The initial exposure of an individual to an antigen is referred to as
   A. hypersensitivity
   B. sensitization
   C. an allergic reaction
   D. none of the above

8. The antibody responsible for producing allergic and anaphylactic responses is
   A. IgA
   B. IgE
   C. IgM
   D. IgG

9. Which of the following is true regarding vaccines?
   A. They stimulate antibody production
   B. They contain antigenic proteins from a virus or bacterium
   C. Some last a lifetime
   D. All of the above

10. Which of the following is NOT considered a hymenopteran insect?
    A. Fire ant
    B. Spider
    C. Wasp
    D. Hornet

11. Histamine receptors are located in the
    A. airways
    B. peripheral blood vessels
    C. digestive tract
    D. all of the above

12. Histamine causes all of the following physiological reactions EXCEPT
    A. bronchodilation
    B. increased peristalsis
    C. capillary leaking
    D. vasodilation

13. The person with anaphylaxis may exhibit all of the following signs and symptoms EXCEPT
    A. hypertension
    B. stridor
    C. urticaria
    D. abdominal cramping

14. Angioedema is best described as
    A. facial swelling
    B. third cranial nerve paralysis
    C. generalized body hives
    D. eczema of the neck

15. In most cases, the signs and symptoms of anaphylaxis begin _____ following exposure to the antigen.
    A. within 1 minute
    B. 5–10 minutes
    C. 10–20 minutes
    D. 1 hour

16. The anaphylactic shock patient should be managed with
    A. aggressive airway management
    B. epinephrine and diphenhydramine
    C. 100% oxygen
    D. all of the above

17. Epinephrine causes all of the following EXCEPT
    A. bronchodilation
    B. peripheral blood vessel constriction
    C. heart rate decrease
    D. contractile force increase

18. Diphenhydramine is given in anaphylaxis because it
    A. blocks histamine receptor sites
    B. enhances the effects of epinephrine
    C. renders the antigen inactive
    D. produces permanent immunity

19. In addition to epinephrine and diphenhydramine, the medical control physician may order corticosteroids because they
    A. slow histamine release
    B. reduce capillary leakage
    C. reduce edema and swelling
    D. all of the above

20. Which of the following best describes the use of PASG in anaphylaxis?
    A. It is no longer recommended
    B. It should be used only in the most severe cases
    C. It will reduce peripheral vascular resistance
    D. It eliminates the need for vasopressors

✓answers & rationales

1.

D. Anaphylaxis is an acute, generalized, violent antigen/antibody reaction that may be rapidly fatal even with prompt and appropriate emergency care. (PCPP 3–346   EPC 1397)

2.

B. An antigen is any substance capable of producing an immune response. Among the many examples are bacteria, viruses, drug molecules, animal secretions or serum, and blood. (PCPP 3–347   EPC 1396)

3.

C. Humoral immunity is a chemical attack on an invading substance by antibodies, also called immunoglobulins (Igs). (PCPP 3–347   EPC 1396)

4.

A. Antibodies are produced by specialized cells of the immune system called B cells. There are five classes of antibodies: IgA, IgD, IgE, IgG, and IgM. (PCPP 3–347   EPC 1396)

5.

D. During the primary response, IgG and IgM are released to help fight the antigen. (PCPP 3–348   EPC 1397)

6.

D. Immunity achieved through vaccination is known as induced active immunity. The vaccine is injected to stimulate development of antibodies to a specific antigen. This is also called artificially acquired immunity. An example is the immunity produced by the diphtheria/pertussis/tetanus (DPT) vaccine. (PCPP 3–348 EPC 1397)

7.

B. The initial exposure of an individual to an antigen is referred to as sensitization. This results in an immune response by which the person begins to develop antibodies. Subsequent exposure produces an allergic reaction. (PCPP 3–349   EPC 1398)

8.

B. The IgE (immunoglobulin E) antibody contributes to allergic and anaphylactic responses. (PCPP 3–350 EPC 1399)

9.

D. A vaccine is an agent that, when injected, will produce an immune response. Most vaccines contain antigenic proteins from a virus or bacterium. Some vaccines, such as that for chicken pox, last a lifetime. Others, such as that for tetanus, must be repeated via boosters. (PCPP 3–348   EPC 1397)

10.

B. Insect stings are the second most frequent cause of fatal anaphylactic reactions. Hymenopterans are insects that produce a unique venom, which causes these severe reactions. These insects include fire ants, hornets, wasps, yellow jackets, and honey bees. (PCPP 3–351   EPC 1399)

11.

D. Histamine 1 receptors are located in the lower airways and peripheral blood vessels. Histamine 2 receptors are located in the stomach. (PCPP 3–351 EPC 1399)

12.

A. Histamine causes bronchoconstriction, capillary leaking from increased permeability, peripheral vasodilation, increased gastric secretion, and increased movement of food through the digestive tract. (PCPP 3–351   EPC 1399)

13.

A. Hypertension does not occur in true anaphylaxis. One of the cardinal effects is massive vasodila-

227

tion, which results in hypotension. (PCPP 3–351 EPC 1399)

14.

A. Peripheral vasodilation and increased capillary permeability cause swelling in the face and mucous membranes. This is called angioedema. (PCPP 3–351   EPC 1399)

15.

A. The signs and symptoms of anaphylaxis usually begin within 1 minute following exposure to the antigen. In a small percentage of patients, it can be delayed over 1 hour. The speed of onset usually predicts the severity of the response. (PCPP 3–352 EPC 1400)

16.

D. The patient in anaphylactic shock should receive aggressive airway management and 100% oxygenation; IV fluid replacement; epinephrine SC or IV; antihistamines, such as diphenhydramine IV; corticosteroids, such as methylprednisolone, hydrocortisone, and dexamethasone; vasopressors, such as dopamine, norepinephrine, and epinephrine, as needed; and beta agonists, such as albuterol. (PCPP 3–354   EPC 1401)

17.

C. Epinephrine is the drug of choice for anaphylaxis because it reverses the effects of histamine by causing bronchodilation and peripheral vasoconstriction. This will reverse the angioedema that threatens the upper airway. It will also increase heart rate and strength of contractions. (PCPP 3–354   EPC 1402)

18.

A. Diphenhydramine is given in anaphylaxis because it competes with histamine at the receptor sites. By blocking the effects of histamine, you stop the life-threatening allergic response. (PCPP 3–355 EPC 1402)

19.

D. Corticosteroids, such as methylprednisolone, hydrocortisone, and dexamethasone play a role in stopping the inflammation response. They slow histamine release from the mast cells and slow capillary leaking, thus reducing tissue edema. Since steroids do not have an immediate effect, they are not considered a first-line medication. (PCPP 3–355   EPC 1402)

20.

A. The use of the PASG in anaphylaxis is no longer recommended. (PCPP 3–354   EPC 1401)

25 Gastroenterology

DIRECTIONS Each of the questions or incomplete statements below is followed by suggested answers or completions. Select the **one answer** that is best in each case.

1. Poorly localized, dull pain that originates in the walls of hollow organs is known as _____ pain.
   A. somatic
   B. referred
   C. visceral
   D. peritoneal

2. Sharp, localized pain that originates in the walls of the body, such as skeletal muscles, is known as _____ pain.
   A. somatic
   B. referred
   C. visceral
   D. peritoneal

3. Pain that originates in a region other than where it is felt is known as _____ pain.
   A. somatic
   B. referred
   C. visceral
   D. peritoneal

4. Upper GI bleeding is defined as bleeding within the GI tract proximal to the
   A. stomach
   B. large intestine
   C. ligament of Treitz
   D. pyloric valve

5. The vast majority of upper GI bleeding is caused by
   A. esophagitis
   B. esophageal varices
   C. peptic ulcer disease
   D. Mallory-Weiss syndrome

6. Signs of upper GI bleeding include
   A. nausea and vomiting
   B. hematemesis

C. melena
D. all of the above

7. A Sengstaken-Blakemore tube is used to
   A. relieve gastric distention
   B. lavage the stomach
   C. control esophageal bleeding
   D. none of the above

8. Your patient, an alcoholic with a long history of liver damage, presents with painless, bright red upper GI bleeding. The most likely cause of the bleeding is
   A. gastritis
   B. peptic ulcer disease
   C. esophageal varices
   D. diverticulosis

9. This condition results from
   A. fatty foods
   B. congenital problems
   C. calcium deposits
   D. portal hypertension

10. Prehospital management of the above patient includes all of the following EXCEPT
    A. hemorrhage control
    B. aggressive fluid replacement
    C. aggressive airway management
    D. rapid transport to the ED

11. Your patient presents with acute onset of diarrhea, fever, nausea and vomiting, and general malaise. He is tachycardic, hypotensive, pale, and cool, with a decreased mental status. Your most likely field diagnosis is
    A. gastritis
    B. acute gastroenteritis
    C. chronic gastroenteritis
    D. ulcerative colitis

12. Which of the following IV solutions is indicated in the prehospital phase?
    A. 0.45% NaCl
    B. 0.9% NaCl
    C. 5% dextrose/lactated Ringer's
    D. 5% dextrose/NaCl

13. In the United States, you are most likely to confront gastroenteritis that was caused by
    A. *H. pylori*
    B. *Salmonella*
    C. *E. coli*
    D. *Shigella*

14. Which of the following contributes to the formation of a peptic ulcer?
    A. Ibuprofen
    B. Smoking
    C. *H. pylori*
    D. All of the above

15. Sometimes a vagotomy is performed to treat severe peptic ulcer that is refractory to medications. This is to
    A. increase mucus production
    B. increase acid production
    C. decrease mucus production
    D. decrease acid production

16. Which of the following statements is true regarding lower GI bleeding?
    A. It often causes hemodynamic instability
    B. Melena indicates a rapid arterial bleed
    C. Bright red blood usually indicates hemorrhoids
    D. Colon polyps are the most common cause

Match the following types of bowel diseases with their respective characteristics:

17. ____ Hernia
18. ____ Intussusception
19. ____ Volvulus
20. ____ Crohn's
21. ____ Ulcerative colitis
22. ____ Adhesions
23. ____ Diverticulosis

    A. Destruction of the mucosal layer of bowel
    B. Outpouchings of mucosa and submucosa
    C. Bowel protruding through the abdominal muscle wall
    D. Inflammatory disease of small bowel
    E. Part of the intestine slips into the part just distal to itself
    F. Twisting of the intestine on itself
    G. Union of separate tissues by fibrous band

24. Your patient presents with severe lower-right abdominal pain at McBurney's point. It began as a vague discomfort around the umbilicus. He also complains of anorexia, nausea, vomiting, and fever and has pronounced rebound tenderness. He may be suffering from
    A. gastritis
    B. acute appendicitis
    C. cholecystitis
    D. pylonephritis

25. An epigastric pain condition characterized by inflammation of the gallbladder is known as
    A. pylonephritis
    B. cholecystitis
    C. gastritis
    D. hepatitis

26. A positive Murphy's sign indicates
    A. gastritis
    B. cholecystitis
    C. hepatitis
    D. pylonephritis

27. Your patient with dull, upper-right quadrant pain (unrelated to eating), malaise, clay-colored stools, and jaundice may be suffering from
    A. cholecystitis
    B. hepatitis
    C. pancreatitis
    D. diverticulitis

Match the following types of hepatitis with their respective characteristics:

28. ____ Hepatitis A
29. ____ Hepatitis B
30. ____ Hepatitis C
31. ____ Hepatitis D
32. ____ Hepatitis E

A. Usually transmitted through blood transfusions
B. Waterborne, third-world infection
C. "Infectious," fecal-oral route
D. "Serum," blood-borne
E. Dormant until activated by HBV

33. Your patient's blood pressure is 120/80, and his pulse is 80 lying down. When you sit him up, his blood pressure drops to 100/60, and his pulse rises to 100. This is known as a

A. hypotensive disorder
B. positive tilt test
C. normal phenomenon
D. rebound mechanism

1.

C. Dull, poorly localized pain that originates in the walls of hollow organs, such as the gallbladder and intestines, is known as visceral pain. Many hollow organs cause visceral pain as they become distended, inflamed, or ischemic. For example, the pain of appendicitis often presents as vague periumbilical pain. (PCPP 3–363   EPC 1408)

2.

A. Sharp, localized pain that originates in the walls of the body, such as skeletal muscles, is known as somatic pain. It travels along definite neural routes determined by dermatomes or tissue blocks developed during the embryonic stage. Bacterial and chemical irritation can cause somatic pain. As the appendix ruptures, it sends its chemical contents into the abdominal cavity, causing irritation and localized pain. (PCPP 3–363   EPC 1408)

3.

B. Pain that originates in a region other than where it is felt is known as referred pain. Many neural pathways from various organs pass through areas where the organ was formed during the embryonic stage. For example, splenic injuries and myocardial ischemia often cause left shoulder pain. (PCPP 3–364   EPC 1408)

4.

C. Upper GI bleeding is defined as bleeding within the GI tract proximal to the ligament of Treitz, which supports the duodenojejunal junction. It results in over 300,000 hospitalizations each year, and mortality is 10%. (PCPP 3–369   EPC 1412)

5.

C. Peptic ulcer disease accounts for 50% of all upper GI bleeding. Since gastritis accounts for an-other 25%, stomach lining erosion accounts for 75% of all upper GI bleeding. (PCPP 3–369 EPC 1412)

6.

D. Because blood severely irritates the GI system, patients can present with nausea and vomiting, hematemesis (bloody vomit), and melena (bloody stool). The blood may be bright red (new, fresh), dark brown (old, partially digested), or black and tarry in the stool. (PCPP 3–369   EPC 1413)

7.

C. A Sengstaken-Blakemore tube is used to control esophageal bleeding. It is not a prehospital procedure. (PCPP 3–370   EPC 1414)

8.

C. Esophageal varices are swollen veins in the lower third of the esophagus. They result from increased pressure in the portal circulation. Diseases of the liver, such as alcoholic cirrhosis, can slow portal circulation, causing engorgement of the veins in the lower esophagus and the rectum. The most common presentation is painless, bright red upper GI bleeding. (PCPP 3–370   EPC 1414)

9.

D. Esophageal varices result from increased back pressure in the hepatic arteries and veins. (PCPP 3–370   EPC 1414)

10.

A. Prehospital management of the patient with bleeding esophageal varices includes aggressive airway management, fluid replacement, and rapid transport to the emergency department. There is no way to control the bleeding in the prehospital setting. (PCPP 3–371   EPC 1415)

11.

B. Your patient who presents with acute onset of diarrhea, fever, nausea and vomiting, and general malaise most likely has acute gastroenteritis. That fact that he is tachycardic, hypotensive, pale, and cool, with a decreased mental status, tells you he is in shock from massive GI fluid losses. (PCPP 3–372   EPC 1415)

12.

B. Isotonic solutions, such as normal saline (0.9% NaCl) or lactated Ringer's, should be given in the field. In the hospital, the patient will be switched to hypotonic solutions, such as 5% dextrose with lactated Ringer's or 5% dextrose with normal saline. (PCPP 3–373   EPC 1416)

13.

A. You are most likely to confront gastroenteritis that was caused by *H. pylori*, the most common infectious gastroenteritis in the United States. It is the same bacterium that often causes peptic ulcer disease. (PCPP 3–374   EPC 1417)

14.

D. Peptic ulcers are commonly caused by nonsteroidal anti-inflammatory drugs, such as ibuprofen and aspirin; acid-stimulating products, such as alcohol and nicotine; and the *H. pylori* bacterium. All contribute to the erosion of the protective mucosal lining in the stomach. When this lining is gone, hydrochloric acid used in the digestive process is allowed to erode the stomach lining. (PCPP 3–374   EPC 1417)

15.

D. If medical therapy fails and the problem persists, it may require surgical resection of the vagus nerve to reduce the stimulation for acid secretion. The vagus nerve carries parasympathetic signals that tell the stomach to secrete hydrochloric acid to digest food. (PCPP 3–375   EPC 1418)

16.

C. Rectal lesions, such as hemorrhoids and anal fissures, usually present with bright red bleeding (hematochezia). This finding, while physically startling, does not signify a medical emergency. (PCPP 3–376   EPC 1419)

Matching   (PCPP 3–377–3–381   EPC 1420–1423)

17. **C**   Hernia
18. **E**   Intussusception
19. **F**   Volvulus
20. **D**   Crohn's
21. **A**   Ulcerative colitis
22. **G**   Adhesions
23. **B**   Diverticulosis

A. Destruction of the mucosal layer of bowel
B. Outpouchings of mucosa and submucosa
C. Bowel protruding through the abdominal muscle wall
D. Inflammatory disease of small bowel
E. Part of the intestine slips into the part just distal to itself
F. Twisting of the intestine on itself
G. Union of separate tissues by fibrous band

24.

B. Appendicitis is the inflammation of the appendix. The patient suffering from appendicitis will usually complain of lower-right quadrant abdominal pain, nausea, vomiting, fever, and anorexia. The peritoneum will generally become inflamed, and rebound tenderness will be present. (PCPP 3–385 EPC 1425)

25.

B. Inflammation of the gallbladder is called cholecystitis. It usually occurs when gall stones lodge in the cystic duct that drains the gallbladder. (PCPP 3–386   EPC 1426)

26.

B. Murphy's sign pain is caused when an inflamed gallbladder is palpated by pressing under the right costal margin. (PCPP 3–387   EPC 1427)

27.

B. Hepatitis is an inflammation or infection of the liver. The patient will often complain of dull, upper-right quadrant abdominal tenderness, usually unrelated to the digestion of food, with malaise, decreased appetite, clay-colored stools, and jaundice. (PCPP 3–389   EPC 1428)

Matching   (PCPP 3–389   EPC 1428)

28. **C**   Hepatitis A
29. **D**   Hepatitis B
30. **A**   Hepatitis C
31. **E**   Hepatitis D
32. **B**   Hepatitis E

A. Usually transmitted through blood transfusions
B. Waterborne, third-world infection
C. "Infectious," fecal-oral route
D. "Serum," blood-borne
E. Dormant until activated by HBV

33.

B. The patient with an acute abdomen should be given a tilt test. First, take the patient's blood pressure and pulse in the supine position. Then repeat both with the patient in the seated position. A positive tilt test is an increase in the pulse rate of 15 beats per minute or a drop in the systolic blood pressure of 15 mmHg when the patient is moved from the supine to the sitting position. A positive tilt test indicates relative hypovolemia. (PCPP 3–370   EPC 1413)

26 Urology and Nephrology

DIRECTIONS Each of the questions or incomplete statements below is followed by suggested answers or completions. Select the **one answer** that is best in each case.

1. The functional unit of the kidney is known as the
   A. papilla
   B. pyramid
   C. glomerulus
   D. nephron

2. Bowman's capsule is a cup-shaped capsule that surrounds the
   A. glomerulus
   B. hilum
   C. nephron
   D. loop of Henle

3. Trace a drop of blood from the renal artery, through the kidney, to the urethral opening by placing the following structures in order:
   A. Proximal tubule
   B. Descending loop of Henle
   C. Hilum
   D. Renal artery
   E. Collecting duct
   F. Ascending loop of Henle
   G. Distal tubule
   H. Glomerulus
   I. Ureter
   J. Urethra
   K. Arteriole
   L. Urinary bladder

4. The kidney's major function(s) include(s)
   A. maintaining blood volume
   B. balancing electrolytes
   C. excreting urea
   D. all of the above

5. During the filtration process, which of the following passes through the capillaries and into Bowman's capsule?
   A. Plasma
   B. Red blood cells
   C. White blood cells
   D. Proteins

6. The normal glomerular filtration rate is about _____ liters per day.
   A. 50–60
   B. 100
   C. 180
   D. 240

7. A waste product created by metabolism within the muscle cells is
   A. urea
   B. erythropoietin
   C. creatinine
   D. renin

8. Which of the following hormones directly produces powerful vasoconstriction?
   A. Renin
   B. Angiotensin I
   C. Angiotensin II
   D. B and C

9. People with chronic kidney failure are at risk for developing
   A. anemia
   B. hypoglycemia
   C. dehydration
   D. all of the above

10. Urine flow may be obstructed in the male by the presence of
    A. epididymis
    B. prostatitis
    C. testitis
    D. testicular torsion

11. Women are more prone to bladder infections than men because
    A. their urethras are shorter
    B. their urethras are longer
    C. their ureters are shorter
    D. their ureters are longer

12. Prerenal acute kidney failure is most often caused by
    A. hypoperfusion
    B. hyperglycemia
    C. renal artery thrombosis
    D. overhydration

13. Renal acute kidney failure is caused by
    A. microangiopathy
    B. acute tubular necrosis
    C. interstitial nephritis
    D. all of the above

14. Postrenal acute kidney failure is most often caused by obstruction in
    A. one ureter
    B. both ureters
    C. the urethra
    D. the ejaculatory duct

15. Classic signs of acute renal failure include
    A. hot, flushed skin
    B. peripheral edema
    C. bradycardia
    D. polyuria

16. Which of the following statements is true regarding chronic kidney failure?
    A. End-stage renal failure occurs when 50% of nephrons are destroyed
    B. Anuria is always present in end-stage renal failure
    C. Most cases are caused by diabetes and hypertension
    D. Metabolic instability occurs even in the early stages

17. Uremia is a condition manifested by
    A. blood in the urine
    B. uric acid in the blood
    C. fluid in the abdominal cavity
    D. calculi in the urine

18. Which of the following is a complication of chronic renal failure?
    A. Fluid volume overload
    B. Hypokalemia
    C. Polyuria
    D. All of the above

19. Your patient in chronic renal failure may present with
    A. ascites
    B. rales in the lung bases
    C. jugular venous distention
    D. all of the above

20. The process of hemodialysis is based on the principle of
    A. diffusion
    B. osmosis
    C. homeostasis
    D. all of the above

21. Possible complications from hemodialysis include
    A. disequilibrium syndrome
    B. hypotension
    C. air embolism
    D. all of the above

22. Renal calculi are most often caused by
    A. calcium salts
    B. struvite
    C. uric acid
    D. cystine

23. Which of the following presentations is most suggestive of a kidney stone?
    A. Quiet patient in fetal position

B. Distended abdomen, supine with knees drawn up

C. Gross hematuria, severe peritonitis

D. Squirming, uncomfortable patient

24. Your nontrauma patient presents with percussion tenderness at the costovertebral angle. Your most likely field diagnosis is

A. nephrolithiasis

B. pylonephritis

C. cystitis

D. lower UTI

25. Prehospital management of all the urinary system problems presented in this chapter can be characterized by

A. very invasive techniques

B. varied pharmacological interventions

C. supportive care

D. intensive lab testing

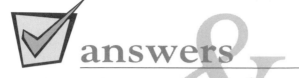

answers & rationales

1.

D. The functional unit of the kidney is the nephron. It is a microscopic structure within the kidney that produces urine. A healthy kidney contains about 1 million nephrons. (PCPP 3–397   EPC 246)

2.

A. Bowman's capsule is a cup-shaped capsule that contains the glomerulus, a tuft of capillaries from which blood is filtered into a nephron. (PCPP 3–397   EPC 247)

3.

D. Renal artery, C. Hilum, K. Arteriole, H. Glomerulus, A. Proximal tubule, B. Descending loop of Henle, F. Ascending loop of Henle, G. Distal tubule, E. Collecting duct, I. Ureter, L. Urinary bladder, J. Urethra. (PCPP 3–397   EPC 248)

4.

D. The major functions of the kidneys are to maintain blood volume by balancing electrolyte, water, and pH levels; retain key compounds, such as glucose; and excrete waste, such as urea. They also help maintain blood pressure and regulate erythrocyte production. (PCPP 3–398   EPC 249)

5.

A. During the filtration process, the only blood products that do not diffuse into Bowman's capsule are blood cells and proteins. The filtrate, therefore, resembles plasma except for the absence of proteins. (PCPP 3–398   EPC 249)

6.

C. The normal filtration rate for a healthy adult is 180 liters per day. This means that our entire blood volume is filtered 60 times through the kidneys each day. (PCPP 3–398   EPC 249)

7.

C. Creatinine is a waste product caused by metabolism of muscle cells. It has large molecules and is not reabsorbed into the bloodstream. Since all filtered creatinine will be excreted in the urine, the blood concentration of creatinine is a direct indicator of glomerular blood flow. (PCPP 3–401   EPC 251)

8.

C. Cells adjacent to the glomerular capillaries respond to low blood pressure by releasing renin, which, in turn, causes the secretion of angiotensin I. As angiotensin I flows through the lungs, it is changed to angiotensin II, a potent vasoconstrictor. People with hypertension often are prescribed either angiotensin converting enzyme (ACE) inhibitors or angiotensin II blockers. (PCPP 3–401   EPC 252)

9.

A. The kidneys produce erythropoietin, a hormone that stimulates the maturation of red blood cells. Patients with chronic kidney failure are at high risk for becoming anemic, due to a low red blood cell count. (PCPP 3–401   EPC 252)

10.

B. Urine flow may be obstructed in the male by the presence of prostatitis, benign prostatic hypertrophy, or renal calculi. The prostrate, a small gland at the base of the bladder, is responsible for production of fluid to transport sperm. In older men, it can become enlarged and, at certain times, obstruct urine flow. (PCPP 3–396   EPC 1432)

11.

A. Urinary tract infections (UTIs) occur frequently. UTIs occur more often in females because of their relatively short urethras, compared to those in males. (PCPP 3–402   EPC 1451)

12.

A. Prerenal acute kidney failure (AKF) is most often caused by a decrease in blood supply to the kidneys, or hypoperfusion. Fortunately this problem is treatable by restoring renal perfusion via IV fluid infusion and inotropic drugs. (PCPP 3–409   EPC 1439)

13.

D. Renal acute kidney failure is due to pathology within the kidney tissue itself. Causes include microangiopathy (small blood vessel injury), acute tubular necrosis (sudden death of the tubular cells), and interstitial nephritis (inflammation within the tissue surrounding the nephrons). (PCPP 3–410   EPC 1440)

14.

C. Postrenal acute kidney failure is due to obstruction distal to the kidney. This is most often caused by obstruction of the urinary bladder neck or the urethra. (PCPP 3–411   EPC 1440)

15.

B. Classic signs of acute renal failure include cool, clammy, pale skin; oliguria; peripheral edema; and, if the patient is in circulatory collapse, tachycardic hypotension, hypotensive, with an altered mental status. (PCPP 3–411   EPC 1441)

16.

C. End-stage renal failure occurs when 80% of nephrons are destroyed. Anuria is not necessarily present in end-stage renal failure. Most cases are caused by diabetes and hypertension. Metabolic instability occurs in end-stage failure. At this stage, only dialysis or a transplant will keep the patient alive. (PCPP 3–413   EPC 1443)

17.

B. Uremia is a condition characterized by increased uric acid in the blood. This is a common complication from chronic renal failure. (PCPP 3–414   EPC 1444)

18.

A. Complications of chronic renal failure include fluid overload, hyperkalemia, uremic pericarditis, pericardial tamponade, and uremic encephalopathy. (PCPP 3–414   EPC 1444)

19.

D. The patient in chronic renal failure may present with severe dyspnea, neck vein distention, ascites, and rales at the lung bases. (PCPP 3–414   EPC 1444)

20.

D. The process of hemodialysis is based on the principles of diffusion, osmosis, and homeostasis. (PCPP 3–417   EPC 1447)

21.

D. Possible complications from hemodialysis include hypotension caused by dehydration, sepsis or blood loss, chest pain or dysrhythmias caused by potassium intoxication, disequilibrium syndrome, and air embolism, which may occur when negative pressure develops in the venous side of the dialysis tubing. (PCPP 3–417   EPC 1447)

22.

A. By far, calcium salts are the most common cause of renal calculi (kidney stones). (PCPP 3–420   EPC 1449)

23.

D. Due to extreme pain and an inability to get into a position of comfort, patients who are passing a kidney stone usually squirm continuously. (PCPP 3–420   EPC 1450)

24.

B. Tenderness to percussion at the costovertebral angle (Lloyd's sign) is a classic sign of pylonephritis (kidney infection). (PCPP 3–423   EPC 1453)

25.

C. Prehospital management of urinary system problems consists mainly of supportive care—managing the ABCs: Maintain a patent airway, ensure adequate ventilation and oxygenation, and support circulation. (PCPP 3–423   EPC 1453)

27

Toxicology and Substance Abuse

DIRECTIONS
Each of the questions or incomplete statements below is followed by suggested answers or completions. Select the **one answer** that is best in each case.

1. The most common route of entry for toxic exposure is
   A. inhalation
   B. ingestion
   C. surface absorption
   D. injection

2. Toxic gases, such as methyl chloride, chlorine, and carbon monoxide, enter the bloodstream through the
   A. blood-brain barrier
   B. skin
   C. alveolar-capillary membrane
   D. intestinal tract

3. Hymenopterans deliver their poisonous substances through the
   A. blood-brain barrier
   B. skin
   C. alveolar-capillary membrane
   D. intestinal tract

4. Which of the following is an advantage of having a poison control center?
   A. It is staffed by poison control specialists
   B. It is available 24 hours a day
   C. It offers the most current information
   D. All of the above

5. Which of the following decontamination processes is contraindicated in a poisoning emergency?
   A. Gastric lavage
   B. Whole bowel irrigation
   C. Syrup of ipecac
   D. Activated charcoal

6. The poison antidote that works by absorbing large amounts of poisonous molecules in the stomach is

A. syrup of ipecac
B. naloxone
C. activated charcoal
D. amyl nitrite

7. The "coma cocktail" consists of
   A. 5% dextrose and 0.45% NS
   B. naloxone, thiamine, 50% dextrose
   C. 50% dextrose and diazepam
   D. naloxone, thiamine, Narcan

8. Which of the following describes the pathophysiology of cyanide poisoning?
   A. Cyanide binds with hemoglobin, preventing oxygen transport
   B. Cyanide paralyzes the central nervous system
   C. Cyanide prevents cellular use of oxygen
   D. Cyanide can only be inhaled

9. A cyanide antidote kit should contain
   A. amyl nitrite ampules
   B. sodium nitrate solution
   C. a sodium thiosulfate solution
   D. all of the above

SCENARIO
Questions 10–11 refer to the following scenario.

Your patient is a 26-year-old male who was barbecuing in his garage with the overhead door half closed. His wife called 911 because he began acting strangely and vomited. You find him walking around the house, disoriented, complaining of a severe headache and nausea.

10. This man is most likely suffering from
    A. carbon monoxide poisoning
    B. acute methanol intoxication
    C. cyanide poisoning
    D. organophosphate poisoning

11. Management of this patient includes
    A. removal from the toxic environment
    B. oxygen administration
    C. transport to a hyperbaric chamber
    D. all of the above

12. Which of the following statements is true regarding caustic agents?
    A. Strong acids tend to cause deeper burns than strong alkalis
    B. Eschar is the result of coagulation from an alkali burn
    C. Strong alkalis produce liquefaction necrosis
    D. Strong alkaline agents tend to pass quickly through the esophagus

SCENARIO

Questions 13–14 refer to the following scenario.

Your patient is a 56-year-old man who presents on the floor with an altered mental status. He is confused and is hallucinating. His heart rate is 180 and he is hypotensive. He shows torsade de pointes on the monitor. You learn that he has no cardiac history, but he is being treated for clinical depression.

13. You suspect he may have taken an overdose of what type of medication?
    A. Beta blockers
    B. Calcium channel blockers
    C. Tricyclics
    D. Benzodiazepines

14. The most important part of your field management of this patient is to
    A. administer flumazenil
    B. administer thiamine
    C. monitor for cardiac dysrhythmias
    D. induce emesis

15. Prozac, Paxil, and Zoloft all belong to a class of drugs known as
    A. monoamine oxidase inhibitors (MAOIs)
    B. selective serotonin reuptake inhibitors (SSRIs)

C. tricyclic antidepressants (TCAs)
D. phenothiazines

16. Your patient takes lithium. He most likely is being treated for
    A. manic-depressive disorder
    B. obsessive-compulsive disorder
    C. hallucinations
    D. chronic pain

17. Sodium bicarbonate is used to alkalinize the urine in all of the following drug overdoses **EXCEPT**
    A. theophylline
    B. tricyclic antidepressants
    C. lithium
    D. salicylates

18. A lethal type of food poisoning caused by improper food storage methods is
    A. *Clostridium botulinum*
    B. *Salmonella*
    C. *E. coli*
    D. scomboid

19. For which of the following bites or stings is there no antivenin?
    A. Black widow spiders
    B. Scorpions
    C. Pit vipers
    D. Brown recluse spiders

SCENARIO

Questions 20–22 refer to the following scenario.

Your patient is a 25-year-old rock climber who was bitten by a rattlesnake and walked to call for help (1 mile). She presents on the ground complaining of weakness, dizziness, and pain at the injection site. She has fang marks on her left leg with oozing. She is nauseated and has vomited twice. Her BP is 80/50; pulse 120 and weak; and skin cool, pale, and clammy to the touch.

20. Rattlesnakes are members of what class of snakes?
    A. *Hymenoptera*

B. Pit vipers

C. Elapidae

D. Coral

21. Which of the following statements is true regarding rattlesnakes?

A. Their bites can result in death within 30 minutes

B. Their bites seldom cause systemic reactions

C. All rattlesnakes have rattles

D. All rattlesnake bites inject poisonous venom

22. Management of a rattlesnake bite includes all of the following EXCEPT

A. applying a constricting band proximal to the wound

B. keeping the patient calm

C. applying ice and compression and elevating the wound

D. immobilizing the extremity

23. Your patient is a 63-year-old homeless male who is a habitual ambulance customer. This evening you find him slumped against a tree in the park, seemingly unconscious. He is alive but responds neither to voice nor to deep pain. Next to him you find a jar labeled "wood alcohol." His BP is 150/90, pulse 90, and respirations 40. He lies in a pool of vomit and reeks of alcohol. This patient is most likely suffering from

A. alcohol intoxication

B. acute methanol poisoning

C. cyanide poisoning

D. none of the above

24. Your patient is a 35-year-old chronic alcoholic who calls you 2 days after leaving the detox unit. He presents with general weakness, tremors of the hands, and sweating and is very anxious. He complains of nausea and vomiting and inability to sleep. His skin is cool and clammy, BP 140/70, pulse 90, and respirations 20. He claims he sees pink elephants behind you and generally acts very strangely. This patient is most likely suffering from

A. acute psychosis

B. delusions

C. acute alcohol withdrawal

D. ethylene glycol poisoning

25. Another name for Rohypnol is

A. ecstasy

B. "date rape" drug

C. MDMA

D. antifreeze

Match the following toxicological emergencies with their respective antidotes:

26. ____ Acetaminophen

27. ____ Atropine

28. ____ Benzodiazepines

29. ____ Nitrates

30. ____ Opiates

A. Flumazenil

B. Naloxone

C. Mucomyst

D. Methylene blue

E. Physostigmine

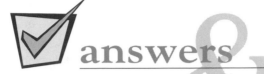

answers & rationales

1.

B. Ingestion is the most common route of entry for toxic exposure. Frequently ingested poisons include household products, petroleum-based agents (gasoline and paint), cleaning agents (alkalis and soaps), cosmetics, prescribed drugs, plants, and foods. (PCPP 3–430   EPC 1457)

2.

C. Inhalation of a poison results in rapid absorption of the toxic agent through the alveolar-capillary membrane. Commonly inhaled poisons include toxic gases; carbon monoxide; ammonia; chlorine; freon; toxic vapors, fumes, or aerosols; carbon tetrachloride; methyl chloride; tear gas; mustard gas; and nitrous oxide. (PCPP 3–430   EPC 1457)

3.

B. Most poisonings by injection result from the bites and stings of insects and animals. Most insects that sting and bite belong to the class *Hymenoptera*, which includes bees, hornets, yellow jackets, wasps, and ants. (PCPP 3–431   EPC 1458)

4.

D. Poison control centers have been set up across the United States and Canada to assist in the treatment of poison victims and to provide information on new products and new treatment recommendations. Centers are usually staffed by physicians, pharmacists, nurses, or poison control specialists trained in toxicology and are available to callers 24 hours a day. (PCPP 3–429   EPC 1456)

5.

C. Once a mainstay (even mothers were told to use it), syrup of ipecac is no longer a recommended method of emergency decontamination. At best, it reduces absorption by only 30%, increases the risk of aspi-ration, and reduces the effectiveness of other oral decontamination agents. (PCPP 3–433   EPC 1460)

6.

C. Activated charcoal promotes gastrointestinal decontamination via its large surface area, which can absorb molecules from the offending poison. (PCPP 3–433   EPC 1460)

7.

B. The "coma cocktail" consists of naloxone, thiamine, and 50% dextrose. (PCPP 3–436   EPC 1463)

8.

C. Cyanide inflicts its damage by inhibiting cytochrome oxidase, an enzyme vital to cellular use of oxygen. Once cyanide enters the body, it acts as a cellular asphyxiant. (PCPP 3–438   EPC 1465)

9.

D. A cyanide antidote kit should contain amyl nitrite ampules, a sodium nitrite solution, and a sodium thiosulfate solution. (PCPP 3–439   EPC 1468)

10.

A. Carbon monoxide is an odorless, tasteless gas that is often the by-product of incomplete combustion. It has more than 200 times the affinity of oxygen to bind with hemoglobin, producing carboxyhemoglobin. Once this molecule has bound with hemoglobin, it is very resistant to removal and causes hypoxia. (PCPP 3–439   EPC 1468)

11.

D. Management of carbon monoxide poisoning includes removing the patient from the toxic environment, administering high concentrations of oxygen, and transporting the victim as soon as possible to a hyperbaric chamber. (PCPP 3–439   EPC 1469)

12.

C. Strong alkaline agents cause injury by inducing liquefaction necrosis, which allows deeper penetration and more extensive burns. Strong acids, on the other hand, produce coagulation, which acts as a protective barrier to further burns. (PCPP 3–443 EPC 1470)

13.

C. Tricyclic antidepressants were once used to treat depression but are on the decline due to their narrow therapeutic index and the availability of safer drugs. However, they are still prescribed. Signs of tricyclic toxicity include an altered mental status, hallucinations, hypotension, and cardiac dysrhythmias, such as torsade de pointes. A severe overdose of tricyclics can result in PEA—pulseless electrical activity. (PCPP 3–445 EPC 1472)

14.

C. Field management of a tricyclic overdose requires standard toxicological therapy, such as managing the ABCs and determining the need for GI decontamination. In addition, sodium bicarbonate may be required. But it is crucial that you perform cardiac monitoring because dysrhythmias are the most common cause of death. (PCPP 3–446 EPC 1473)

15.

B. Paxil, Zoloft, and Prozac belong to a new class of drugs known as selective serotonin reuptake inhibitors (SSRIs). They are prescribed for clinical depression. While the true mechanism of action is unclear, they prevent the reuptake of serotonin, making it more available for the brain. (PCPP 3–447 EPC 1474)

16.

A. Even though its mechanism of action is unclear, lithium remains the drug of choice for treating manic-depressive disorder. (PCPP 3–447 EPC 1474)

17.

A. Sodium bicarbonate is used in the treatment of overdoses of tricyclic antidepressants, lithium, and salicylates to alkalinize the urine to hasten the elimination process. (PCPP 3–448 EPC 1475)

18.

A. *Clostridium botulinum*, the world's most toxic poison, occurs in cases of improper food storage methods, such as canning. (PCPP 3–451 EPC 1478)

19.

D. Since there is no antivenin for a brown recluse spider bite, treatment is mostly supportive. While antivenin exists and is available for the bites and stings of scorpions, black widow spiders, and pit vipers, these all may produce severe reactions themselves. (PCPP 3–455 EPC 1482)

20.

B. Rattlesnakes are members of the pit viper class. Pit vipers are so named because of the intinctive pit between the eye and the nostril on each side of the head. (PCPP 3–458 EPC 1485)

21.

A. A severe bite of a pit viper, such as a rattlesnake, can result in death from shock within 30 minutes. (PCPP 3–458 EPC 1485)

22.

C. Management of a rattlesnake bite includes applying a constrictive band proximal to the wound on the extremity, keeping the patient calm, and immobilizing the extremity. (PCPP 3–459 EPC 1486)

23.

B. Methanol, which is used in a variety of automotive products and cooking fuel, is toxic when ingested. Consumption of as little as 4 cc of methanol has produced blindness, while 10 cc has caused death. It is used occasionally by chronic alcoholics trying to get intoxicated. (PCPP 3–466 EPC 1492)

24.

C. The alcoholic may suffer a withdrawal reaction from either abrupt discontinuence of ingestion after prolonged use or a rapid fall in the blood alcohol level after acute intoxication. Withdrawal symptoms can occur several hours after sudden abstinence and can last up to 5–7 days. (PCPP 3–467 EPC 1494)

25.

B. Rohypnol is a drug used for sexual purposes. It causes sedation and amnesia, like the benzodiazepines. It is commonly known as the "date rape" drug. (PCPP 3–463   EPC 1492)

Matching   (PCPP 3–464–3–465   EPC 1490–1491)

26. **C**   Acetaminophen
27. **E**   Atropine
28. **A**   Benzodiazepines

29. **D**   Nitrates
30. **B**   Opiates

A. Flumazenil
B. Naloxone
C. Mucomyst
D. Methylene blue
E. Physostigmine

28 Hematology

1. Aplastic anemia is caused by
   A. an abnormally high rate of red cell destruction
   B. hemorrhage
   C. failure to produce red cells
   D. hemolysis

2. Most anemic patients will be asymptomatic until their hematocrit drops below _____ %.
   A. 10
   B. 20
   C. 30
   D. 40

3. Sickle cell patients normally will develop which of the following types of crisis?
   A. Vascular occlusions
   B. A drop in hemoglobin
   C. Infections
   D. All of the above

4. Patients suffering from a sickle cell crisis should receive
   A. high-flow oxygen
   B. analgesia
   C. crystalloid fluid challenge
   D. all of the above

5. Which of the following is NOT a complication of polycythemia?
   A. Anemia
   B. Thrombosis
   C. Bleeding abnormalities
   D. Congestive heart failure

6. The most common presenting sign of non-Hodgkin's lymphoma is
   A. anorexia
   B. painless, enlarged lymph nodes
   C. pruritus
   D. fatigue

7. The majority of Hodgkin's lymphoma patients present with
   A. no symptoms
   B. fatigue and anorexia
   C. painful, enlarged lymph nodes
   D. fever

8. You are on a routine transfer and you read that your patient has thrombocytopenia. This means you should watch out for
   A. congestive heart failure
   B. abnormal bleeding and bruising
   C. acute hypoxemia
   D. severe nausea and vomiting

9. A cancerous disorder of plasma cells is known as
   A. DIC
   B. von Willebrand's disease
   C. multiple myeloma
   D. idiopathic thrombocytopenia

10. A white cell count of 19,500 would suggest
   A. leukemia
   B. non-Hodgkin's lymphoma
   C. bacterial infection
   D. leukocytopenia

answers & rationales

1.

C. Aplastic anemia is caused by a failure to produce red blood cells. This can be the result of an iron deficiency, a vitamin B_{12} deficiency, or a chronic disease, such as renal failure. (PCPP 3–493 EPC 1507)

2.

C. Anemia is typically classified as a hematocrit of less than 37% in women and 40% in men. However, most anemic patients will be asymptomatic until their hematocrit drops below 30%. (PCPP 3–492 EPC 1506)

3.

D. Patients with sickle cell disease will develop three types of problems. They will suffer vascular occlusions (because the abnormally shaped cells get stuck), drops in hemoglobin, and infections (because they are immunosuppressed). (PCPP 3–494 EPC 1508)

4.

D. Patients suffering from a sickle cell crisis should receive high-flow oxygen (to maximize oxygen saturation), analgesia (for moderate to severe pain), and crystalloid fluid challenge (to combat dehydration). (PCPP 3–494 EPC 1508)

5.

A. Polycythemia is an abnormally high hematocrit, over 50%, due to abnormally high red cell production. It can cause thrombosis; platelet dysfunction, leading to abnormal bleeding; and, in the most severe cases, congestive heart failure. (PCPP 3–494 EPC 1508)

6.

B. The most common presenting sign of non-Hodgkin's lymphoma is painless, enlarged lymph nodes. (PCPP 3–496 EPC 1510)

7.

A. The majority of Hodgkin's lymphoma patients present with no symptoms. (PCPP 3–496 EPC 1510)

8.

B. Thrombocytopenia is an abnormal decrease in the number of platelets. For this reason, handle your patient carefully and watch for abnormal bleeding or bruising. (PCPP 3–497 EPC 1511)

9.

C. Multiple myeloma is a cancerous disorder of the plasma cells in the bone marrow, which begin to crowd out the healthy cells, leading to a reduction of blood cell production. The patient becomes anemic and prone to infection. (PCPP 3–499 EPC 1513)

10.

C. A normal white cell count is from 5000 to 9000 per cubic millimeter of blood. A count of 10,800 to 23,000 per cubic millimeter suggests a bacterial infection. A count greater than 30,000 per cubic millimeter is called a leukemoid reaction and is suggestive of leukemia. (PCPP 3–495 EPC 1509)

29 Environmental Emergencies

1. The body can generate heat by
   A. shivering
   B. increasing cellular metabolism
   C. exercising strenuously
   D. all of the above

2. Which of the following affects the thermal gradient?
   A. Ambient air temperature
   B. Infrared radiation
   C. Relative humidity
   D. All of the above

3. Heat loss in the form of infrared rays is known as
   A. radiation
   B. convection
   C. conduction
   D. evaporation

4. Heat flows from the skin to the air because of
   A. radiation
   B. convection
   C. conduction
   D. evaporation

5. Heat is carried away from the body by a process known as
   A. radiation
   B. convection
   C. conduction
   D. evaporation

6. The key heat-regulating center is located in the
   A. thymus gland
   B. thalamus
   C. cerebral cortex
   D. hypothalamus

7. When the body becomes too hot, which of the following happens?
   A. Peripheral vasodilation
   B. Decreased cardiac output
   C. Decreased respiratory rate
   D. Increased thermogenesis

8. When the body becomes too cold, which of the following does NOT happen?
   A. Sympathetic stimulation
   B. Piloerection
   C. Vasodilation
   D. Thermogenesis

9. Fever differs from hyperthermia in that
   A. it lowers body temperature
   B. it is a compensatory mechanism
   C. it does not involve the hypothalamus
   D. cooling mechanisms are activated

10. Heat cramps are caused by
    A. a rapid change in extracellular osmolarity
    B. potassium and water losses
    C. increased thermogenesis (shivering)
    D. decreased perfusion of abdominal muscles

11. Heat exhaustion is caused by
    A. increased sodium and water losses
    B. a rapid, dangerous elevation of body temperature
    C. peripheral vasoconstriction
    D. increased circulating blood volume

12. Prehospital management of the heat stroke patient includes all of the following EXCEPT
    A. rapid cooling
    B. oxygen administration
    C. dopamine IV
    D. IV access

13. In which of the following conditions is pre-hospital cooling of the fever patient contraindicated?
   A. Altered mental status
   B. Imminent febrile seizures
   C. Fever >105°F
   D. Fever due to epiglottitis

14. Initial signs of hypothermia include
   A. cool, pale skin
   B. tachycardia
   C. tachypnea
   D. all of the above

15. Prehospital management of the frostbite victim includes all of the following EXCEPT
   A. immersing the frozen part in 102–104°F water
   B. gently massaging the frozen part
   C. elevating the thawed part
   D. covering the thawed part with loose sterile dressings

16. The primary cause of death from drowning is
   A. acid-base abnormality
   B. asphyxia
   C. pulmonary edema
   D. hemodilution

17. Which of the following factors has an impact on drowning survival?
   A. Cleanliness of water
   B. Length of submersion
   C. Age and health of victim
   D. All of the above

18. Which of the following is a result of the mammalian diving reflex?
   A. Tachypnea
   B. Bradycardia
   C. Vasodilation
   D. All of the above

19. Prehospital management of the drowning victim includes all of the following EXCEPT
   A. C-spine management and oxygenation
   B. the Heimlich maneuver
   C. defibrillation as indicated
   D. CPR as indicated

Match the following terms of basic nuclear physics with their respective definitions:

20. ____ Protons
21. ____ Neutrons
22. ____ Electrons
23. ____ Isotopes
24. ____ Alpha particles
25. ____ Gamma rays

   A. Unstable atoms emitting ionizing radiation
   B. Positively charged particles present in all elements
   C. Particles lacking an electrical charge
   D. Negatively charged minute particles
   E. Low-energy particles, easily blocked by clothing
   F. Dangerous, high-energy particles, requiring lead shielding

26. Which of the following is an effect of long-term radiation exposure?
   A. Decreasing leukocytes
   B. Bone marrow damage
   C. Birth defects
   D. All of the above

27. Which of the following factors will have a major effect on the amount of radiation a person absorbs?
   A. Length of time exposed
   B. Shielding
   C. Distance from the source
   D. All of the above

28. According to Boyle's law, 1 liter of air at sea level will be compressed to _____ at a depth of 33 feet of water.
    A. 1000 ml
    B. 500 ml
    C. 333 ml
    D. 250 ml

29. According to Henry's law, at 33 feet below the surface, the quantity of nitrogen and oxygen dissolved in the tissues will be _____ that at sea level.
    A. one-half
    B. three times
    C. two times
    D. four times

30. A person experiencing sinus headache pain, dizziness, and hearing loss after diving too fast may be suffering from
    A. barotrauma
    B. eustachian tube rupture
    C. middle ear infection
    D. all of the above

31. A diver who appears to be intoxicated and takes unnecessary risks may be experiencing
    A. carbon monoxide poisoning
    B. barotrauma
    C. the bends
    D. nitrogen narcosis

32. A diver who holds his breath during ascent may experience
    A. air embolism
    B. pneumothorax
    C. alveoli rupture
    D. all of the above

33. A diver who ascends without allowing time for gradual recompression may experience
    A. air embolism
    B. pneumomediastinum
    C. eustachian tube rupture
    D. the bends

SCENARIO

Questions 34–35 refer to the following scenario.

Your patient is a 23-year-old construction worker who collapsed on the job. The temperature is 88°F with 78% humidity. He presents on the ground, with skin that is hot, wet, and red. He has no medical history according to his coworkers, and there is no Medic-Alert identification. His BP is 90/60, pulse 120, respirations 30 and shallow, lungs clear, chemstrip 100, and axillary temperature 107°F.

34. This patient is most likely suffering from
    A. heat cramps
    B. heat exhaustion
    C. heat stroke
    D. heat prostration

35. Immediate prehospital management of this patient includes all of the following EXCEPT
    A. rapid cooling
    B. oxygenation
    C. IV fluids
    D. vasopressors

36. Glass thermometers are not recommended for prehospital use because
    A. they are easily broken
    B. they do not measure as high or low as necessary
    C. they are difficult to calibrate during long transport times
    D. none of the above

SCENARIO

Questions 37–40 refer to the following scenario.

Your patient is a 38-year-old female who got lost in the woods on a hiking trip. She spent the night in a small cave with overnight temperatures dropping to the mid-twenties. It had rained earlier in the day, and she had no time to dry off before settling in the cave. She was found by searchers at around 10 A.M. the next day. She presents awake but confused and disoriented. She appears very stiff, and her movements are uncoordinated. Her BP is 100/60, pulse 80, respirations slow and shallow, skin cool and pale, chemstrip 120, and axillary temperature 86°F.

37. This person is suffering from
    A. mild hypothermia
    B. mild hyperthermia
    C. severe hypothermia
    D. hyperpyrexia

38. In severe hypothermia, the patient's ECG may show the presence of
    A. delta waves
    B. J waves
    C. coving
    D. ST segment depression

39. Since the nearest hospital is 1 hour by car, which of the following statements is true regarding the prehospital management of this patient?
    A. Rewarming should not be attempted
    B. Heated oxygen should not be administered
    C. External heat should never be applied
    D. The patient must be handled gently

40. If the patient loses consciousness and arrests, prehospital management should include all of the following EXCEPT
    A. CPR
    B. defibrillation
    C. medication administration
    D. heated and humidified oxygen

answers & rationales

1.

D. The human body can generate heat by shivering, by increasing cellular metabolism, and by exercising strenuously. (PCPP 3–506   EPC 1517)

2.

D. Several factors affect a thermal gradient. They include ambient air temperature (the temperature of the surrounding air), infrared radiation (radiation with a wavelength longer than that of visible light), and relative humidity (the percentage of water vapor present in the air). (PCPP 3–506 EPC 1517)

3.

A. Heat loss in the form of infrared rays is called radiation. All objects not at absolute zero temperature will radiate heat. (PCPP 3–507   EPC 1517)

4.

C. Direct contact of the body surface with another, cooler object causes the body to lose heat by conduction. Heat flows from higher-temperature matter to lower-temperature matter. If the ambient air temperature is cooler than the skin temperature, then heat will flow from the skin to the air. (PCPP 3–506   EPC 1517)

5.

B. Heat loss to air currents passing over the body is called convection. (PCPP 3–506   EPC 1517)

6.

D. The temperature-regulating centers are located in the hypothalamus at the base of the brain. This area functions like a thermostat. It produces neurosecretions important in the control of many metabolic activities, including temperature regulation. (PCPP 3–508   EPC 1519)

7.

A. When the body becomes too hot, it attempts to eliminate body heat through five mechanisms: vasodilation, perspiration, decreased heat production, increased cardiac output, and increased respiratory rate. (PCPP 3–508   EPC 1519)

8.

C. When the body becomes too cold, it attempts to preserve heat by engaging the following mechanisms: vasoconstriction, piloerection, increased heat production by shivering, and sympathetic stimulation. (PCPP 3–509   EPC 1520)

9.

B. Fever differs from hyperthermia in that fever is a compensatory mechanism. It is the body's attempt to clear itself of the infectious agent by raising the body temperature. (PCPP 3–516 EPC 1526)

10.

A. Heat cramps are caused primarily by a rapid change in extracellular fluid osmolarity, resulting from sodium and water losses. This causes intermittent painful contractions of various skeletal muscles. (PCPP 3–511   EPC 1522)

11.

A. Heat exhaustion results from excessive water and salt losses due to sweating. Deficiencies in water and sodium combine to cause electrolyte volume and vasomotor regulatory disturbances. (PCPP 3–513   EPC 1523)

12.

C. Prehospital management of the heat stroke patient includes rapid cooling, oxygen administration, IV access, ECG monitoring, and core temperature monitoring. Vasopressors and anti-cholinergic drugs should be avoided. (PCPP 3–514   EPC 1524)

13.

D. Fever should not be treated in the field unless it is extremely high (greater than 105°F), changes in mental status exist, or febrile seizures appear imminent. (PCPP 3–516   EPC 1526)

14.

D. Initial signs of hypothermia are peripheral vasoconstriction and increased cardiac output and respiratory rates. (PCPP 3–517   EPC 1528)

15.

B. Prehospital management of the frostbite victim includes immersing the frozen part in water heated to 102–104°F, elevating the thawed part, and covering the thawed part with loose sterile dressings. (PCPP 3–524   EPC 1534)

16.

B. Deaths due to drowning and near-drowning are primarily caused by asphyxia from airway obstruction in the lungs secondary to the aspirated water or laryngospasm. (PCPP 3–525   EPC 1535)

17.

D. Factors that have an impact on drowning and near-drowning survival rates include the cleanliness of the water, the length of time the victim is submerged, and the age and general health of the victim. (PCPP 3–527   EPC 1537)

18.

B. When a person dives into cold water, he or she reacts to the submersion of the face. This is known as the mammalian diving reflex. As a result of this reflex, breathing is inhibited, the heart rate becomes slower, and vasoconstriction develops in the tissues. (PCPP 3–527   EPC 1537)

19.

B. Prehospital management of the drowning victim includes C-spine management, oxygenation, defibrillation, and CPR as indicated. (PCPP 3–527   EPC 1537)

Matching   (PCPP 3–540   EPC 1550)

20. B   Protons
21. C   Neutrons
22. D   Electrons
23. A   Isotopes
24. E   Alpha particles
25. F   Gamma rays

A. Unstable atoms emitting ionizing radiation
B. Positively charged particles present in all elements
C. Particles lacking an electrical charge
D. Negatively charged minute particles
E. Low-energy particles, easily blocked by clothing
F. Dangerous, high-energy particles, requiring lead shielding

26.

D. Cell damage due to ionizing radiation is cumulative over a lifetime. If a person is exposed to ionizing radiation long enough, he will exhibit a decreased number of white blood cells, possible defects in offspring, an increased incidence of cancer, and various degrees of bone marrow damage. (PCPP 3–541   EPC 1551)

27.

D. The amount of radiation received by a person depends on the source of the radiation, the length of time exposed, the distance from the source, and the shielding between the exposed person and the source. (PCPP 3–542   EPC 1552)

28.

B. Air is compressible. Boyle's law states that for every 33 feet below the surface you dive, the pressure of gas in your lungs doubles, while the volume decreases by one-half. One liter of air at the surface, therefore, is compressed to 500 milliliters at 33 feet below the surface. (PCPP 3–529   EPC 1539)

29.

C. Henry's law states that the amount of gas dissolved in a given volume of fluid is proportional to the pressure of the gas with which it is in equilibrium. Since the body is made up primarily of liquid, gases that are inhaled will be dissolved in the body in proportion to the partial pressure of each breath. The body uses oxygen, but it does not use nitrogen.

Therefore, the primary gas dissolved in the body is nitrogen because it is inert and not used by the body. At 33 feet below the surface, the quantity of oxygen and nitrogen dissolved in the tissues will be two times that at sea level. (PCPP 3–529   EPC 1539)

30.

A. Barotrauma, commonly called "the squeeze," becomes a concern during descent. If the diver cannot equilibrate the pressure between the nasopharynx and the middle ear through the eustachian tube, he can experience middle ear pain. (PCPP 3–530 EPC 1540)

31.

D. Major diving emergencies while at the bottom of the dive involve nitrogen narcosis, commonly called "raptures of the deep." This is due to nitrogen's effect on cerebral function. (PCPP 3–530 EPC 1540)

32.

D. The most serious barotrauma can occur if a diver holds his breath during ascent. As a diver ascends, the air in the lungs, which has been compressed, expands. If it is not exhaled, the alveoli may rupture. If this occurs, the result may be structural damage to the lung and air embolism. This may also produce mediastinal and subcutaneous emphysema or pneumothorax. (PCPP 3–531   EPC 1541)

33.

D. A diver who ascends without allowing time for gradual recompression may experience "the bends." This is a condition that develops in divers subjected to a rapid reduction of air pressure after ascending to the surface following exposure to compressed air. Nitrogen bubbles enter the tissue spaces in small blood vessels. Bubbles produced by rapid decompression are thought to obstruct blood flow and lead to local ischemia, subjecting tissues to anoxia stress. (PCPP 3–532   EPC 1541)

34.

C. This patient is most likely suffering from heat stroke. Heat stroke occurs when the body's hypo-

thalamic temperature regulation is lost, causing uncompensated hyperthermia, which, in turn, causes cell death and physiologic collapse. (PCPP 3–514 EPC 1534)

35.

D. Immediate prehospital management of the heat stroke patient includes cooling the patient rapidly, administering oxygen, establishing IVs, and monitoring the ECG and core temperature. Vasopressors and anticholinergic drugs are contraindicated, since they may inhibit sweating. (PCPP 3–514 EPC 1524)

36.

B. Glass thermometers are not recommended because they usually do not measure above 106°F or below 95°F. (PCPP 3–515   EPC 1525)

37.

C. With a core temperature of less than 90°F, this patient is suffering from severe hypothermia. (PCPP 3–518   EPC 1528)

38.

B. The typical hypothermic ECG shows the presence of J waves, also called Osborne waves. (PCPP 3–520   EPC 1530)

39.

D. Rewarming of this patient should be attempted, since transportation to the hospital will take more than 15 minutes. External application of heat by warm blankets is a safe and effective means of rewarming the hypothermic patient. Another excellent means of rewarming the hypothermic patient is by administering heated and humidified oxygen. Of course, the hypothermic patient should be moved gently. (PCPP 3–520   EPC 1532)

40.

C. Prehospital management of the hypothermic cardiac arrest includes CPR, defibrillation, and administration of heated and humidified oxygen. (PCPP 3–521   EPC 1532)

30 Infectious Disease

DIRECTIONS Each of the questions or incomplete statements below is followed by suggested answers or completions. Select the **one answer** that is best in each case.

1. Which of the following is a government agency that monitors for infectious diseases?
   A. CDC
   B. NIOSH
   C. NFPA
   D. OSHA

2. Normal flora are best described as
   A. highly contagious bacteria
   B. host defenses
   C. opportunistic pathogens
   D. B and C

3. A small, unicellular organism that causes an infection that is treatable by antibiotics is a
   A. bacterium
   B. virus
   C. fungus
   D. parasite

4. Which of the following statements is true regarding infectious agents?
   A. Some bacteria have developed resistance to antibiotics
   B. Secondary infections following antibiotic therapy may be more serious than the original infection
   C. Exotoxins may become deactivated in the presence of heat or light
   D. All of the above

5. A microscopic agent of infection that invades cells and is not treatable by antibiotics is a
   A. bacterium
   B. virus
   C. fungus
   D. parasite

6. Biological agents such as yeasts and molds are examples of
   A. bacteria
   B. viruses
   C. fungi
   D. parasites

7. The parasite that is contracted by eating inadequately cooked pork products is the
   A. pinworm
   B. hook worm
   C. trichina
   D. ascarid

8. Examples of blood-borne diseases include all of the following EXCEPT
   A. hepatitis A
   B. hepatitis B
   C. AIDS
   D. syphilis

9. Examples of airborne diseases include all of the following EXCEPT
   A. meningitis
   B. tuberculosis
   C. measles
   D. hepatitis A

10. Which of the following microorganisms is considered virulent?
    A. HBV
    B. HIV
    C. Syphilis
    D. All of the above

Match the following phases of the infectious process with their respective definitions:

11. ____ Latent period
12. ____ Communicable period
13. ____ Incubation period
14. ____ Seroconversion

15. ____ Window phase
16. ____ Disease period

A. Exposure to appearance of symptoms
B. Onset of symptoms to resolution
C. Cannot transmit infectious agent
D. Exposure to seroconversion
E. Creation of antibodies
F. Transmission of infectious agent is possible

17. In order to test a paramedic for immunity to hepatitis B, it is necessary to
    A. test for the presence of antigens
    B. wait for symptoms to occur
    C. test for the presence of antibodies
    D. none of the above

18. The paramedic should be concerned about infection control procedures
    A. before the incident
    B. during the incident
    C. after the incident
    D. all of the above

19. Appropriate universal precautions include
    A. never recapping needles
    B. wearing gloves during all patient contact
    C. isolating all body fluids
    D. all of the above

20. Which of the following decontamination methods is appropriate for laryngoscope blades and Magill forceps?
    A. EPA-approved disinfectant spray
    B. 1:10 water and bleach solution
    C. EPA-approved germicide
    D. Hot water immersion (200°F)

21. Which of the following statements is true regarding AIDS?
    A. It is transmitted via most body fluids
    B. Paramedics are included in the high-risk group for contracting this disease

C. The disease weakens the body's immune system by affecting T lymphocytes
D. All of the above

22. The most frequent source of AIDS infection in health care workers is
    A. airborne droplets
    B. accidental needle stick
    C. endotracheal intubation
    D. mouth-to-mask ventilation

23. The type of hepatitis transmitted from restaurant workers who fail to wash their hands before handling food is
    A. A
    B. B
    C. C
    D. D

24. A yearly PPD test is necessary to monitor for the presence of which disease?
    A. Hepatitis B
    B. Meningitis
    C. Tuberculosis
    D. AIDS

25. Chicken pox, a childhood disease, may manifest itself later in life in a disease called
    A. varicella
    B. shingles
    C. rubeola
    D. rubella

26. Your patient who presents with general malaise, low-grade fever, headache, and a stiff or sore neck may be suffering from
    A. hepatitis A
    B. meningitis
    C. tuberculosis
    D. AIDS

27. Meningitis is spread primarily by which of the following methods?

A. A needle stick

B. Consumption of contaminated food

C. Blood transfusion

D. A sneeze or cough

28. The childhood disease characterized by fever and salivary gland swelling is

A. mumps

B. rubeola

C. varicella

D. chicken pox

Match the following airborne diseases with their respective characteristics:

29. ____ Influenza

30. ____ Rhinovirus

31. ____ Rubella

32. ____ RSV

33. ____ Pertussis

A. Whooping cough

B. Childhood respiratory infection

C. German measles

D. Common cold

E. Types A, B, and C

34. Cold sores are a form of

A. chlamydia

B. gonorrhea

C. herpes

D. syphilis

Match the following respiratory infections with their respective characteristics:

35. ____ Epiglottitis

36. ____ Croup

37. ____ Pharyngitis

38. ____ Sinusitis

39. ____ Hantavirus

A. Sore throat

B. Caused by *H. influenza*

C. Carried by rodents

D. Laryngotracheobronchitis

E. Inflammation of paranasal sinuses

40. Which of the following statements is true regarding rabies?

A. It is a bacterial disorder

B. The incubation period is less than 1 week

C. Once it invades the brain, it is usually fatal

D. In the past 20 years, rabid squirrels have been the cause of reported cases

41. The classic "bull's-eye" rash is an early sign of

A. Lyme disease

B. tetanus

C. trichomoniasis

D. chancroid

42. The sexually transmitted disease characterized by lower abdominal pain, yellowish vaginal discharge, and pain with intercourse is

A. syphilis

B. gonorrhea

C. AIDS

D. herpes

Match the following sexually transmitted diseases with their respective characteristics:

43. ____ Herpes simplex II

44. ____ Chlamydia

45. ____ Trichomoniasis

46. ____ Chancroid

47. ____ Syphilis

A. Vesicle lesions

B. Four distinct stages

C. Highly contagious ulcer

D. Intracellular parasites

E. Protozoan parasite, main cause of vaginitis

48. The parasitic infestation of the skin of the scalp, trunk, or pubic area transmitted by sharing combs is known as

A. pediculosis

B. lice

C. scabies

D. A and B

49. Nosocomial infections are
   A. caused by rodent bites
   B. caused by mite infestation
   C. acquired in the hospital
   D. highly contagious

50. To minimize your personal risk when caring for a patient with a suspected infectious disease, you should consider
   A. the infectious agent
   B. the host
   C. the environment
   D. all of the above

answers & rationales

1.

A. The U.S. Department of Health and Human Services (DHHS) Centers for Disease Control (CDC) in Atlanta, Georgia, monitors for and tracks the morbidity and mortality rates of infectious diseases. (PCPP 3–550   EPC 1557)

2.

D. Normal flora, also known as host defenses, are organisms that live inside our bodies without ordinarily causing disease. They help keep us disease-free by creating environmental conditions that are not conducive to disease-producing microorganisms, or pathogens. (PCPP 3–550   EPC 1557)

3.

A. Bacteria are small, unicellular organisms that live throughout the environment and frequently cause infection. Most bacterial infections respond to treatment with drugs called antibiotics. (PCPP 3–551   EPC 1558)

4.

D. In recent years, some bacterial strains have developed resistance to antibiotics. Secondary infections following antibiotic therapy may be more serious than the original infection because the protective flora have been eliminated. Exotoxins may become deactivated in the presence of heat or light. This is why the body's normal response to a bacterial infection is fever. (PCPP 3–552   EPC 1559)

5.

B. Most infections are caused by biological agents called viruses. Viruses are referred to as intracellular parasites, since they must invade the cells of the organism they infect. Once inside a cell, they use the various cellular enzymes to replicate and produce more viruses. They cannot produce outside of the host cell, and unlike bacteria, they are very difficult to treat. Once a virus infects a cell, it can be killed only by destroying the infected cell. Drugs have not yet been developed that can selectively destroy cells infected by viruses, while simultaneously leaving uninfected cells unharmed. (PCPP 3–553   EPC 1559)

6.

C. Biological agents such as yeasts and molds are examples of fungi. Fungi are biological agents that can cause human infection, usually found on the skin. (PCPP 3–554   EPC 1561)

7.

C. The trichina is a parasite that is contracted by eating inadequately cooked pork products, such as sausage. (PCPP 3–554   EPC 1561)

8.

A. Blood-borne diseases are those transmitted by contact with the blood or body fluids of an infected person. Blood-borne diseases include AIDS, hepatitis B, hepatitis C, hepatitis D, and syphilis. (PCPP 3–555   EPC 1562)

9.

D. Airborne diseases are those transmitted through the air on droplets expelled during a productive cough or sneeze. Examples of airborne diseases include tuberculosis, meningitis, mumps, measles, rubella, and chicken pox. (PCPP 3–555   EPC 1562)

10.

A. Virulence is the microorganism's strength or ability to infect or overcome the body's defenses. Some organisms, such as the hepatitis B virus (HBV), are very virulent and can remain infectious on a surface for weeks. Some, such as HIV and syphilis, die when exposed to air. (PCPP 3–556 EPC 1563)

Matching (PCPP 3–557 EPC 1564)

11. **C** Latent period
12. **F** Communicable period
13. **A** Incubation period
14. **E** Seroconversion
15. **D** Window phase
16. **B** Disease period

A. Exposure to appearance of symptoms
B. Onset of symptoms to resolution
C. Cannot transmit infectious agent
D. Exposure to seroconversion
E. Creation of antibodies
F. Transmission of infectious agent is possible

17.
C. In order to test a paramedic for immunity to hepatitis B, it is necessary to test for the presence of antibodies. This is known as a titer. (PCPP 3–560)

18.
D. There are four phases of infection control in prehospital care. These include preparations before, response to, patient contact during, and recovery from emergency incidents. (PCPP 3–561 EPC 1565)

19.
D. Appropriate universal precautions include never recapping needles, wearing gloves during all patient contact, and isolating all body fluids. (PCPP 3–562 EPC 1566)

20.
D. Laryngoscope blades and Magill forceps come into contact with the patient's mucous membranes and require high-level decontamination. Use an EPA-approved chemical sterilizing agent, or immerse the object in hot water (176–212°F) for 30 minutes. (PCPP 3–566 EPC 1569)

21.
D. AIDS, a worldwide epidemic and a virtual threat to every individual on this planet, is caused by the human immunodeficiency virus (HIV). It is transmitted through most body secretions and by most body fluids. It weakens the body's immune system by affecting the T lymphocytes. Paramedics are in-

cluded in the high-risk group for contracting this disease. (PCPP 3–570 EPC 1572)

22.
B. The most frequent source of AIDS infection of health care workers is the accidental needle stick. (PCPP 3–571 EPC 1574)

23.
A. Hepatitis A is the most common form of hepatitis. The route of transmission is usually fecal-oral. Patients usually become infected by eating food contaminated with stool from another person infected with the disease. (PCPP 3–574 EPC 1576)

24.
C. A purified protein derivative (PPD) test is necessary to monitor for tuberculosis. It consists of placing a small amount of protein from tuberculosis bacteria into the skin. After 48 hours, the site is examined. If there is a firm, raised area greater than 10 millimeters in diameter, the patient is said to have converted, indicating prior exposure to tuberculosis. (PCPP 3–577 EPC 1579)

25.
B. Chicken pox, a childhood disease, may manifest itself later in life in a disease called shingles. Once a person has been infected, he is usually immune for life, but the virus may remain dormant in the body for many years, generally living in nerves along the back. In later life, the virus may become active, causing shingles. (PCPP 3–581 EPC 1583)

26.
B. Meningitis is the most common central nervous system infection encountered in prehospital care. The disease infects the lining of the brain and spinal cord. It occurs more frequently in children, but adults can also be victims. It is caused by bacteria, viruses, and occasionally fungi. (PCPP 3–582 EPC 1584)

27.
D. Meningitis is primarily transmitted through airborne droplets expelled by a productive cough or sneeze. (PCPP 3–582 EPC 1584)

28.
A. The childhood disease characterized by fever and salivary gland swelling is called mumps. The in-

fection results from the mumps virus, which is transmitted usually through the saliva of an infected person. (PCPP 3–585   EPC 1587)

Matching   (PCPP 3–584   EPC 1588)

29. **E**   Influenza
30. **D**   Rhinovirus
31. **C**   Rubella
32. **B**   RSV
33. **A**   Pertussis

A. Whooping cough
B. Childhood respiratory infection
C. German measles
D. Common cold
E. Types A, B, and C

34.
C. Cold sores are a form of the herpes simplex type one virus. These sorcs are usually found around the mouth and lips. (PCPP 3–588   EPC 1590)

Matching   (PCPP 3–588   EPC 1590)

35. **B**   Epiglottitis
36. **D**   Croup
37. **A**   Pharyngitis
38. **E**   Sinusitis
39. **C**   Hantavirus

A. Sore throat
B. Caused by *H. influenza*
C. Carried by rodents
D. Laryngotracheobronchitis
E. Inflammation of paranasal sinuses

40.
C. Rabies is a viral disorder that affects the nervous system. The incubation period is highly variable, from 9 days to 8 weeks. Once the virus invades the brain, it is usually fatal. In the past 20 years, rabid bats have been the cause of reported cases. (PCPP 3–593   EPC 1594)

41.
A. Lyme disease is transmitted by the infected deer tick. Its bite leaves a ring-like rash, which spreads outward. This is an early sign that disappears with time. (PCPP 3–595   EPC 1597)

42.
B. Gonorrhea is a common sexually transmitted disease. It is characterized by burning urination, yellowish vaginal discharge, and pain with walking or movement such as intercourse. (PCPP 3–596   EPC 1598)

Matching   (PCPP 3–596   EPC 1600)

43. **A**   Herpes simplex II
44. **D**   Chlamydia
45. **E**   Trichomoniasis
46. **C**   Chancroid
47. **B**   Syphilis

A. Vesicle lesions
B. Four distinct stages
C. Highly contagious ulcer
D. Intracellular parasites
E. Protozoan parasite, main cause of vaginitis

48.
D. Lice, or pediculosis, is a parasitic infestation of the skin of the scalp, trunk, or pubic area transmitted by sharing combs. Since they infest rather than break the skin, lice do not causc infcction. (PCPP 3–600   EPC 1602)

49.
C. Nosocomial infections are acquired while in the hospital, especially by patients with compromised immune function. (PCPP 3–601   EPC 1603)

50.
D. To minimize your personal risk when caring for a patient with a suspected infectious disease, you should consider the infectious agent, the host, and the environment. (PCPP 3–603   EPC 1604)

31 Behavioral and Psychiatric Disorders

DIRECTIONS
Each of the questions or incomplete statements below is followed by suggested answers or completions. Select the **one answer** that is best in each case.

1. Which of the following can cause a behavioral emergency?
   A. The patient's personality
   B. Structural changes in the brain
   C. The patient's social place
   D. All of the above

2. Which of the following interviewing techniques is considered appropriate for the behavioral emergency patient?
   A. Using a formal checklist of questions
   B. Never allowing the patient to lead the interview
   C. Pressing the patient for specific answers
   D. Communicating honestly and firmly

3. During long periods of silence, you should
   A. press the patient to keep talking
   B. keep talking yourself
   C. stay calm and relaxed
   D. leave the patient alone

4. If the behavioral emergency patient believes that there are large pink elephants in the room, you should
   A. tell him you see them too
   B. understand they are real for him
   C. tell him there are no pink elephants
   D. tell him he has an obvious psychiatric problem

5. If the distraught patient says he wants to "end it all," you should
   A. let him
   B. try to stop him from talking about it
   C. tell him everything will be all right
   D. try to get him to talk more about it

6. Your priority in any behavioral emergency is
   A. your safety
   B. the patient's safety
   C. the underlying reason for the patient's behavioral problem
   D. the patient's life-threatening injuries

7. Which of the following is **NOT** a cause of delirium?
   A. Parkinson's disease
   B. Substance intoxication
   C. Substance withdrawal
   D. Medical condition

Match the following behavioral terms with their respective definitions:

8. ____ Aphasia
9. ____ Apraxia
10. ____ Agnosia
11. ____ Catatonia
12. ____ Dementia

   A. Failure to recognize objects
   B. Gradual memory and cognitive impairment
   C. Impaired ability to speak
   D. Immobility and stupor
   E. Impaired ability to carry out motor activities

13. The patient who believes he is Jimmy Hoffa and is being chased by mobsters is probably suffering from
   A. manic-depression
   B. paranoid schizophrenia
   C. acute anxiety
   D. none of the above

14. A mood disorder characterized by feelings of helplessness and hopelessness is
   A. anxiety
   B. depression
   C. mania
   D. schizophrenia

15. Which of the following organic causes can mimic depression?
    A. Hyperthyroidism
    B. Hypothyroidism
    C. Cushing's disease
    D. Graves' disease

16. A patient with bipolar disorder usually suffers from
    A. frequent hallucinations
    B. wide mood swings
    C. delusional behavior
    D. altered disorganization

17. Lithium (Lithobid) is often prescribed for _____ patients.
    A. schizophrenic
    B. suicidal
    C. organic brain syndrome
    D. manic-depressive

18. Which of the following statements best describes somatoform disorders?
    A. Patients are preoccupied with physical symptoms
    B. Patients exaggerate common physical symptoms as serious illness
    C. Patients complain of pain unexplained by a physical ailment
    D. All of the above

19. Munchausen syndrome is a type of _____ disorder.
    A. factitious
    B. somatoform
    C. hypochondriasis
    D. dissociative

20. Psychogenic amnesia, multiple personality disorder, depersonalization, and fugue state are all examples of _____ disorder.
    A. factitious
    B. somatoform

C. hypochondriasis
D. dissociative

Match the following types of personality disorders with their respective characteristics:

21. ____ Paranoid
22. ____ Schizoid
23. ____ Schizotypal
24. ____ Antisocial
25. ____ Depersonalizing
26. ____ Histrionic
27. ____ Narcissistic
28. ____ Avoidant
29. ____ Dependent
30. ____ Obsessive-compulsive
31. ____ Kleptomanic
32. ____ Pyromanic
33. ____ Trichotillomanic
34. ____ Bulimic
35. ____ Anorexic

A. Voluntary refusal to eat
B. Social inhibition, inadequacy
C. Distrust and suspicion
D. Impulse to pull out one's hair
E. Disregard for rights of others
F. Recurrent episodes of binge eating/abnormal elimination
G. Feeling detached from oneself
H. Impulse to steal objects not for immediate use
I. Excessive emotions and attention seeking
J. Detachment from social relationships
K. Acute discomfort in close relationships
L. Impulse to set fires
M. Preoccupation with orderliness, perfectionism, control
N. Submissive and clinging behavior
O. Need for admiration, lack of empathy

36. Which of the following is a major suicide risk factor?
    A. Previous attempts

B. Depression

C. Widowed spouses

D. All of the above

37. Headache, palpitations, insomnia, and hyperventilation may be signs of
    A. depression
    B. schizophrenia
    C. anxiety
    D. extrapyramidal symptoms

38. Diazepam (Valium) and lorazepam (Ativan) are examples of _____.
    A. phenothiazines
    B. benzodiazepines
    C. tricyclic antidepressants
    D. antihistamines

39. Haloperidol (Haldol) and chlorpromazine (Thorazine) are examples of _____ medications.
    A. antipsychotic
    B. antianxiety
    C. antidepressant
    D. anti-Parkinson

40. A patient, after receiving chlorpromazine, suddenly presents with dystonia, dyskinesia, and akathisia. Prehospital management of this condition includes
    A. diphenhydramine
    B. diazepam
    C. more chlorpromazine
    D. haloperidol

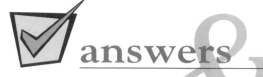

answers & rationales

1.

D. Behavioral emergencies can be caused by a number of underlying problems. These include psychosocial problems (the patient's personality style), sociosocial problems (how the patient acts within society), and organic problems (alcohol, drug abuse, trauma, medical illnesses, dementia, etc.). (PCPP 3–609   EPC 1608)

2.

D. Certain interviewing techniques are appropriate for the behavioral patient. These include communicating self-confidence as well as honesty, firmness, and a reasonable attitude about issues important to the patient and the situation. (PCPP 3–612   EPC 1610)

3.

C. A paramedic should not be afraid of long silent periods during the interview. During this time, the paramedic should remain relaxed and attentive. (PCPP 3–612   EPC 1610)

4.

B. Some behavioral patients have delusions. Avoid being judgmental. When a patient exhibits delusional behavior, understand that this behavior is reality for this patient. (PCPP 3–612   EPC 1612)

5.

D. If your patient expresses suicidal thoughts, stay calm and do not appear uncomfortable. Instead, try to get him to talk more about it and be frank. Ask him if he has ever tried to kill himself or if he has a plan, the means, and the opportunity. (PCPP 3–612   EPC 1611)

6.

A. Your top priority in any behavioral emergency is your own personal safety. (PCPP 3–610   EPC 1609)

7.

A. Delirium is a condition characterized by rapid onset of widespread disorganized thought or confusion. It is caused by medical problems, substance intoxication, or withdrawal, or it may have multiple etiologies. (PCPP 3–615   EPC 1614)

Matching   (PCPP 3–615   EPC 1614)

  8. C   Aphasia
  9. E   Apraxia
10. A   Agnosia
11. D   Catatonia
12. B   Dementia

A. Failure to recognize objects
B. Gradual memory and cognitive impairment
C. Impaired ability to speak
D. Immobility and stupor
E. Impaired ability to carry out motor activities

13.

B. The patient suffering from paranoid schizophrenia often feels that someone, such as the FBI or CIA, is after him. Such paranoia often results from the patient's feeling of self-importance. Some paranoid-schizophrenics become delusional and believe that they are famous figures, such as Jesus Christ or Napoleon. (PCPP 3–616   EPC 1615)

14.

B. Depression is a common psychiatric disorder. It is characterized by feelings of helplessness and hopelessness. (PCPP 3–618   EPC 1617)

15.

B. Certain conditions such as substance abuse, medications, organic brain syndrome, hypothyroidism, and chronic steroid use may mimic depression. (PCPP 3–618   EPC 1607)

16.

B. Bipolar disorder, also called manic-depressive disorder, is a condition characterized by tremendous mood swings from euphoria to debilitating depression. (PCPP 3–619   EPC 1618)

17.

D. Lithium is a drug often prescribed for patients with manic-depressive disorder, also known as bipolar disorder. (PCPP 3–619   EPC 1618)

18.

D. Somatoform disorders are characterized by physical symptoms that have no apparent physiological cause. There are many forms of this disorder. Patients may be preoccupied with physical symptoms. They may exaggerate common physical symptoms as serious illness or complain of pain unexplained by a physical ailment. (PCPP 3–620 EPC 1619)

19.

A. Munchausen syndrome is the severe form of factitious disorder. A factitious disorder is characterized by three criteria: an intentional production of physical signs or symptoms, motivation to assume the "sick role," and external incentives for the behavior. (PCPP 3–621   EPC 1620)

20.

D. Psychogenic amnesia, multiple personality disorder, depersonalization, and fugue state are all examples of dissociative disorder, in which the patient attempts to avoid stress by separating from his core personality. (PCPP 3–621   EPC 1620)

Matching (PCPP 3–622   EPC 1621)

21. **C** Paranoid
22. **J** Schizoid
23. **K** Schizotypal
24. **E** Antisocial
25. **G** Depersonalizing
26. **I** Histrionic
27. **O** Narcissistic
28. **B** Avoidant

29. **N** Dependent
30. **M** Obsessive-compulsive
31. **H** Kleptomanic
32. **L** Pyromanic
33. **D** Trichotillomanic
34. **F** Bulimic
35. **A** Anorexic

A. Voluntary refusal to eat
B. Social inhibition, inadequacy
C. Distrust and suspicion
D. Impulse to pull out one's hair
E. Disregard for rights of others
F. Recurrent episodes of binge eating/abnormal elimination
G. Feeling detached from oneself
H. Impulse to steal objects not for immediate use
I. Excessive emotions and attention seeking
J. Detachment from social relationships
K. Acute discomfort in close relationships
L. Impulse to set fires
M. Preoccupation with orderliness, perfectionism, control
N. Submissive and clinging behavior
O. Need for admiration, lack of empathy

36.

D. Some major suicidal risk factors include previous attempts, history of depression, and widowed spouses. (PCPP 3–624   EPC 1623)

37.

C. Headache, palpitations, insomnia, and hyperventilation may be signs of an acute anxiety attack. Anxiety is a normal response to stress. However, it can build up to such a point that it overwhelms the patient, who then feels helpless and becomes unable to function normally. (PCPP 3–616   EPC 1615)

38.

B. Benzodiazepines such as diazepam (Valium) and lorazepam (Ativan) are prescribed for patients who suffer from acute anxiety attacks because of their sedative effects. (PCPP 3–617   EPC 1616)

39.

A. Haloperidol (Haldol) and chlorpromazine (Thorazine) are examples of antipsychotic medications. They are often used to chemically restrain a violent patient. (PCPP 3–631   EPC 1629)

40.

A. Antipsychotic medications are associated with many side effects. The most common of these are extrapyramidal symptoms. They include dystonia (impaired muscle tone), dyskinesia (a defect in voluntary movement), and akathisia (inability to sit still). Prehospital management of a patient suffering from extrapyramidal symptoms should include the administration of oxygen, establishment of an IV of normal saline, and administration of 50 mg of diphenhydramine IV. (PCPP 3–631   EPC 1629)

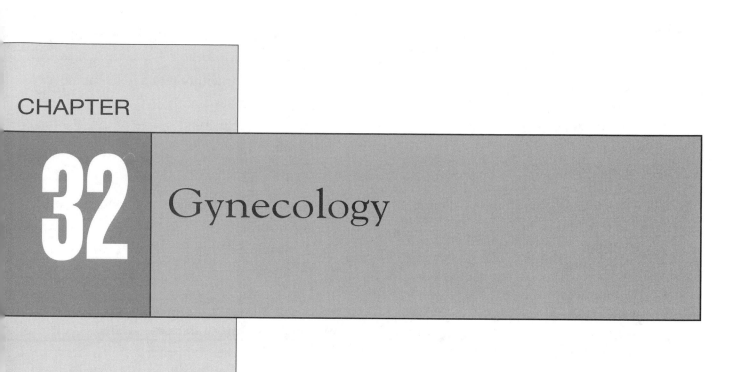

Gynecology

DIRECTIONS Each of the questions or incomplete statements below is followed by suggested answers or completions. Select the **one answer** that is best in each case.

1. Fertilization normally occurs in the
   A. ovaries
   B. fallopian tubes
   C. uterus
   D. vagina

2. The uterine lining that sloughs off during the menstrual period is the
   A. perineum
   B. endometrium
   C. myometrium
   D. perimetrium

3. The function of the ovaries is to produce
   A. estrogen
   B. progesterone
   C. eggs for reproduction
   D. all of the above

4. A fertilized egg normally implants on the
   A. uterine wall
   B. cervix
   C. perineum
   D. urethra

5. The neck of the uterus that dilates to allow passage of the baby is the
   A. perineum
   B. fallopian opening
   C. cervix
   D. endometrium

6. The area surrounding the vagina that sometimes tears during childbirth is the
   A. perineum
   B. endometrium
   C. urethra
   D. cervix

7. A woman's gravidity refers to her number of
   A. pregnancies
   B. viable deliveries
   C. abortions
   D. cesarean sections

8. A woman's parity refers to her number of
   A. pregnancies
   B. viable deliveries
   C. abortions
   D. cesarean sections

9. The beginning of menses is called
   A. menopause
   B. menarche
   C. ovulation
   D. menstruation

10. Physical examination of the gynecological patient includes all of the following EXCEPT
    A. palpating for masses
    B. inspecting for distention and guarding
    C. asking about tenderness
    D. performing an internal vaginal exam

11. Common complications of pelvic inflammatory disease include
    A. sepsis
    B. ectopic pregnancies
    C. pelvic organ adhesions
    D. all of the above

12. The most common site for ectopic pregnancies is
    A. the uterus
    B. a fallopian tube
    C. the cervix
    D. the abdomen

Match the following gynecological problems with their respective definitions:

13. _____ Cystitis
14. _____ Mittelschmerz
15. _____ Endometritis
16. _____ Endometriosis
17. _____ Ruptured ovarian cyst

A. Urinary bladder infection
B. Infection of uterine lining
C. Ovulation pain
D. Fluid-filled pocket left after ovulation
E. Endometrium tissue found in abdomen

18. Prehospital management of female gynecological trauma includes
    A. vaginal packing
    B. IV D₅W run wide open
    C. direct pressure on the external genitalia
    D. none of the above

19. Which of the following statements is true regarding sexual assault?
    A. Most victims are female

B. Paramedics should not question the victim about the incident in the field
C. Paramedics should not perform physical examination of the genitalia
D. All of the above

20. Which of the following statements is true regarding the preserving of evidence in sexual assault cases?
    A. Place all clothing items in the same bag
    B. Use plastic bags for blood-soaked articles
    C. Do not allow the patient to clean her fingernails
    D. Clean the patient's wounds

21. Your female patient who complains of lower abdominal pain while walking and during sexual intercourse, fever, and vaginal discharge may be suffering from
    A. ovarian cyst
    B. mittelschmerz
    C. epididymitis
    D. pelvic inflammatory disease

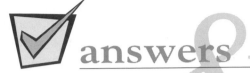

answers & rationales

1.

B. The fallopian tubes are hollow tubes that transport the egg from the ovary to the uterus. Fertilization usually occurs in a fallopian tube. (PCPP 3–641 EPC 257)

2.

B. The endometrium is the lining of the uterus. Each month, under the influence of estrogen and progesterone, the endometrium builds up in preparation for a fertilized ovum. If fertilization does not occur, the lining simply sloughs off. The sloughing off of the uterine lining is referred to as the menstrual period. (PCPP 3–641 EPC 255)

3.

D. The ovaries are the female gonads. They produce estrogen, progesterone, and eggs for reproduction. (PCPP 3–641 EPC 257)

4.

A. The uterus is a small, pear-shaped organ that connects with the vagina. The fertilized egg normally implants on the uterine wall. (PCPP 3–641 EPC 255)

5.

C. The cervix or neck of the uterus is visible through the vagina. During labor, the cervix dilates from its closed state to a diameter of approximately 10 centimeters or more, allowing for passage of the baby. (PCPP 3–641 EPC 255)

6.

A. The perineum is the area surrounding the vagina and anus. This area is sometimes torn during childbirth. (PCPP 3–637 EPC 253)

7.

A. A woman's gravidity refers to her number of pregnancies. A nulligravida has never been pregnant. A primigravida is pregnant for the first time. A multigravida has been pregnant more than once.

Common Obstetrical Terminology

Term	Meaning
antepartum	the time interval prior to delivery of the fetus
postpartum	the time interval after delivery of the fetus
prenatal	the time interval prior to birth, synonymous with antepartum
natal	literally means birth
gravidity	the number of times a woman has been pregnant
primigravida	a woman who is pregnant for the first time
multigravida	a woman who has been pregnant more than once
nulligravida	a woman who has not been pregnant
parity	the number of times a woman has delivered a viable fetus
primipara	a woman who has delivered her first child
multipara	a woman who has delivered more than one baby
nullipara	a woman who has yet to deliver her first child
grand multipara	a woman who has delivered at least seven babies

The gravidity and parity of a woman are expressed in the following convention: G_4P_2. "G" refers to the gravidity, and "P" refers to the parity. (PCPP 3–644 EPC 1631)

8.

B. A woman's parity refers to her number of viable deliveries. A nullipara has never delivered a viable infant. A primipara has delivered one child. A multipara has delivered many babies. (PCPP 3–644 EPC 1632)

9.

B. The female undergoes a monthly hormonal cycle that prepares the uterus to receive a fertilized egg. A girl's menses or menstrual period usually begins when she is between 12 and 14 years old. The beginning of the menses is called menarche. (PCPP 3–641   EPC 257)

10.

D. Physical examination of the gynecological patient should be limited to taking a good history and palpating for masses, distention, and guarding. Never perform an internal vaginal exam in the field. (PCPP 3–645   EPC 1632)

11.

D. Pelvic inflammatory disease (PID) is an infection of the female reproductive tract. Common complications of PID include sepsis, pelvic organ adhesions, and future ectopic pregnancies. (PCPP 3–647   EPC 1634)

12.

B. Ectopic pregnancy is the implantation of a growing fetus in a place where it does not belong. The most common site is within a fallopian tube. (PCPP 3–649   EPC 1636)

Matching   (PCPP 3–648   EPC 1635)

13. A   Cystitis
14. C   Mittelschmerz
15. B   Endometritis
16. E   Endometriosis
17. D   Ruptured ovarian cyst

A. Urinary bladder infection
B. Infection of uterine lining
C. Ovulation pain
D. Fluid-filled pocket left after ovulation
E. Endometrium tissue found in abdomen

18.

C. Prehospital management of female gynecological trauma includes managing a laceration by direct pressure on the external genitalia, maintaining intravascular blood volume by starting an IV of lactated Ringer's, and treating for shock. Never pack the vagina with any material or dressing, regardless of the severity of the bleeding. (PCPP 3–650   EPC 1638)

19.

D. Sexual assault is one of the fastest-growing crimes in the United States. Most victims are female and know their assailants. The victim should not be questioned about the incident in the field, since it is not important from the standpoint of prehospital care to determine whether penetration took place. A medic should never perform a physical examination of the genitalia in a possible sexual abuse case. (PCPP 3–650   EPC 1637)

20.

C. There are certain things a paramedic can do to preserve physical evidence in a sexual assault case: Do not use plastic bags for blood-stained articles; bag each item separately if it must be bagged; handle clothing as little as possible, if at all; do not allow the patient to comb her hair or clean her fingernails; do not allow her to change her clothes, bathe, or douche before the medical exam; and do not clean wounds, if at all possible. (PCPP 3–651   EPC 1638)

21.

D. Pelvic inflammatory disease is an infection of the female reproductive organs. It is usually sexually transmitted. The patient presents with fever, chills, lower abdominal pain, and vaginal bleeding or discharge. In addition, the patient may complain of pain on walking or pain with intercourse. (PCPP 3–647   EPC 1634)

33 Obstetrics

DIRECTIONS Each of the questions or incomplete statements below is followed by suggested answers or completions. Select the **one answer** that is best in each case.

1. Which of the following events occurs 14 days before the beginning of the next menstrual period?
   A. Ovulation
   B. Fertilization
   C. Implantation
   D. Effacement

2. Fertilization normally occurs in the
   A. uterus
   B. placenta
   C. cervical opening
   D. fallopian tubes

3. The umbilical cord contains
   A. one artery and one vein
   B. two arteries and two veins
   C. one artery and two veins
   D. two arteries and one vein

4. The EDC refers to
   A. the date of conception
   B. the due date
   C. the date the mother will be admitted to the hospital
   D. the date of implantation

5. Immediately following birth, which of the following happens?
   A. The ductus arteriosus closes, diverting blood to the lungs
   B. The ductus venosus closes, stopping blood flow from the placenta
   C. The foramen ovale closes, stopping blood flow between the atria
   D. All of the above

6. A woman with a fundal height of 18 centimeters has been pregnant approximately _____ weeks.
   A. 6
   B. 9
   C. 18
   D. 36

7. Which of the following statements is true regarding vital sign changes in the pregnant woman?
   A. The blood pressure rises and the pulse rate falls
   B. The blood pressure falls and the pulse rate rises
   C. The blood pressure and the pulse rate rise
   D. The blood pressure and the pulse rate fall

8. The bulging of the baby's head past the opening of the vagina is called
   A. effacement
   B. primipara
   C. prolapsing
   D. crowning

Match the following types of abortions with their respective definitions:

9. ____ Spontaneous
10. ____ Incomplete
11. ____ Criminal
12. ____ Therapeutic
13. ____ Elective

A. Abortion performed to save the mother's life
B. Some fetal tissue passed
C. Miscarriage
D. Abortion performed by nonlicensed person
E. Abortion requested by mother

14. The first stage of labor begins with the
   A. crowning of the infant's head
   B. dilation of the cervix
   C. delivery of the baby
   D. onset of uterine contractions

15. The second stage of labor begins with the
    A. crowning of the infant's head
    B. dilation of the cervix
    C. delivery of the baby
    D. onset of uterine contractions

16. The third stage of labor begins with the
    A. crowning of the infant's head
    B. dilation of the cervix
    C. delivery of the baby
    D. onset of uterine contractions

17. Complete dilation of the cervix is considered to be
    A. 5 cm
    B. 10 cm
    C. 15 cm
    D. 20 cm

18. Management of a patient with postpartum hemorrhage includes all of the following EXCEPT
    A. fundal massage
    B. pitocin IV
    C. PASG
    D. vaginal packing

19. Which of the following distinguishes preeclampsia from eclampsia?
    A. Vaginal bleeding
    B. Visual disturbances
    C. Grand mal seizures
    D. Peripheral edema

20. Magnesium IV may be ordered for which of the following situations?
    A. Lower abdominal pain
    B. Postpartum hemorrhage
    C. Eclamptic seizures
    D. Preterm labor pains

SCENARIO

Questions 21–23 refer to the following scenario.

Your patient is a 19-year-old woman who presents with severe lower abdominal pain and vaginal bleeding. She claims she is not pregnant but has not had her period for at least 7 weeks. She also complains of weakness, nausea, and vomiting. She admits to being sexually active with multiple partners. She was seen in the ED for several cases of PID in the past 2 years. Her BP is 90/60, pulse 110, respirations 24, and skin cool and clammy.

21. You should suspect
    A. abruptio placenta
    B. placenta previa
    C. PID
    D. ruptured ectopic pregnancy

22. Her problem was caused by
    A. the premature separation of the placenta from the uterine wall
    B. the uterus covering the cervical opening
    C. an inflamed appendix
    D. implantation of the fertilized ovum in a fallopian tube

23. Management of this patient includes all of the following EXCEPT
    A. IV fluids
    B. vaginal packing
    C. PASG
    D. high-flow oxygen

SCENARIO

Questions 24–27 refer to the following scenario.

Your patient is a 26-year-old 30-weeks-pregnant patient who complains of severe, tearing abdominal pain and some minor vaginal bleeding. Upon palpation, her abdomen is very tender, and her uterus seems to be tightly contracted. Fetal heart tones are absent. She is multigravida, but nullipara.

24. You should suspect
    A. abruptio placenta
    B. placenta previa
    C. miscarriage
    D. ectopic pregnancy

25. Her problem was caused by
    A. the premature separation of the placenta from the uterine wall
    B. the uterus covering the cervical opening
    C. a spontaneous abortion
    D. implantation of the fertilized ovum in a fallopian tube

26. This patient's pregnancy history includes
    A. one pregnancy and one birth
    B. many pregnancies and one birth
    C. one pregnancy and no births
    D. many pregnancies and no births

27. Management of this patient includes all of the following EXCEPT
    A. IV fluids
    B. vaginal packing
    C. PASG
    D. high-flow oxygen

SCENARIO

Questions 28–30 refer to the following scenario.

Your patient is a 30-year-old multigravida in her thirtieth week. She presents with bright red vaginal bleeding but denies any abdominal pain. Her uterus is soft and feels "out of place." Her problem began following sexual intercourse with her husband.

28. You should suspect
    A. abruptio placenta
    B. placenta previa
    C. miscarriage
    D. ectopic pregnancy

29. Her problem was caused by
    A. the premature separation of the placenta from the uterine wall
    B. the uterus covering the cervical opening
    C. a spontaneous abortion
    D. implantation of the fertilized ovum in a fallopian tube

30. Management of this patient includes all of the following EXCEPT
    A. IV fluids
    B. vaginal exam
    C. PASG
    D. high-flow oxygen

31. Which of the following statements is true regarding the pregnant trauma patient?
    A. Overt signs of shock are seen early
    B. The earlier the pregnancy, the greater the likelihood for fetal injury
    C. The mother's body will shunt blood to the fetus following acute blood loss
    D. None of the above

32. The proper treatment for a normovolemic patient with supine-hypotensive syndrome is
    A. Trendelenburg positioning
    B. left lateral recumbent positioning
    C. furosemide 40 mg IV
    D. dopamine 5 mcg/kg/min IV

33. Which of the following statements is true regarding gestational diabetes?
    A. It normally occurs in the first trimester
    B. Prehospital management of diabetic emergencies is the same as in the non-pregnant patient
    C. The younger the mother, the higher the incidence
    D. All of the above

34. The difference between Braxton-Hicks contractions and true labor is
    A. cervical changes
    B. intensity of pain
    C. presence of blood discharge
    D. none of the above

35. Airway maintenance of the infant during a breech birth is accomplished by
    A. inserting an endotracheal tube
    B. using a meconium aspirator
    C. using a nasopharyngeal airway
    D. inserting two fingers into the vagina

36. If the umbilical cord is prolapsed, you should
    A. push it back into the vagina
    B. attempt to deliver the baby
    C. pull on the cord
    D. transport immediately

37. If the baby presents with thick meconium staining around the mouth and nose, you should
    A. intubate and suction the trachea after initial ventilation
    B. intubate and suction the trachea before initial ventilation
    C. suction the oropharynx with a bulb syringe and ventilate
    D. use a high-pressure demand valve to ventilate

38. A few days following delivery of the baby, the mother complains of sudden onset of sharp chest pain and severe shortness of breath. The most likely cause of her condition is
    A. acute myocardial infarction
    B. uterine rupture
    C. uterine inversion
    D. pulmonary embolism

39. For which of the following complications of delivery should you NOT attempt to deliver the baby in the field?
    A. Shoulder dystocia
    B. Cephalopelvic disproportion
    C. Precipitous delivery
    D. Multiple births

40. A baby whose body is pink, whose extremities are blue, who has a pulse rate of 88, and who is crying strongly and actively moving receives an APGAR score of
    A. 4
    B. 6
    C. 8
    D. 10

answers & rationales

1.

A. Fourteen days before the beginning of the next menstrual period, the ovum is released from the ovary into the abdominal cavity. This is known as ovulation.   (PCPP 3–656   EPC 1641)

2.

D. Fertilization is the combination of the female ovum and the male spermatozoa. This usually takes place in a fallopian tube.   (PCPP 3–657   EPC 1642)

3.

D. The placenta is attached to the developing fetus by the umbilical cord. This cord normally contains two arteries and one vein. (PCPP 3–657   EPC 1642)

4.

B. The estimated date of confinement (EDC) is the mother's due date. (PCPP 3–661   EPC 1645)

5.

D. The fetal circulation changes immediately at birth. As soon as the baby takes a breath, the ambient pressure in the lungs decreases dramatically. Because of this pressure change, the ductus arteriosus closes, diverting blood to the lungs. In addition, the ductus venosus closes, stopping blood flow from the placenta. The foramen ovale also closes as a result of pressure changes in the heart, stopping blood flow from the right to the left atrium. (PCPP 3–662   EPC 1646)

6.

C. The fundal height is the distance from the pubis to the top of the uterine fundus. Each centimeter of fundal height roughly corresponds to a week of gestation. Therefore, a women with a fundal height of 18 centimeters has been pregnant approximately 18 weeks. (PCPP 3–666   EPC 1650)

7.

B. Because of normal changes occurring in the cardiovascular system of the pregnant woman, her blood pressure tends to be lower and her pulse rate tends to be faster during pregnancy. (PCPP 3–659 EPC 1644)

8.

D. Crowning is the bulging of the fetal head past the opening of the vagina during a contraction. It is an indication of an impending delivery. (PCPP 3–667 EPC 1664)

Matching   (PCPP 3–670)

9. C Spontaneous
10. B Incomplete
11. D Criminal
12. A Therapeutic
13. E Elective

A. Abortion performed to save the mother's life
B. Some fetal tissue passed
C. Miscarriage
D. Abortion performed by nonlicensed person
E. Abortion requested by mother

14.

D. The first stage of labor begins with the onset of uterine contractions and ends with the complete dilation of the cervix. It lasts approximately 8 hours in nulliparous women and 5 hours in multiparous women. (PCPP 3–680   EPC 1663)

15.

B. The second stage of labor begins with the complete dilation of the cervix and ends with the delivery of the fetus. In nulliparous patients, the second stage lasts approximately 50 minutes, and in multiparous women, it lasts approximately 20 minutes. (PCPP 3–680   EPC 1663)

16.

C. The third stage of labor begins with the delivery of the fetus and ends with the delivery of the placenta. The delivery of the placenta usually occurs within 30 minutes after birth. (PCPP 3–681   EPC 1664)

17.

B. Complete dilation of the cervix is considered to be 10 centimeters. (PCPP 3–680   EPC 1663)

18.

D. Postpartum hemorrhage is the loss of 500 milliliters or more of blood in the first 24 hours following delivery. Prehospital management of the postpartum hemorrhage patient includes administering oxygen and beginning external fundal massage, administering large-bore IVs of normal saline or lactated Ringer's, and applying antishock trousers. Never pack the vagina. (PCPP 3–694 EPC 1675)

19.

C. Eclampsia is the most serious manifestation of hypertensive disorders of pregnancy. It is characterized by grand mal seizure activity. (PCPP 3–675 EPC 1657)

20.

C. Magnesium sulfate may be ordered for eclamptic seizures. (PCPP 3–675   EPC 1658)

21.

D. Ectopic pregnancy is difficult to diagnose in the field. However, any woman of childbearing age who presents with lower abdominal pain, vaginal bleeding, and a late menstrual period should be suspected of having a ruptured ectopic pregnancy. (PCPP 3–671   EPC 1654)

22.

D. Ectopic pregnancy is the implantation of a fertilized ovum outside of the uterus, most commonly in a fallopian tube. The ovum, however, can implant anywhere else in the abdominal cavity. (PCPP 3–671   EPC 1654)

23.

B. Management of the patient with a suspected ruptured ectopic pregnancy includes treatment for shock, IV fluids, pneumatic antishock garment, and high-flow oxygen. (PCPP 3–672   EPC 1655)

24.

A. Any pregnant patient in her third trimester who complains of tearing abdominal pain and vaginal bleeding should be suspected of having an abruptio placenta. (PCPP 3–673   EPC 1656)

25.

A. Abruptio placenta is the premature separation of the placenta from the wall of the uterus. The separation can be either partial or complete. (PCPP 3–673   EPC 1656)

26.

D. This patient is multigravida and nullipara. Gravida refers to her number of pregnancies (many). Her parity refers to her number of viable births (none). (PCPP 3–664   EPC 1648)

27.

B. Management of this patient includes IV fluids, pneumatic antishock garment (legs only), and high-flow oxygen, generally treating for shock. (PCPP 3–674   EPC 1657)

28.

B. This patient probably has placenta previa. Her history of third-trimester pregnancy, multigravida, and bleeding following intercourse is consistent with this diagnosis. (PCPP 3–672 EPC 1655)

29.

B. Placenta previa is the attachment of the placenta very low in the uterus so that it partially or completely covers the internal cervical opening. (PCPP 3–672   EPC 1655)

30.

B. Treatment for this patient is aimed at treating for shock: IV fluids, pneumatic antishock garment, and high-flow oxygen. (PCPP 3–673   EPC 1656)

31.

D. During pregnancy, overt signs of shock are late and often inconsistent. The later the pregnancy, the larger the gravid uterus, and the greater the likelihood of fetal injury. The mother's body will shunt blood away from the fetus following acute blood loss. (PCPP 3–668   EPC 1652)

32.

B. Supine-hypotensive syndrome usually occurs late in pregnancy when the large uterus compresses the inferior vena cava when the mother lies in a supine position. If she is normovolemic and shows no signs of dehydration, place her in the left lateral position or elevate her right hip to decompress the vena cava. This is known as caval decompression. (PCPP 3–668   EPC 1661)

33.

B. Gestational diabetes usually occurs in the last 20 weeks of pregnancy, when placental hormones cause an increased resistance to insulin and a decreased glucose tolerance. Prehospital management of a diabetic emergency (hypoglycemia or hyperglycemia) is the same as with the nonpregnant patient. (PCPP 3–677   EPC 1660)

34.

A. In true labor contractions, the cervix effaces (thins and shortens). During Braxton-Hicks contractions, also known as false labor, there are no cervical changes. (PCPP 3–678   EPC 1660)

35.

D. During a breech birth, the baby's face may be pressed against the vaginal wall as he attempts to take a breath. In this case, you must insert two fingers in a "V" shape into the vagina and push the vaginal wall away from the infant's nose. (PCPP 3–690   EPC 1670)

36.

D. If the umbilical cord is prolapsed, you should not try to push it back into the vagina, attempt to deliver the baby, or pull on the cord. Simply place the mother in Trendelelburg or knee-chest position, administer high-flow oxygen, apply a moist dressing to the presenting part, and transport immediately. (PCPP 3–692   EPC 1672)

37.

B. Meconium is a sign of fetal distress. The thicker and darker it is, the worse it is and the higher the infant mortality rate is. If the meconium is thin and watery, merely suction it with a bulb syringe and allow the infant to breathe as you normally would. If it is thick and dark (some describe it as axle grease), you must remove as much of it as possible before the infant aspirates it into the lungs. Immediately intubate the infant and suction the trachea prior to allowing ventilation. (PCPP 3–694   EPC 1675)

38.

D. Pulmonary embolism is the presence of a blood clot in the pulmonary vasculature system. It is most often caused by a thrombus that developed during pregnancy and appears to occur more frequently following cesarean section than vaginal delivery. (PCPP 3–696   EPC 1677)

39.

B. Cephalopelvic disproportion occurs when the infant's head is too big to pass through the maternal pelvis easily. There may be strong contractions but generally labor does not progress. The usual management of this condition is cesarean section. Administer oxygen, establish IV access, and transport the mother immediately to the hospital. (PCPP 3–693   EPC 1675)

40.

C. The APGAR score table is as follows: (PCPP 3–689   EPC 1670)

Element	0	1	2
Appearance	Body and extremities blue, pale	Body pink, extremities blue	Completely pink
Pulse rate	Absent	<100	>100
Grimace	No response	Grimace	Cough, cry, sneeze
Activity	Limp	Some flexion	Active
Respiratory effort	Absent	Slow and irregular	Strong cry

34

Trauma and Trauma Systems

DIRECTIONS Each of the questions or incomplete statements below is followed by suggested answers or completions. Select the **one answer** that is best in each case.

1. Serious and life-threatening injuries occur in _____% of trauma patients.
   A. <10
   B. 15–25
   C. 30–40
   D. >50

2. In 1990, the American College of Surgeons worked to pass the _____, which helped develop trauma systems.
   A. Highway Safety Act
   B. EMS Systems Act
   C. COBRA
   D. Trauma Care Systems Act

3. Guidelines to aid the prehospital provider in determining which patients require immediate transport to a trauma center are known as
   A. mechanism of injury standards
   B. injury severity indexes
   C. standing orders
   D. trauma triage criteria

4. Which of the following adult patients require rapid transport to a trauma center?
   A. Adult who falls 10 feet
   B. Passenger in a car in which driver died
   C. Patient ejected from vehicle
   D. Motorcycle driver thrown from bike
   E. Passenger in a compartment intruded by 24 inches
   F. Victim with flail chest
   G. Victim with femur fracture
   H. Victim with respirations of 24, systolic BP of 98, pulse of 110
   I. Victim shot in the wrist
   J. Patient with systolic BP of 88 and pulse of 130
   K. Ambulatory patient from rollover with no signs of serious impact
   L. Patient with extrication time of 35 minutes
   M. Patient with unstable pelvis
   N. Patient with facial burns
   O. Patient with lower extremity paralysis

5. Which of the following children requires rapid transport to a trauma center?
   A. Child who fell from 12-foot roof
   B. Child in bicycle/vehicle collision
   C. Unrestrained child in vehicle collision at medium speed
   D. All of the above

6. The Golden Hour begins at the time of _____ and ends at the time of _____.
   A. dispatch, arrival at the hospital
   B. injury, surgery
   C. arrival at the scene, departure to the hospital
   D. none of the above

7. Disdvantages to using an air medical service (helicopter) include
   A. limited space for inflight care
   B. distracting engine noise
   C. expense
   D. all of the above

8. "Let's Not Meet by Accident" is a/an
   A. ad campaign by NHTSA
   B. public television documentary
   C. public education program for high schools
   D. pamphlet denouncing drunk driving

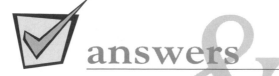
1.

A. Serious and life-threatening injuries occur in fewer than 10% of trauma patients. That's the good news. The bad news is that prehospital care providers can do little to stabilize these patients because they involve major head injury or body cavity hemorrhage. In these cases, the best care includes rapid transport to a trauma center. (PCPP 4–5   EPC 815)

2.

D. In 1990, the American College of Surgeons worked to achieve passage of the Trauma Care Systems Act, which helped establish guidelines, funding, and state-level leadership and support for the development of trauma systems. (PCPP 4–6   EPC 816)

3.

D. Trauma triage criteria are guidelines that help prehospital personnel determine which patients require immediate transportation to a trauma center. They identify the mechanism of injury that can cause serious internal trauma, and they establish the physical or clinical findings that reflect serious internal injury. (PCPP 4–9   EPC 819)

4.

The following mechanisms of injury and physical findings indicate rapid transportation to a trauma center: B, C, D, E, F, I, J, L, M, N, O (PCPP 4–12   EPC 822)

Falls greater than 20 feet
Death of a car occupant
Pedestrian/bicyclist struck by a vehicle traveling over 5 mph
Ejection from the vehicle
Severe vehicle impact
Rollover with signs of serious impact
Motorcycle impact greater than 40 mph
Extrication time greater than 20 minutes
Revised trauma score less than 11
Glasgow Coma Score less than 14
Pulse greater than 120 or less than 50

Systolic blood pressure less than 90
Respiratory rate less than 10 or greater than 29
Penetrating trauma except for distal extremities
2 or more proximal long bone fractures
Flail chest
Pelvic fractures
Limb paralysis
Burns to more than 15% of body surface area
Burns to the face or airway

5.

D. Significant mechanism of injury considerations with infants and children include the following: (PCPP 4–12   EPC 822)

Falls of greater than 10 feet
Bicycle/vehicle collisions
Vehicle collisions at medium speed
Unrestrained child in vehicle collisions

6.

B. The Golden Hour begins at the time of injury and ends with the time of surgery. Trauma research done at the University of Maryland concluded that critical trauma victims survived if surgical repair of their injuries occurred within 1 hour. (PCPP 4–10   EPC 820)

7.

D. Air medical services are a valuable patient transportation option, but there are disdvantages. These include limited space for inflight care, engine noise, expense, adverse weather conditions, and the unpredictable nature of combative patients. (PCPP 4–10   EPC 820)

8.

C. "Let's Not Meet by Accident" is a public education program aimed at high school children that reinforces safe driving. The program is taught in hospital emergency departments by paramedics, nurses, and physicians, who stress the results of unsafe driving practices. (PCPP 4–12   EPC 822)

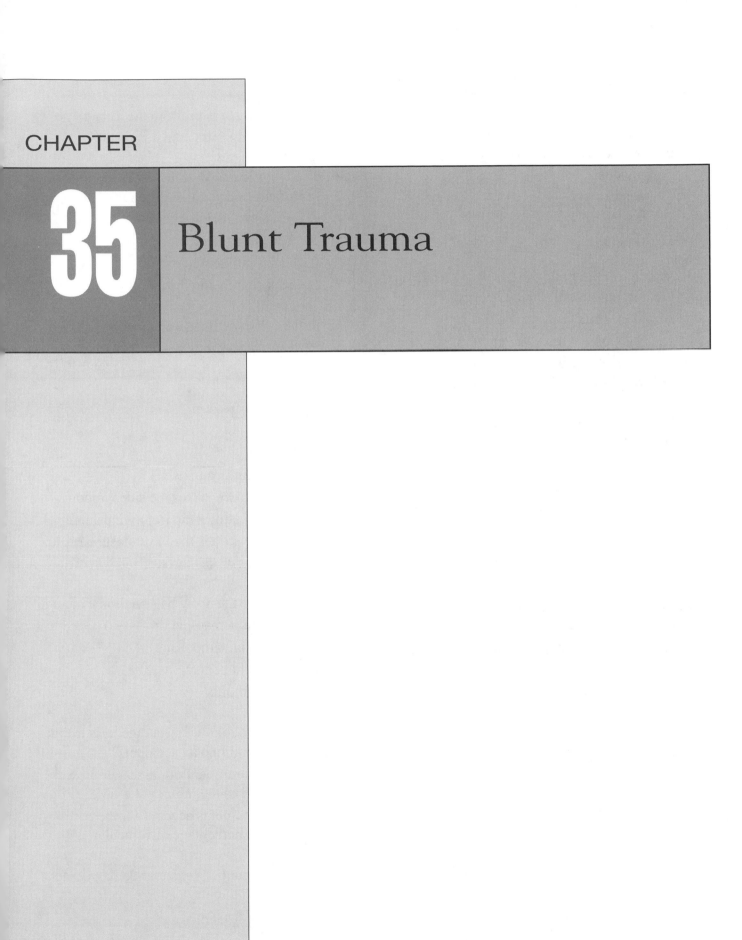

DIRECTIONS Each of the questions or incomplete statements below is followed by suggested answers or completions. Select the **one answer** that is best in each case.

1. A car traveling at 55 mph will tend to remain traveling at 55 mph until something stops it or slows it down. This is known as the law of
   A. kinetics
   B. inertia
   C. energy
   D. motion

2. Which of the following will generate the greatest amount of kinetic energy?
   A. 20 lb. object traveling at 50 mph
   B. 30 lb. object traveling at 40 mph
   C. 40 lb. object traveling at 30 mph
   D. 50 lb. object traveling at 20 mph

3. In an automobile collision, there are five events that occur. Place them in chronological order:
   A. body collision
   B. additional impacts
   C. secondary collision
   D. organ collision
   E. vehicle collision

4. During your scene assessment, you learn that the driver wore a lap belt only. Based on this information, what types of injuries would you expect?
   A. Head and neck
   B. Chest
   C. Intra-abdominal or lower spine
   D. Pelvic and femur fractures

5. Your patient was a restrained driver in a two-car frontal impact collision. You notice also that his airbag was deployed. He complains only of a burning in his eyes. What is the most likely cause of his complaint?
   A. A preexisting eye problem
   B. Residue from the airbag

C. Corneal abrasion from the airbag
D. Increasing intracranial pressure

6. The recommended child safety seat position for infants and small children is the
   A. front seat facing the front
   B. front seat facing the rear
   C. back seat facing the front
   D. back seat facing the rear

7. In the urban setting, which of the following types of impact is most common?
   A. Frontal
   B. Lateral
   C. Rotational
   D. Rear end

8. Axial loading occurs when
   A. the shoulder strikes the side window
   B. the head strikes the front windshield
   C. the knee strikes the lower dashboard
   D. the chest strikes the steering wheel

9. Injuries from the paper bag syndrome include
   A. subdural hematoma
   B. pericardial tamponade
   C. lacerated trachea
   D. pneumothorax

10. Which of the following statements is true regarding lateral impact accidents?
    A. A greater amount of passenger protection lessens the injury pattern
    B. These accidents account for the smallest percentage of vehicular deaths
    C. The amount of vehicular damage exaggerates the injury pattern
    D. None of the above

11. The most commonly seen injury associated with rear-impact accidents is
    A. kidney laceration
    B. lumbar spine fracture
    C. cervical spine injuries
    D. cardiac contusion

12. Figures from states that require mandatory alcohol-level testing after fatal automobile collisions reveal that _____ % of the drivers were intoxicated.
    A. <10
    B. 25
    C. 40
    D. >50

13. Which body area is associated with the highest mortality from motor vehicle trauma?
    A. Head
    B. Chest/abdomen
    C. Lower extremities
    D. Pelvis

14. Which of the following injury patterns is most associated with frontal motorcycle accidents in which the driver is ejected?
    A. Lateral pelvis dislocations
    B. Bilateral femur fractures
    C. Spleen and liver lacerations
    D. Crushing injuries

15. Which of the following statements is true regarding pedestrian accidents?
    A. Adults tend to turn away from the oncoming car prior to impact
    B. Children tend to face the oncoming car prior to impact

C. Adults are often thrown up and over the bumper
D. All of the above

16. Primary injuries from a blast include
    A. extremity fractures
    B. liver lacerations
    C. lung injuries
    D. impaled objects

17. Secondary injuries from a blast include
    A. extremity fractures
    B. liver lacerations
    C. lung injuries
    D. impaled objects

18. Tertiary injuries from a blast include
    A. extremity fractures
    B. liver lacerations
    C. lung injuries
    D. impaled objects

19. When assessing falls, you should focus your attention on
    A. the height of the fall
    B. the surface the victim fell onto
    C. the body part that hit first
    D. all of the above

20. The recommended method for immobilizing a football player's head and neck on a long board is to
    A. keep both helmet and shoulder pads on
    B. remove helmet, keep shoulder pads on
    C. remove shoulder pads, keep helmet on
    D. remove both helmet and shoulder pads
    E. A or D

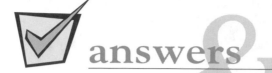

answers & rationales

1.

B. Sir Isaac Newton described the law of inertia. It states that an object at rest tends to remain at rest, while an object in motion tends to remain in motion unless acted on by an external force. Therefore, a car traveling at 55 mph will tend to remain traveling at 55 mph until something stops it (i.e., another car, tree, telephone pole, wall) or slows it down (i.e., brakes, road friction, gravity). (PCPP 4–20   EPC 826)

2.

A. Kinetic energy is the energy of motion. It can be measured by the following formula:

$$\frac{\text{Mass (weight)} \times \text{Velocity}^2}{2}$$

Using this formula, speed becomes the most important factor. Even the lightest object (20 lbs.) traveling at the fastest speed (50 mph) will generate the greatest amount of kinetic energy. (PCPP 4–20   EPC 826)

3.

First, you have the vehicle collision (car hits tree), then the body collision (body hits dash and windshield), then the organ collision (internal organs hit sternum and rib cage), then the secondary collisions (back-seat grocery bags hit front-seat passengers), and, finally, any additional impacts (another car fails to break and hits you). E, A, D, C, B (PCPP 4–23   EPC 829)

4.

C. When the lap belt is worn without the shoulder straps, the victim suffers a sudden folding of the body at the waist, resulting in intra-abdominal and lower spine injuries. (PCPP 4–26   EPC 832)

5.

B. The residue from the airbag deployment may cause eye irritation. This can be relieved by gentle irrigation with sterile water. (PCPP 4–27   EPC 833)

6.

D. With infants and very small children, the child safety seat should be positioned in the back seat facing the rear. As the child grows, the seat can be turned to face the front. (PCPP 4–28   EPC 834)

7.

C. In a rotational impact, the auto is struck from an oblique angle and rotates as the collision forces are expended. Rotational impacts account for 38% of all motor vehicle collisions in the urban setting. In the rural setting, anticipate a greater percentage of frontal impacts. (PCPP 4–28   EPC 834)

8.

B. Axial loading is the application of forces of trauma along the axis of the spine. When the head hits the windshield, that force is transmitted down the cervical spine, often causing compressions of those vertebrae. (PCPP 4–31   EPC 837)

9.

D. The paper bag syndrome is a common injury process associated with steering wheel impact. The driver takes a deep breath in anticipation of the collision. When the chest impacts the steering wheel, lung tissue ruptures, much like an inflated paper bag caught between clapping hands. Pneumothorax and pulmonary contusion may result. (PCPP 4–29   EPC 835)

10.

D. Lateral impacts account for 15% of all auto accidents, yet they are responsible for 22% of vehicular fatalities. The amount of structural steel between the impact side and the vehicle interior is greatly reduced. When a lateral impact occurs, the index of suspicion for serious internal injuries should be higher than vehicle damage alone suggests. (PCPP 4–32   EPC 837)

11.

C. In rear-end impact, the collision force pushes the auto forward, while the vehicle seat propels the occupant forward. If the headrest is not up, the head is unsupported and remains stationary. The neck extends severely, while the head rotates backwards. Cervical spine injuries are common with rear-end collisions. (PCPP 4–34   EPC 839)

12.

D. In states with mandatory alcohol testing after fatal auto collisions, figures reveal that over 50% of the drivers were intoxicated. (PCPP 4–37   EPC 842)

13.

A. Trauma to the head (47.7%) and body cavity (37.3%) accounts for 85% of vehicular mortality. This is why you focus on the head, neck, chest, abdomen, and pelvis during your rapid trauma assessment. (PCPP 4–37   EPC 842)

14.

B. In frontal or head-on motorcycle accidents, the impact often propels the rider upward and forward. Occasionally the rider traps both femurs at the handlebars, causing bilateral fractures. (PCPP 4–38   EPC 843)

15.

B. In contrast to adults, children turn toward an oncoming vehicle. Because they are smaller, the injury is located anatomically higher, as the bumper fractures the femur or pelvis. (PCPP 4–40   EPC 845)

16.

C. Primary blast injuries are caused by the initial air blast and pressure wave. Injuries resulting from the compression of hollow organs, such as the lungs, include pneumothorax and alveolar rupture. (PCPP 4–46   EPC 851)

17.

D. Secondary blast injuries are caused by flying debris propelled by the force of the blast. Impacting debris may produce blunt or penetrating trauma. (PCPP 4–46   EPC 851)

18.

A. Tertiary blast injuries propel the victim away from the blast and into objects or the ground. Injuries are similar to those found in auto ejection. (PCPP 4–46 EPC 851)

19.

D. When assessing the mechanism of injury of falls, you should evaluate the following aspects: the height of the fall, the landing surface, and the part of the body that impacted first. (PCPP 4–51   EPC 856)

20.

E. When immobilizing the head and neck of a football player, you should either remove both helmet and shoulder pads or leave them both on in order to maintain the head and neck in a neutral position. (PCPP 4–51   EPC 856)

36

Penetrating Trauma

DIRECTIONS Each of the questions or incomplete statements below is followed by suggested answers or completions. Select the **one answer** that is best in each case.

1. If you double the speed of an object, its kinetic energy increases by
   A. half
   B. double
   C. fourfold
   D. eightfold

2. The study of projectiles in motion and their interactions with the gun, the air, and the objects they contact is known as
   A. trajectory
   B. ballistics
   C. profile
   D. caliber

Match the following ballistics terms with their respective definitions:

3. _____ Trajectory
4. _____ Cavitation
5. _____ Drag
6. _____ Profile
7. _____ Caliber
8. _____ Yaw

A. The size and shape of a bullet as it contacts a target
B. The path a bullet follows
C. Swing or wobble around the axis of a bullet's travel
D. The diameter of a bullet
E. Forces acting on a bullet to slow it down
F. A temporary vacuum created by a bullet's passage

9. As a rifle bullet hits the body, what generally happens to its profile?
   A. It stays on the same straight path
   B. It tumbles and rotates 180°
   C. It breaks apart like shrapnel
   D. It remains in a gyroscopic motion

10. You are treating a police officer who was shot in the chest at close range with a handgun. He was wearing a Kevlar vest. As you remove the vest and examine him, you expect to find
    A. a large entrance wound but no exit wound
    B. a small entrance wound and a large exit wound
    C. no entrance wound but erythema where the entrance wound would be
    D. a small entrance wound and small exit wound

11. A hunting rifle produces much greater kinetic energy because of its
    A. heavy projectile
    B. high speed
    C. bullets that expand upon impact
    D. all of the above

12. The M-16 and AK-47 are examples of
    A. automatic handguns
    B. domestic hunting rifles
    C. assault weapons
    D. shotguns

13. Which of the following statements is true regarding knife injuries?
    A. Men attackers usually stab downward
    B. Women attackers usually stab upward and outward
    C. Impaled knives should always be removed in the field
    D. None of the above

14. According to the projectile injury process, which tissue suffers the most damage?
    A. Tissue that is stretched from the cavitational wave
    B. Tissue in the direct pathway
    C. Adjacent tissue
    D. All of the above

15. Which of the following impaled objects should be removed?
    A. Lodged in the cheek, causing airway obstruction
    B. Lodged in the trachea, causing airway obstruction
    C. Lodged in such a way as to prevent CPR
    D. All of the above

16. Which of the following statements is true regarding penetrating injuries?
    A. Solid organs have the resiliency of muscle and other connective tissues
    B. Muscles, the skin, and other connective tissues are thin and delicate
    C. When muscle is penetrated, the wound track closes and serious injury is limited
    D. Penetrating injury to the lung is generally less extensive than in other body tissue

17. Which of the following statements is true regarding penetrating trauma to a hollow organ?
    A. If the organ is filled with fluid, it can tear apart explosively
    B. If it is filled with fluid, the energy is dissipated in the fluid with minimal damage
    C. Injury to an air-filled organ results in explosive tissue damage and hemorrhage
    D. Pericardial tamponade results from rupture of the heart's contents into the thorax

18. Which of the following statements is true regarding penetrating trauma to the abdomen?
    A. The area is well-protected by skeletal structures
    B. Projectiles rarely produce a cavitational wave
    C. The intestines tolerate stretching and compression well
    D. Serious peritoneal irritation may result from bowel perforation with immediate signs and symptoms

19. Which of the following statements is true regarding a bullet's entrance wound?
    A. It matches the size of the bullet's profile
    B. It will often have a "blown out" appearance
    C. If the bullet is fired at close range, subcutaneous emphysema will be present
    D. It accurately portrays the potential for damage

20. Which of the following statements is true regarding damage caused by a low-velocity object?
    A. It can create a pressure shock wave
    B. It is limited to the object's path of travel
    C. It may include a "blow-out" exit wound
    D. It is generally very obvious by the size of the entrance wound

answers & rationales

1.

C. The speed of an object has a squared relationship to its kinetic energy. If you double the speed of an object, its kinetic energy increases by fourfold ($2^2 = 4$). As in blunt trauma, speed kills. (PCPP 4–57 EPC 859)

2.

B. The study of projectiles in motion and their interactions with the gun, the air, and the object they contact is known as ballistics. (PCPP 4–58 EPC 860)

Matching (PCPP 4–58 EPC 860)

3. B Trajectory
4. F Cavitation
5. E Drag
6. A Profile
7. D Caliber
8. C Yaw

A. The size and shape of a bullet as it contacts a target
B. The path a bullet follows
C. Swing or wobble around the axis of a bullet's travel
D. The diameter of a bullet
E. Forces acting on a bullet to slow it down
F. A temporary vacuum created by a bullet's passage

9.

B. Since a rifle bullet has its center of gravity farther back from the leading edge, it is likely to tumble once it hits the body. It generally rotates 180° and continues its travel base-first, causing massive damage. (PCPP 4–59 EPC 861)

10.

C. A Kevlar vest protects the wearer from most medium-energy projectiles, such as a handgun. The vest absorbs the impact, but some energy is transferred to the wearer and may cause significant blunt trauma, as evidenced by an area of erythema (redness) over the impacted area. (PCPP 4–61 EPC 863)

11.

D. High-powered rifles produce tremendous kinetic energy because of their high muzzle velocity (speed) and their heavy projectiles (bullets) that expand dramatically upon impact. Domestic hunting ammunition is especially lethal. (PCPP 4–62 EPC 864)

12.

C. The M-16 (American made) and the AK-47 (Russian made) are examples of assault rifles used by infantry soldiers. Their ammunition is generally fully jacketed so they will not expand upon impact, actually making them less dangerous than the domestic hunting rifle. (PCPP 4–62 EPC 864)

13.

D. Knife-wielding males usually strike with a forward, outward, or crosswise stroke. Females usually strike with an overhand and downward blow. (PCPP 4–67 EPC 869)

14.

B. Tissue in the direct pathway of the bullet suffers most. It is severely contused and likely to have been torn from its attachments. (PCPP 4–64 EPC 866)

15.

D. In general, you want to immobilize an impaled object to prevent further injury, except in the following cases: an object lodged in the cheek or trachea, causing an airway obstruction, or one preventing you from performing CPR. (PCPP 4–75 EPC 877)

16.

D. Because the lung tissue consists of millions of small, air-filled sacs that slow down and limit the transmission of the cavitational wave, penetrating trauma to the lungs generally causes less damage than trauma to other body tissues. (PCPP 4–68 EPC 870)

17.

A. Since fluid is noncompressible and rapidly transmits the impact energy outward, the energy released can tear the organ apart explosively. This is true of the bladder, stomach, intestines, and heart. (PCPP 4–68   EPC 870)

18.

C. The major occupant of the abdomen, the bowel, is very tolerant of compression and stretching. The liver, kidneys, spleen, and pancreas, however, are highly susceptible to injury and life-threatening hemorrhage. (PCPP 4–69   EPC 871)

19.

A. Entrance wounds are generally the size of the bullet's profile and quickly close due to the skin's natural elasticity. (PCPP 4–71   EPC 873)

20.

B. Low-velocity weapons, such as knives, ice picks, and blast debris, have a limited kinetic energy exchange rate as they enter the victim's body. Injury in these cases is usually limited to the tissue actually contacted by the penetrating object. (PCPP 4–66   EPC 868)

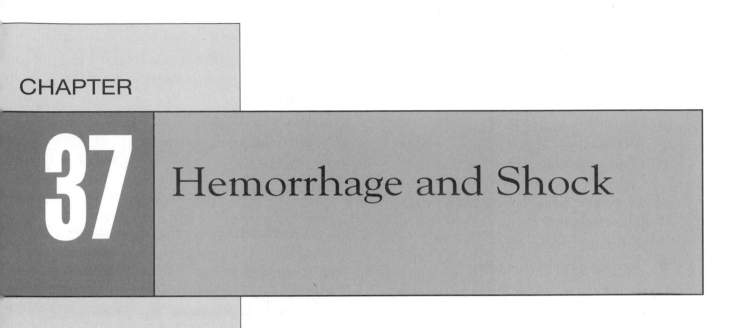

CHAPTER

37

Hemorrhage and Shock

DIRECTIONS Each of the questions or incomplete statements below is followed by suggested answers or completions. Select the **one answer** that is best in each case.

1. Which of the following factors does NOT affect the heart's stroke volume?
   A. Heart rate
   B. Preload
   C. Afterload
   D. Contractile force

2. Stroke volume could be increased by all of the following EXCEPT
   A. increasing venous return
   B. increasing contractile force
   C. decreasing afterload
   D. promoting venodilation

3. The amount of blood pumped from the heart in one contraction is called
   A. preload
   B. afterload
   C. stroke volume
   D. tidal volume

4. Which of the following statements best illustrates the Frank-Starling mechanism?
   A. The greater the afterload, the greater the stroke volume
   B. The less the stroke volume, the less the afterload
   C. The greater the preload, the greater the stroke volume
   D. The less the preload, the greater the afterload

5. The amount of blood pumped by the heart in 1 minute is called
   A. minute volume
   B. stroke volume
   C. cardiac output
   D. contractile volume

6. The amount of resistance against which the heart must pump in order to eject blood is called
   A. stroke volume
   B. end-diastolic volume
   C. afterload
   D. pulse pressure

7. The muscular layer of an artery is called the tunica
   A. intima
   B. media
   C. adventitia
   D. arteriole

8. Which of the following blood vessels has the greatest ability to vary the size of its internal lumens?
   A. Artery
   B. Arteriole
   C. Capillary
   D. Venule

9. Which of the following statements is true regarding capillaries?
   A. They lack tunica media
   B. Their tunica adventitia is very thin
   C. The walls are only two cells thick
   D. They contain over 20% of the vascular volume

10. The majority of blood volume consists of
    A. red blood cells
    B. plasma
    C. platelets
    D. white blood cells

11. The percentage of red blood cells in the blood is called
    A. homeostasis
    B. hematocrit
    C. hemoglobin
    D. hematoma

12. Red blood cells make up what percentage of total blood volume in the healthy adult?
    A. 20
    B. 45
    C. 55
    D. 60

13. Which of the following is NOT a phase of clotting?
    A. Vascular phase
    B. Platelet phase
    C. Coagulation phase
    D. Autonomic phase

14. Clotting normally takes _____ minutes.
    A. 7–10
    B. 10–20
    C. 20–30
    D. >30

15. Your patient has attempted suicide by slitting his wrists. You notice that he has run the knife across his wrist, perpendicular to the arm, and that the wound is rather deep. Which of the following statements is true regarding the likelihood for serious blood loss?
    A. You should expect severe blood loss
    B. There is most likely tremendous internal blood loss
    C. Blood loss is probably not life-threatening
    D. A tourniquet will probably be necessary

16. Which of the following would NOT adversely affect the clotting process?
    A. Aggressive fluid therapy
    B. Immobilization of the wound site
    C. Hypothermia
    D. Administration of an NSAID

17. Which of the following techniques is NOT recommended for external hemorrhage control?
    A. Venous constricting band
    B. Direct pressure
    C. Pressure points
    D. Tourniquet

18. Epistaxis can be caused by
    A. hypertension
    B. a strong sneeze
    C. direct trauma
    D. all of the above

19. Hemoptysis is best described as
    A. coughing up bright red blood
    B. vomiting up dark brown blood
    C. blood in the urine
    D. blood in the stool

20. Your patient presents with melena. This is best described as
    A. bright red blood from rectal hemorrhoids
    B. massive vaginal hemorrhage
    C. anemic blood
    D. black, tarry stools

21. Your patient presents with profound hypotension from external and internal hemorrhage. How much blood do you estimate he has already lost?
    A. <15%
    B. 15–25%
    C. 25–35%
    D. >35%

22. Which of the following factors renders the elderly more susceptible to the adverse effects of hemorrhage?
    A. Lower fluid volume reserve
    B. Beta blockers and anticoagulant medications
    C. Less responsive compensatory mechanisms
    D. All of the above

23. Pelvic fractures can account for blood loss of _____ ml.
    A. up to 500
    B. 500–750
    C. up to 1500
    D. more than 2000

24. Your patient complains of rectal bleeding. Upon examination of the toilet immediately following his bowel movement, you note the presence of bright red blood in the water. This type of bleeding is known as
    A. hematochezia
    B. melena
    C. hematemesis
    D. hemostasis

25. A positive tilt test occurs when the pulse rate _____ by 20 beats per minute or the BP _____ by 20 mmHg when a patient moves from a supine position to a sitting position.
    A. increases, increases
    B. decreases, increases
    C. increases, decreases
    D. decreases, decreases

26. The process known as glycolysis requires _____ oxygen and generates _____ energy.
    A. no, a small amount of
    B. a small amount of, no
    C. adequate, normal
    D. adequate, a great amount of

27. In the second stage of cellular metabolism, what is added to complete the Krebs cycle?
    A. Fats
    B. Glucose
    C. Oxygen
    D. Carbohydrates

28. Which of the following increases the flow of blood through a capillary bed?
    A. Histamine release
    B. A rise in pH
    C. An increase in oxygen supply
    D. A decrease in carbon dioxide

29. The body can quickly increase its circulating blood volume by _____ the precapillary sphincters and _____ the postcapillary sphincters.
    A. opening, closing
    B. opening, opening
    C. closing, closing
    D. closing, opening

30. Blood is returned to the heart via the venous system. This flow is aided by
    A. skeletal muscle contractions
    B. respirations
    C. valves in the veins
    D. all of the above

31. Baroreceptors constantly monitor for changes in
    A. oxygen levels
    B. carbon dioxide levels
    C. heart rate
    D. blood pressure

32. Stimulation of the baroreceptors causes all of the following EXCEPT
    A. peripheral vasodilation
    B. increased cardiac output
    C. increased heart rate
    D. bronchodilation

Match the following agents and hormones with their respective roles in influencing operations of the cardiovascular system:

33. _____ Epinephrine
34. _____ ADH
35. _____ Angiotensin II
36. _____ Aldosterone
37. _____ Glucagon
38. _____ ACTH
39. _____ Growth hormone
40. _____ Erythropoietin

A. Increases red blood cell production
B. Reduces inflammation, increases clotting time
C. Increases cardiac output, vasoconstricts
D. Reduces urine output
E. Promotes glucose uptake and protein synthesis
F. Potent vasoconstrictor
G. Converts glycogen to glucose
H. Maintains ion balance in the kidneys

41. Anaerobic metabolism results in which of the following?
    A. Inefficient energy
    B. Increased pyruvic acid formation
    C. Glycolysis
    D. All of the above

42. Tachycardia; cool, clammy, and pale skin; and a stable blood pressure describe a patient in

A. compensated shock
B. decompensated shock
C. irreversible shock
D. none of the above

43. Which of the following happens in decompensated shock?
    A. Precapillary sphincters open
    B. Rouleaux are formed
    C. Blood pressure falls
    D. All of the above

Match the following types of shock with their respective examples:

44. _____ Hypovolemic
45. _____ Anaphylactic
46. _____ Septic
47. _____ Obstructive
48. _____ Cardiogenic
49. _____ Respiratory
50. _____ Neurogenic

A. Pulmonary embolus
B. Spinal cord injury
C. Third spacing
D. Flail chest
E. Myocardial infarction
F. Massive infection
G. Massive histamine release

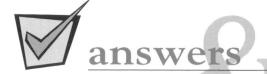

answers & rationales

1.

A. The amount of blood ejected by the heart at one contraction is referred to as the stroke volume. Stroke volume is determined by preload, afterload, and contractile force. (PCPP 4–79   EPC 222)

2.

D. Preload could be increased by increasing venous return, by increasing the contractile force of the heart, and by decreasing the afterload. (PCPP 4–80 EPC 222)

3.

C. The amount of blood pumped from the heart in one contraction is called stroke volume. (PCPP 4–79 EPC 222)

4.

C. The greater the volume of the preload is, the more the ventricles are stretched. The greater the stretch, up to a certain point, the greater the subsequent cardiac contraction. This is referred to as the Frank-Starling mechanism. (PCPP 4–80   EPC 223)

5.

C. The amount of blood pumped from the heart in 1 minute is called cardiac output. Cardiac output is calculated by stroke volume times heart rate. (PCPP 4–80   EPC 223)

6.

C. The amount of resistance against which the heart must pump is called afterload. The heart must overcome this resistance in order to eject blood. Afterload is determined by the degree of peripheral vascular resistance. Peripheral resistance is determined by the degree of vasoconstriction present on the arterial side. (PCPP 4–80   EPC 223)

7.

B. Arteries consist of three distinct layers: the tunica intima (innermost), tunica media (muscular), and tunica adventitia (outer covering). The tunica media allows the vessel to regulate blood flow by increasing or decreasing its lumen through muscle constriction and dilation. In fact, arterioles can change their size by a factor of 6. (PCPP 4–81 EPC 218)

8.

B. Arterioles have the greatest ability to vary the size of their inner lumen via constriction or dilation. (PCPP 4–81   EPC 218)

9.

A. The capillaries are microscopic vessels that lack the muscular and connective layers of arteries and veins. They are one cell thick and contain 7% of the vascular volume. (PCPP 4–81   EPC 218)

10.

B. Plasma makes up approximately 55% of the total blood volume. It consists of 92% water, 6–7% proteins, and a small portion consisting of electrolytes, lipids, enzymes, clotting factors, glucose, and other dissolved substances. (PCPP 4–81   EPC 120)

11.

B. The percentage of blood occupied by red blood cells is referred to as the hematocrit. Normal hematocrit in the healthy person is approximately 45%. (PCPP 4–81   EPC 121)

12.

B. Red blood cells account for approximately 45% of the total blood volume. This percentage is known as the patient's hematocrit. (PCPP 4–81   EPC 121)

13.

D. There are three phases of clotting: the vascular phase (where the vessel constricts), the platelet phase (where platelets adhere to blood vessel walls), and the coagulation phase (where fibrin forms a network around the wound for protection). (PCPP 4–83   EPC 880)

14.

A. The clotting mechanism normally takes between 7 and 10 minutes to stop the flow of blood. The nature of the wound and other factors affect how rapidly and well the clotting mechanisms respond to hemorrhage. (PCPP 4–84   EPC 880)

15.

C. A clean, lateral cut of a blood vessel allows the vessel to retract and thicken its wall. This reduces the lumen, reduces blood flow, and assists in the clotting mechanism. In this type of case, blood loss usually will not be life-threatening. A longitudinal cut is an entirely different matter. (PCPP 4–84   EPC 880)

16.

B. The clotting process normally works very well unless inhibited by the following factors: movement of the wound site (tears the clot loose), aggressive fluid therapy (increases pressure and dilutes clotting factors), hypothermia (slows the process), and medications (such as aspirin, NSAIDs, warfarin). (PCPP 4–85   EPC 882)

17.

A. External hemorrhage should be controlled in the following manner: direct pressure over the wound site and elevation, pressure point compression, and, as a last resort, application of an artery-constricting tourniquet. (PCPP 4–86   EPC 882)

18.

D. A moderate to severe nosebleed, known as epistaxis, can be caused by direct trauma, hypertension, a strong sneeze, or dry air. (PCPP 4–88 EPC 885)

19.

A. Hemoptysis, coughing up bright red blood, is due to a disruption in the alveolar-capillary membrane. This is caused by certain degenerative diseases, such as tuberculosis or cancer, or by chest trauma. (PCPP 4–89   EPC 885)

20.

D. Melena is black, tarry feces due to gastrointestinal bleeding, usually indicating digested blood. (PCPP 4–89   EPC 886)

21.

D. At greater than 35% blood loss, a person will present with profound hypotension because he has lost the massive vasoconstriction that helped maintain the blood pressure. As the precapillary sphincters reopened, the blood pressure dropped. This marks the beginning of decompensated shock. (PCPP 4–90   EPC 887)

22.

D. The elderly are more adversely affected by blood loss due to their lower fluid volume reserve, slower and less responsive compensatory mechanisms, reduced perception of pain, and lower levels of mental acuity and due to the presence of medications such as beta blockers and anticoagulants. (PCPP 4–91   EPC 888)

23.

D. Pelvic fractures can account for more than 2 liters of blood loss. If you suspect a fracture, always maintain the stability and integrity of the pelvic ring to minimize the possibility of lacerating a major blood vessel. (PCPP 4–94   EPC 891)

24.

A. Hematochezia is the passage of stools containing red blood. This usually represents active bleeding in the colon or rectum or internal hemorrhoids. (PCPP 4–95   EPC 892)

25.

C. A positive tilt test occurs when the pulse rate increases by 20 beats per minute or the BP decreases by 20 mmHg when a patient moves from a supine to a sitting position. This is known as orthostatic hypotension and is the result of relative hypovolemia. (PCPP 4–95   EPC 892)

26.

A. Glycolysis is the first stage of the process in which the cell breaks apart an energy source and releases a small amount of energy. It requires no oxygen at this stage. (PCPP 4–100   EPC 285)

27.

C. The Krebs cycle, also known as the citric acid cycle, is the second stage of metabolism, requiring the presence of oxygen, in which the breakdown of glucose yields a great amount of energy. This is also known as aerobic metabolism. (PCPP 4–100 EPC 285)

28.

A. The precapillary sphincters regulate the flow of blood into a capillary bed. They will open when the oxygen supply decreases, the carbon dioxide level increases, the pH falls, or histamine is released. This process is just one component of the homeostatic control process. (PCPP 4–102 EPC 224)

29.

D. The interstitial and intracellular spaces represent 88% of the body's total fluid volume. In a crisis, the body can draw on this reservoir by closing the precapillary sphincters, drawing fluid from the interstitial spaces and cells into the capillary bed, and returning this fluid to the general circulation through the opened postcapillary sphincters. (PCPP 4–103   EPC 104)

30.

D. Venous return is aided by skeletal muscle contractions (help push the blood against gravity), valves in the veins (prevent backflow), and respirations (create negative pressure in the chest). (PCPP 4–103   EPC 224)

31.

D. Baroreceptors are located in the carotid bodies and the arch of the aorta. These baroreceptors closely monitor pressure. (PCPP 4–104   EPC 223)

32.

A. Baroreceptors are stretch receptors that stretch with increased pressure. When they detect reduced flow and pressure, they send messages to the brain to stimulate the sympathetic nervous system. This results in increased heart rate and cardiac output to increase circulation and bronchodilation. (PCPP 4–104   EPC 223)

Matching   (PCPP 4–105   EPC 287)

33. **C**	Epinephrine	**A.**	Increases red blood cell production
34. **D**	ADH		
35. **F**	Angiotensin II	**B.**	Reduces inflammation, increases clotting time
36. **H**	Aldosterone		
37. **G**	Glucagon	**C.**	Increases cardiac output, vasoconstricts
38. **B**	ACTH		
39. **E**	Growth hormone	**D.**	Reduces urine output
		E.	Promotes glucose uptake and protein synthesis
40. **A**	Erythropoietin		
		F.	Potent vasoconstrictor
		G.	Converts glycogen to glucose
		H.	Maintains ion balance in the kidneys

41.

D. During periods of inadequate tissue perfusion, cell metabolism switches from aerobic to an aeroabic mode. Results of this process are inefficient energy, an increase in pyruvic acid formation, and glycolysis. (PCPP 4–108   EPC 879)

42.

A. Following the onset of inadequate tissue perfusion, various compensatory mechanisms of the body are stimulated. The heart rate and strength of cardiac contractions increase. There will be an increase in systemic vascular resistance to assist in maintaining the blood pressure. These compensatory changes will continue until the body is unable to maintain blood pressure and tissue perfusion. Your patient in compensatory shock will exhibit tachycardia, cool, clammy, and pale skin with a stable blood pressure. (PCPP 4–108   EPC 898)

43.

D. In the later stages of shock the blood pressure begins to fall and blood supply to essential organs diminishes. As a result, the precapillary sphincters open while the postcapillary sphincters remain closed. This results in sludging of red blood cells and the formation of rouleaux. (PCPP 4–109   EPC 899)

Matching   (PCPP 4–105   EPC 287)

44. **C**	Hypovolemic	**A.**	Pulmonary embolus
45. **G**	Anaphylactic	**B.**	Spinal cord injury
46. **F**	Septic	**C.**	Third spacing
47. **A**	Obstructive	**D.**	Flail chest
48. **E**	Cardiogenic	**E.**	Myocardial infarction
49. **D**	Respiratory	**F.**	Massive infection
50. **B**	Neurogenic	**G.**	Massive histamine release

38

Soft Tissue Trauma

DIRECTIONS Each of the questions or incomplete statements below is followed by suggested answers or completions. Select the **one answer** that is best in each case.

1. The outermost layer of the skin, consisting of dead or dying cells, is the
   A. epidermis
   B. dermis
   C. subcutaneous layer
   D. sebaceous layer

2. The fatty secretion that helps keep the skin pliable and waterproof is called
   A. intima
   B. cilia
   C. mucous
   D. sebum

3. The skin layer containing blood vessels and nerves is the
   A. epidermis
   B. dermis
   C. subcutaneous layer
   D. sebaceous layer

4. The skin layer containing adipose fat and connective tissue is the
   A. epidermis
   B. dermis
   C. subcutaneous layer
   D. sebaceous layer

5. The smooth interior layer of the blood vessels is the tunica
   A. intima
   B. media
   C. adventitia
   D. lumina

6. The middle muscular layer of the blood vessels is the tunica
   A. intima
   B. media
   C. adventitia
   D. lumina

7. The outer fibrous layer of the blood vessels is the tunica
   A. intima
   B. media
   C. adventitia
   D. lumina

8. The functions of the skin include
   A. protecting the body from environmental pathogens
   B. providing a barrier against infection
   C. perceiving temperature, pain, and pressure
   D. all of the above

9. A closed wound in which the skin is unbroken, but the tissue underneath is damaged, is a/an
   A. abrasion
   B. concussion
   C. contusion
   D. amputation

10. General reddening of the skin due to dilation of the superficial capillaries is
    A. ecchymosis
    B. erythema
    C. hyphema
    D. contusion

11. A scraping away of the superficial layers of the skin is a/an
    A. erythema
    B. ecchymosis
    C. contusion
    D. abrasion

12. A collection of blood trapped within a body compartment is a/an
    A. hyphema
    B. erythema
    C. hematoma
    D. contusion

13. Black-and-blue discoloration of the skin due to the leakage of blood into the tissues is
    A. hyphema
    B. ecchymosis
    C. erythema
    D. contusion

14. Which of the following blood vessels cannot stop bleeding by constricting?
    A. Arteries
    B. Capillaries
    C. Venules
    D. Arterioles

15. Which of the following is **NOT** a component of the wound-healing process?
    A. Gluconeogenesis
    B. Inflammation
    C. Epithelialization
    D. Neovascularization

16. Your patient cut his foot 4 days ago and failed to seek medical attention for it. He now presents with pain, tenderness, erythema, warmth, and thick, pale yellow pus oozing from the wound site. Your field diagnosis includes
    A. allergic reaction
    B. bacterial infection
    C. viral infection
    D. compartment syndrome

17. Which of the following preexisting conditions can increase the likelihood of infection of an open wound?
    A. COPD
    B. AIDS
    C. Smoking
    D. All of the above

18. Which of the following drugs detracts from the body's ability to fight infection?
    A. Albuterol
    B. Nifedipine
    C. Ibuprofen
    D. Furosemide

19. Your patient is a homeless street person who presents with an old foot wound that appears infected. You also note some subcutaneous emphysema surrounding the wound site and a foul odor when you squeeze the wound edges. You suspect
    A. tetanus
    B. lockjaw
    C. gangrene
    D. sepsis

20. The classic sign of tetanus is
    A. greenish exudate from the wound
    B. mandibular trismus
    C. compartment syndrome
    D. abnormal scar formation

21. Muscular ischemia caused by rising pressures within an anatomical fascial space is known as
    A. compartment syndrome
    B. tetanus
    C. keloidosis
    D. rhabdomyolysis

22. Rhabdomyolysis is usually the result of
    A. severe wound infection
    B. impaired hemostasis
    C. crush injury
    D. severe bed sores

23. The proper care for an amputated part includes placing the part
    A. directly on ice
    B. in warm saline
    C. in a sealed dry bag, then into cold water
    D. directly into cold water

24. Which of the following is a standard treatment for an entrapped victim with a crush injury?
    A. Crystalloid IV infusion
    B. Sodium bicarbonate
    C. Mannitol
    D. All of the above

25. The single most effective prehospital treatment for compartment syndrome is
    A. needle decompression of the compartment
    B. elevation of extremity
    C. administration of a diuretic
    D. immobilization of the extremity and the adjacent joints

✓ answers & rationales

1.

A. The outermost layer of skin is the epidermis. It is composed of dead or dying cells that are pushed outward by new cells growing underneath. As these cells reach the surface, they wear away with everyday activity. (PCPP 4–126 EPC 117)

2.

D. Sebum is the fatty secretion from the sebaceous gland. This oil lubricates the epidermis and helps make it both pliable and watertight. (PCPP 4–127 EPC 117)

3.

B. The dermis is the layer of tissue that contains blood vessels, nerves, sweat glands, sebaceous glands, and hair follicles. (PCPP 4–127 EPC 118)

4.

C. The subcutaneous layer is comprised of fat and connective tissue and serves to insulate the body. (PCPP 4–127 EPC 118)

5.

A. The tunica intima is the smooth, thin lining of blood vessels. It allows the free flow of blood and promotes the exchange of nutrients and waste products between the tissues and the bloodstream. (PCPP 4–129 EPC 218)

6.

B. The tunica media is the muscular part of the tube. It regulates the inner diameter of the blood vessel by either dilating or constricting to meet the body's demands. These involuntary muscles are under the control of the autonomic nervous system. (PCPP 4–129 EPC 218)

7.

C. The tunica adventitia is the outer fibrous layer of the blood vessels. This layer consists of connective tissue and provides protection. (PCPP 4–129 EPC 218)

8.

D. The functions of the skin are many. It protects the human body from many dangers found in the environment; functions as an organ of sensation, perceiving temperature and pain; contains vital fluids; aids in temperature regulation by secreting sweat and shunting blood; and provides a barrier against infection and insulation from trauma. (PCPP 4–125 EPC 912)

9.

C. A contusion is a closed wound in which the skin is unbroken although damage has occurred to the immediate tissue beneath. It is usually caused by blunt, nonpenetrating injuries that crush and damage small blood vessels. (PCPP 4–131 EPC 913)

10.

B. An erythema is general reddening of the skin due to dilation of the superficial capillaries. This situation is often caused by a contusion. (PCPP 4–131 EPC 913)

11.

D. An abrasion is the scraping away of the superficial layers of the skin, often by an open soft tissue injury. An abrasion removes the layers of the epidermis and upper reaches of the dermis. Bleeding is usually limited because the injury involves only superficial capillaries. (PCPP 4–133 EPC 915)

12.

C. A hematoma is a collection of blood beneath the skin or trapped within a body compartment. Hematomas can contribute significantly to hypovolemia. For example, the thigh can contain over a liter of fluid before swelling becomes apparent. (PCPP 4–132   EPC 914)

13.

B. Ecchymosis is the black-and-blue discoloration of the skin caused by the leakage of blood into the tissues. It is a delayed sign in wound progression. (PCPP 4–131   EPC 913)

14.

B. Capillaries do not possess the muscular layer that reflexively constricts the vessel in response to local injury. For this reason, capillaries continue to bleed until the clotting process is successful. (PCPP 4–138   EPC 920)

15.

A. The wound-healing process consists of a number of phases. These include hemostasis (controlling hemorrhage), inflammation (repairing cells), epithelialization (restoring the skin layer), neovascularization (promoting new capillary growth), and collagen synthesis (strengthening the healed tissue). (PCPP 4–138   EPC 920)

16.

B. If bacteria have invaded an open wound, an infection can occur, and symptoms appear approximately 2–3 days after the event. Signs of infection include pain, tenderness, erythema, warmth, and thick pus oozing from the wound site. (PCPP 4–140   EPC 923)

17.

D. Risk factors for wound infection include chronic disease (decreased ability to heal), AIDS and HIV (reduced immune response), and smoking (vasoconstriction). Patients with these preexisting conditions are at an increased risk for developing a wound infection. (PCPP 4–141   EPC 924)

18.

C. Certain drugs detract from the body's ability to fight infection. These include corticosteroids (prednisone and cortisone), NSAIDS (ibuprofen), antigout medications (colchicine), and some antineoplastic (anticancer) drugs. (PCPP 4–141   EPC 924)

19.

C. Gangrene is a deep-space infection caused by the anaerobic bacterium *Clostridium perfringens*. The subcutaneous emphysema and odor are the result of the gas generated by the infection. A combination of antibiotics, surgery, and hyperbaric medicine is effective if used early. (PCPP 4–142   EPC 925)

20.

B. Tetanus is a rare, but life-threatening, complication from a wound infection. It is caused by the bacterium *Clostridium tetani* and manifests itself by mandibular trismus, or jaw clenching (lockjaw). Routine immunization every 10 years can reduce the incidence. (PCPP 4–142   EPC 925)

21.

A. Compartment syndrome is the result of rising pressure within a fascial space, such as in the deep, muscular regions of the extremities. Usually the result of a closed injury, the swelling and bleeding cannot escape and are entrapped within the muscle fascia. Irreversible damage can occur if not reversed within a few hours. (PCPP 4–143   EPC 926)

22.

C. Rhabdomyolysis is an acute disease that involves the destruction of skeletal muscle due to ischemia. This is usually the result of a crush injury in which body parts are trapped for at least 4 hours. By-products from the anaerobic metabolism and from muscle disintegration can reach the central circulation when the body part is freed. (PCPP 4–145   EPC 928)

23.

C. Amputated parts should be put into a dry bag, sealed, and placed in cool water that contains a few ice cubes. (PCPP 4–153   EPC 944)

24.

D. In addition to standard management of the ABCs, treatment for an entrapped victim with a suspected crush injury includes crystalloid IV infusion (to maintain fluid volume), sodium bicarbonate IV (to prevent acidosis), and an osmotic diuretic such as mannitol (to maintain kidney function). (PCPP 4–164   EPC 947)

25.

B. The best prehospital treatment for compartment syndrome is to elevate the affected extremity. This reduces edema, increases venous return, lowers compartment pressure, and helps prevent ischemia. Sometimes the simplest answer is the correct one. (PCPP 4–166   EPC 948)

39 Burns

DIRECTIONS Each of the questions or incomplete statements below is followed by suggested answers or completions. Select the **one answer** that is best in each case.

1. The extent of burn injury depends on which of the following factors?
   A. Temperature
   B. Concentration of heat energy
   C. Length of contact time
   D. All of the above

2. According to Jackson's theory of thermal wounds, which of the following zones suffers the greatest amount of tissue damage?
   A. Zone of stasis
   B. Zone of coagulation
   C. Zone of hyperemia
   D. Zone of emergence

3. Which of the following lists the phases of a thermal burn in their proper chronological order?
   A. Resolution, emergent, hypermetabolic, fluid shift
   B. Hypermetabolic, fluid shift, resolution, emergent
   C. Emergent, fluid shift, hypermetabolic, resolution
   D. Fluid shift, resolution, emergent, hypermetabolic

Match the following electrical terms with their respective definitions:

4. _____ Voltage
5. _____ Current
6. _____ Amperes
7. _____ Resistance
8. _____ Ohm

A. An opposing force against electrical flow
B. The measure of current
C. The measure of resistance
D. An electrical gradient
E. Electrical flow rate

9. Liquefaction necrosis is caused by
   A. acid burns
   B. alkali burns
   C. either A or B
   D. neither A nor B

10. Which of the following types of radiation emits the most powerful rays?
    A. Alpha
    B. Beta
    C. Delta
    D. Gamma

11. The extent of radiation depends on which of the following factors?
    A. Duration of exposure
    B. Distance from the source
    C. Shielding from the source
    D. All of the above

12. Cumulative radiation exposure is measured with a/an
    A. dosimeter
    B. radmeter
    C. Gray device
    D. Geiger counter

13. Any patient who has been in an enclosed area during combustion should be suspected of having
    A. pulmonary embolism
    B. pulmonary edema
    C. carbon monoxide poisoning
    D. hyponatremia

14. Which of the following is most likely to cause subglottic burns?
    A. Hot air
    B. Flame
    C. Steam
    D. Hot gases

15. Your patient who presents with dyspnea and hoarseness, following the inhalation of superheated steam, is in danger of developing
    A. pulmonary embolism
    B. complete upper airway obstruction
    C. anaphylaxis
    D. bronchospasm

16. A burn involving the epidermis and dermis, producing blisters and pain, is classified as
    A. first degree
    B. second degree
    C. superficial
    D. full thickness

17. An adult with burns to both arms, chest, abdomen, and entire back has a _____% BSA burn.
    A. 36
    B. 45
    C. 54
    D. 63

18. An infant with burns to both legs has a _____% BSA burn.
    A. 9
    B. 14
    C. 18
    D. 27

19. Which of the following is a complication of a burn injury?
    A. Hypothermia
    B. Hypovolemia
    C. Eschar
    D. All of the above

20. The major complication of circumferential burns is the
    A. fluid loss in the burn area
    B. loss of a barrier against infection
    C. tourniquet effect, cutting off distal circulation
    D. anaerobic metabolism proximal to the burn site

21. According to the American Burn Association, which of the following patients should be evaluated in a burn center?
    A. Partial thickness burn to >15% of BSA
    B. Full thickness burn to >5% of BSA
    C. High-voltage electrical injuries
    D. All of the above

22. What percentage of partial thickness burns can be safely cooled with water?
    A. <15%
    B. 15–20%
    C. 20–25%
    D. 25–50%

23. Partial thickness burns over 15% or full thickness burns over 5% of BSA should be managed by
    A. rapid cooling with water
    B. water and fanning
    C. applying ice to the burned area
    D. dry, sterile dressings

24. Your patient has sustained moderate to severe burns to 30% BSA. According to the Parkland formula, how much fluid should he receive in the first 4 hours? He weighs 154 lbs.
    A. 8400 ml
    B. 4200 ml
    C. 2100 ml
    D. 280 ml

25. In the above patient with a short travel time, how much of this fluid should be administered during the prehospital phase?
    A. About 1 liter
    B. 2–3 liters

C. 5 liters

D. 500 ml

26. Which of the following treatments is indicated for a patient suspected of cyanide poisoning?

A. Aggressive airway management

B. A nitrite compound

C. A sulfur-containing compound

D. All of the above

27. Standard management of chemical burns includes

A. rinsing the area with ice water

B. using a neutralizing agent

C. leaving any corrosive materials on the skin

D. irrigating vigorously with cool water

28. Which of the following substances can you safely irrigate?

A. Sodium

B. Phenol

C. Lye

D. Dry lime

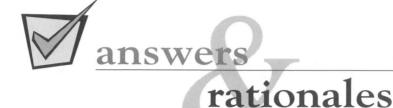
answers & rationales

1.

D. The extent of burn injury depends on the amount of heat energy transferred to the patient's body. When assessing the severity of a burn injury, focus on three important factors: the temperature, the concentration of heat energy, and the length of contact time. (PCPP 4–176   EPC 955)

2.

B. According to Jackson's theory on thermal wounds, the zone of coagulation suffers the most damage because it is the nearest to the source. Cell membranes rupture and are destroyed, blood coagulates, and structural proteins denature. (PCPP 4–176 EPC 955)

3.

C. The body's response to burns includes the following stages in order: emergent (catecholamine release), fluid shift (massive external plasma losses), hypermetabolic (major need for nutrients for tissue repair), and resolution (scarring and rehabilitation). (PCPP 4–176   EPC 955)

Matching   (PCPP 4–177   EPC 956)

4. **D** Voltage
5. **E** Current
6. **B** Amperes
7. **A** Resistance
8. **C** Ohm
A. An opposing force against electrical flow
B. The measure of current
C. The measure of resistance
D. An electrical gradient
E. Electrical flow rate

9.

B. Liquefaction necrosis is the process by which an alkali dissolves and liquefies tissue. The alkali quickly penetrates the skin and causes progressively deeper burns. Acid burns are generally less severe because they result in coagulation necrosis, which forms a protective layer that limits further damage. (PCPP 4–180   EPC 958)

10.

D. Gamma radiation, also known as X-rays, is the most powerful ionizing radiation. It has the ability to travel through the entire body or ionize any atom within. It is the most dangerous and most feared type of radiation because it is difficult to protect against. (PCPP 4–182   EPC 961)

11.

D. The extent of a radiation injury depends on three important factors: the duration of the exposure, the distance from the source, and the shielding from the source. (PCPP 4–182   EPC 961)

12.

A. A Geiger counter measures immediate radiation exposure, while a dosimeter measures cumulative exposure. (PCPP 4–182   EPC 961)

13.

C. Any patient who has been in an enclosed area during combustion should be suspected of having carbon monoxide poisoning. Carbon monoxide is a by-product of incomplete combustion. Poisoning occurs because the hemoglobin of the blood has a much greater affinity for carbon monoxide than it does for oxygen. If your patient inhales carbon monoxide, it will displace oxygen, resulting in hypoxemia. (PCPP 4–183   EPC 962)

14.
C. Superheated steam has a greater heat content than air, flame, or gas and can cause subglottic (below the glottis) burns. (PCPP 4–184   EPC 963)

15.
B. A patient who inhales superheated steam and presents with shortness of breath, difficulty breathing, and hoarseness is in danger of developing a complete airway obstruction. Superheated steam contains enough energy to severely burn the upper airway. If damaged, this tissue will swell rapidly and seriously reduce the size of the airway lumen. The patient who presents with minor hoarseness may develop a complete airway obstruction later on. (PCPP 4–185   EPC 964)

16.
B. A second-degree, or partial thickness, burn involves the epidermis and the dermis. It produces blisters and is extremely painful. (PCPP 4–186 EPC 965)

17.
C. The rule of nines states that in the adult patient the arms are worth 9% each, the chest and abdomen 18%, and the entire back 18%. This patient, therefore, has a 54% body surface area (BSA) burn. (PCPP 4–187   EPC 965)

18.
D. In the child, the rule of nines differs slightly. The head, being larger in proportion to the rest of the body, is worth 18%. The legs, therefore, are 13.5% each. So a child with burns to both legs has a 27% BSA burn. (PCPP 4–187   EPC 965)

19.
D. Some complications of burns include hypothermia (loss of body heat through the burn area), hypovolemia (plasma loss through the burn area), and eschar (destruction of skin cells). (PCPP 4–188 EPC 966)

20.
C. A circumferential burn encircles the complete exterior of an extremity. In these types of burns, the constriction may be severe enough to occlude all blood flow into the distal extremity. In the case of a thoracic burn, it may drastically reduce chest expansion, reducing respiratory tidal volume. (PCPP 4–188   EPC 967)

21.
D. According to the American Burn Association, the following burn injuries should be evaluated in a burn center:

- Partial thickness burn >15% BSA
- Full thickness burn >5% BSA
- Significant face, feet, hands, perineal burns
- High-voltage electrical injuries
- Inhalation injuries
- Chemical burns causing progressive tissue destruction
- Associated significant injuries (PCPP 4–195 EPC 974)

22.
A. Use local cooling to treat minor soft tissue burns that involve only a small portion of the body surface area at partial thickness. Care for only those burns that involve less than 15% of the body surface area in this way. (PCPP 4–196   EPC 975)

23.
D. Use dry sterile dressings to treat partial thickness burns over 30% of the body or full thickness burns over 5% of the body surface area. This will reduce air movement past the sensitive first and second degree burns and provide padding against minor bumping. In the third degree burn, they provide a barrier to possible contamination. (PCPP 4–196   EPC 975)

24.
B. According to the Parkland formula, a moderate to severe burn patient should receive 2 ml times his weight in kg (70) times the BSA burned (30). This calculates to 4200 ml. (PCPP 4–197   EPC 976)

25.
A. The author states that the initial fluid bolus for a patient with a short travel time can be one-fourth the above dose—thus, a little over 1000 ml. (PCPP 4–197   EPC 976)

26.
D. A patient with severe cyanide toxicity normally presents with severe respiratory distress and an

altered mental status. Management includes aggressive airway protection, and cyanide antidote therapy (a nitrite compound such as amyl nitrite or sodium nitrite) and a sulfur-containing compound (such as sodium thiosulfate). (PCPP 4–199   EPC 977)

27.

D. Prehospital management of most chemical burns includes rinsing the area with large volumes of cool water. The water not only rinses away the offending material, but also dilutes any water-soluble agents. The cooling effect of the water also reduces the heat and the rate of chemical reaction. (PCPP 4–202   EPC 981)

28.

C. Some substances either do not dissolve in water or may react violently with it. Phenol, dry lime, and sodium are three of those substances. In these cases, you should try to remove as much of the substance as possible before applying water. All others should be irrigated with copious amounts of water. (PCPP 4–202   EPC 981)

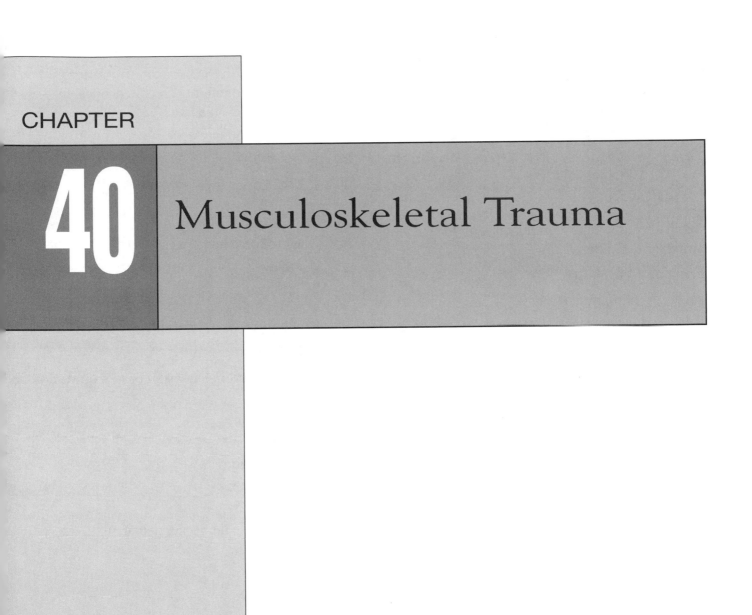

CHAPTER

40

Musculoskeletal Trauma

1. Which of the following is NOT part of the axial skeleton?
   A. Skull
   B. Pelvis
   C. Vertebral column
   D. Thorax

Match the following components of long bones with their definitions:

2. ____ Diaphysis
3. ____ Epiphysis
4. ____ Metaphysis
5. ____ Periosteum
6. ____ Haversian canal

A. Intermediate transition region
B. Passage for blood vessels and nerves
C. The wide end of a long bone
D. Long cylindrical shaft
E. Tough outer bone layer

7. Connective tissue that provides the articular surfaces of the skeletal system is called
   A. cartilage
   B. synovium
   C. ligament
   D. fossa

8. The connective tissue band that holds joints together is called a
   A. fossa
   B. ligament
   C. cartilage
   D. synovium

9. The oily, viscous fluid that lubricates articular surfaces is known as
   A. fossa
   B. ligaments
   C. cartilage
   D. synovium

10. The most commonly fractured bone in the human body is the
    A. scapula
    B. humerus
    C. femur
    D. clavicle

11. The proximal humerus articulates with the
    A. radius
    B. ulna
    C. glenoid fossa
    D. clavicle

12. The act of turning the palm or foot upward is called
    A. pronation
    B. abduction
    C. adduction
    D. supination

13. The metacarpal bones articulate with the
    A. radius
    B. ulna
    C. phalanges
    D. all of the above

14. The hollow surface of the pelvis into which the head of the femur fits is the
    A. glenoid fossa
    B. calcaneus
    C. acetabulum
    D. tibial plateau

15. The distal femur articulates with the
    A. pelvis
    B. tibia
    C. fibula
    D. radius

16. The medial malleolus is formed by the
    A. tibia
    B. fibula
    C. calcaneus
    D. tarsal bones

17. _____ is the only muscle over which we have control.
    A. Cardiac muscle
    B. Smooth muscle
    C. Skeletal muscle
    D. None of the above

18. The Achilles is an example of a
    A. ligament
    B. tendon
    C. cartilage
    D. long bone

19. Blunt trauma causing bleeding and discoloration underneath the skin is a
    A. laceration
    B. contusion
    C. abrasion
    D. subluxation

20. The overstretching of a muscle is called a
    A. strain
    B. sprain
    C. subluxation
    D. dislocation

21. The overstretching of a ligament is known as a/an
    A. strain
    B. sprain
    C. abduction
    D. adduction

22. A partial separation of a joint is called a/an
    A. dislocation
    B. subluxation
    C. pronation
    D. insufflation

23. The biceps/triceps relationship is an example of
    A. opposition
    B. synergism
    C. direct articulation
    D. indirect articulation

24. The origin point for the biceps muscle is the
    A. humerus
    B. radius
    C. clavicle
    D. scapula

25. A grade 2 ankle sprain is characterized by which of the following criteria?
    A. Complete tear of the ligament
    B. Significant incomplete tear with intact but unstable joint
    C. Minor incomplete tear with intact, stable joint
    D. Partial displacement of the bone ends

26. You learn that three days after hip fracture surgery your 34-year-old patient went into cardiac arrest and died. The most likely cause for his sudden death was
    A. acute myocardial infarction
    B. fat embolism
    C. cardiac tamponade
    D. massive hemorrhage and internal blood loss

Match the following types of fractures with their respective definitions:

27. ____ Comminuted
28. ____ Impacted
29. ____ Greenstick
30. ____ Oblique
31. ____ Spiral
32. ____ Transverse
33. ____ Fatigue

    A. A bone broken into several pieces
    B. Incomplete fracture often seen in children
    C. A break straight across the bone

D. A break caused by rotational forces

E. Runs at an angle across the bone

F. The bone is compressed in itself

G. Caused by prolonged or repeated stress

34. In pediatrics, an epiphyseal fracture is especially worrisome because of the
    A. threat of fat embolism
    B. increased incidence of osteomyelitis
    C. damage to the growth plate
    D. increased angulation that inhibits proper healing

35. A common cause for bursitis is
    A. infection
    B. repeated trauma
    C. gout
    D. all of the above

36. Your 74-year-old female patient presents with generalized joint immobility, pain, increased pain on movement, fatigue, and flexion contractures. She claims she has had this problem for years and that it has gotten worse. Your field diagnosis is
    A. rheumatoid arthritis
    B. osteoarthritis
    C. gout
    D. none of the above

37. Gout is an inflammation of the joints caused by
    A. deterioration of osteoblast production
    B. increased uric acid accumulation
    C. irregular bony overgrowth
    D. torn bursa sacs

38. Which of the following is **NOT** one of the six Ps in evaluating a limb injury?
    A. Paralysis
    B. Paresthesia
    C. Pressure
    D. Pruritis

39. Which of the following statements is true regarding the management of musculoskeletal injuries?
    A. Always splint the joints above and below the fracture site
    B. Always splint the bones above and below a dislocated joint
    C. Always perform distal neurovascular tests before and after any splinting
    D. All of the above

40. The best position for an injured limb is
    A. halfway between flexion and extension
    B. fully extended
    C. fully flexed
    D. in the deformed position

41. Which of the following statements best describes the proper use of heat and ice for musculoskeletal injuries?
    A. Ice for the first 24 hours, followed by heat
    B. Heat for the first 24 hours, followed by ice
    C. Ice for the first 48 hours, followed by heat
    D. Ice only

42. In which of the following situations should you attempt to reduce a dislocation in the field?
    A. There is a significant neurovascular deficit
    B. Transport time is very short
    C. You are unsure of your diagnosis
    D. There are other significant injuries

43. The management of a pelvic fracture includes which of the following procedures?
    A. Pneumatic antishock garment
    B. IV fluid replacement
    C. Rapid transport
    D. All of the above

44. Traction splinting is indicated in which of the following conditions?
    A. Isolated midshaft femur fracture

B. Disease-induced proximal femur fracture

C. Bilateral femur fractures with profound shock

D. All of the above

45. A Colles' fracture involves which bone?

A. Proximal ulna

B. Proximal radius

C. Distal radius

D. Distal ulna

46. Often you may not be able to differentiate a proximal femur fracture from a/an

A. posterior hip dislocation

B. anterior hip dislocation

C. pelvic fracture

D. acetabulum fracture

47. Your patient presents with her foot turned outward and the head of her femur palpable in the inguinal area. Your field diagnosis and management include

A. anterior hip dislocation—immediate reduction

B. anterior hip dislocation—immobilization

C. proximal femur fracture—traction splint

D. posterior hip dislocation—reduction

48. Your patient presents with an obvious anterior shoulder dislocation. Because of a long transport time, severe pain, and some distal neurovascular deficits, you decide to reduce the dislocation. Which of the following is a sign that you have been successful?

A. You hear a "pop"

B. The joint moves freely through its normal range of motion

C. Normal shoulder alignment is seen

D. All of the above

49. Your patient has a musculoskeletal injury and complains of moderate to severe pain. Which of the following conditions precludes the use of nitrous oxide in his pain management?

A. COPD

B. Pneumothorax

C. Middle ear infection

D. All of the above

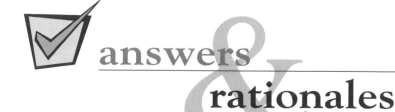

answers & rationales

1.

B. The axial skeleton consists of the skull, the vertebral column, and the thorax. The upper and lower extremities, the shoulder girdle, and the pelvis make up the appendicular skeleton. (PCPP 4–216 EPC 134)

Matching (PCPP 4–212 EPC 134)

2. D	Diaphysis	**A.**	Intermediate transition region
3. C	Epiphysis		
4. A	Metaphysis	**B.**	Passage for blood vessels and nerves
5. E	Periosteum		
6. B	Haversian canal	**C.**	The wide end of a long bone
		D.	Long cylindrical shaft
		E.	Tough outer bone layer

7.

A. A layer of connective tissue called cartilage covers the epiphyseal surface. It is a smooth, strong, flexible material that functions as the actual surface of articulation between bones. It allows for easy movement between the ends of adjacent bones, such as the femur and tibia. It also absorbs some of the impact associated with walking, running, or other jarring activities. (PCPP 4–214 EPC 132)

8.

B. Ligaments are connective tissues connecting bone to bone and holding the joints together. Ligaments will stretch to allow joint movement, while holding the bone ends firmly in place. (PCPP 4–216 EPC 133)

9.

D. The ligaments surrounding a joint form the synovial capsule. This chamber holds a small amount of fluid to lubricate the articular surfaces. The oily, viscous fluid assists joint motion by reducing friction. (PCPP 4–216 EPC 134)

10.

D. The clavicle, which is anterior to the scapula and not very well protected, is the most commonly fractured bone in the human body. (PCPP 4–217 EPC 139)

11.

C. The humerus is the single bone of the proximal upper extremity. It is secured against the glenoid fossa of the shoulder joint proximally. The humerus articulates with the radius and ulna at the elbow. (PCPP 4–218 EPC 140)

12.

D. The act of turning the palm or foot upward is called supination. The opposite movement, turning the hand or foot downward, is called pronation. (PCPP 4–218 EPC 664)

13.

C. The metacarpal bones articulate with the phalanges of the fingers and the carpal bones. (PCPP 4–218 EPC 136)

14.

C. The actual articular surface for the femur is the acetabulum. It is a hollow depression in the lateral pelvis into which the head of the femur fits. (PCPP 4–218 EPC 146)

15.

B. The distal femur articulates with the tibia. (PCPP 4–219 EPC 143)

16.

A. The distal tibia forms the medial malleolus or the protuberance of the ankle, while the fibula forms the lateral malleolus. (PCPP 4–219 EPC 143)

17.

C. Skeletal muscles are muscles over which we have conscious control. They are necessary to move the extremities and the body in general. The largest component of the muscular system, they are the muscles most commonly traumatized. (PCPP 4–222   EPC 148)

18.

B. The Achilles is an example of a tendon. A tendon is a specialized connective tissue band that accomplishes the insertion and in some cases the origin of muscles. They are extremely strong and will not stretch. They often will break an area of bone loose rather than tear. (PCPP 4–224   EPC 152)

19.

B. Trauma frequently causes contusions. As with all contusions, small blood vessels rupture, causing dull pain, leakage of fluid into the interstitial spaces, and the classical discoloration. (PCPP 4–225   EPC 989)

20.

A. A strain is an overstretching of the muscle and presents as pain. (PCPP 4–226   EPC 990)

21.

B. A sprain is a tearing of the connective tissue of the joint capsule—specifically, a ligament or ligaments. This injury causes exquisite pain at the site, followed shortly by inflammation and swelling. (PCPP 4–226   EPC 990)

22.

B. A subluxation is an incomplete dislocation of the joint. The surfaces remain in contact, while the joint is partially deformed. (PCPP 4–226   EPC 990)

23.

A. The biceps muscle group allows us to flex our elbow. The triceps muscle group allows us to extend our elbow. This is known as opposition because while one contracts, the other relaxes. (PCPP 4–223   EPC 137)

24.

D. The origin of a muscle is the point of attachment that remains stationary as the muscle contracts. The origin of the biceps muscle is at two points on the scapula—the acromion and coracoid processes. The other attachment point is known as the insertion. (PCPP 4–223   EPC 151)

25.

B. Ligament sprains are classified according to the following scale: (PCPP 4–226   EPC 990)

Grade	Tear	S&S	Joint Stability
1	Incomplete, minor	Pain, minimal swelling	Stable
2	Incomplete but significant	Moderate to severe pain and swelling	Unstable but intact
3	Complete	Severe pain and spasm	Unstable

26.

B. An infrequent, but serious complication from a fracture is a fat embolism that enters the venous system and travels to the heart and then the lungs, where it lodges. If it is large enough, it can cause cardiac arrest. (PCPP 4–229   EPC 229)

Matching (PCPP 4–229   EPC 993)

27. **A**   Comminuted
28. **F**   Impacted
29. **B**   Greenstick
30. **E**   Oblique
31. **D**   Spiral
32. **C**   Transverse
33. **G**   Fatigue

A. A bone broken into several pieces
B. Incomplete fracture often seen in children
C. A break straight across the bone
D. A break caused by rotational forces
E. Runs at an angle across the bone
F. The bone is compressed in itself
G. Caused by prolonged or repeated stress

34.

C. The epiphyseal plate is another term for the growth plate. Damage to this area may inhibit proper bone growth, usually of the proximal tibia. (PCPP 4–230 EPC 994)

35.

D. Bursitis is the inflammation of the bursa sacs, which reduce friction and cushion ligaments and tendons. Bursitis can be caused by infection, repeated trauma, gout, or unknown etiologies. (PCPP 4–232   EPC 996)

36.

A. Rheumatoid arthritis is a chronic, systemic, progressive, debilitating joint disease caused by inflammation of the synovial joints. It occurs two to three times more frequently in women and is characterized by generalized joint immobility, pain, increased pain on movement, fatigue, and sometimes flexion contractures. (PCPP 4–232 EPC 996)

37.

B. Gout is an inflammation in joints and connective tissue caused by the accumulation of uric acid crystals. Signs and symptoms include peripheral joint pain, swelling, and possible deformity. (PCPP 4–232   EPC 996)

38.

D. The six Ps comprise a helpful mnemonic to remember key elements when evaluating a limb injury. They include Pain (upon palpation or movement), Pallor (pale skin), Paralysis (immobility), Paresthesia (numbness or tingling), Pressure (inner tension), and Pulses (absence or weakness). (PCPP 4–235   EPC 999)

39.

D. Always splint the joints above and below the fracture site and the bones above and below a dislocated joint. Before and after any splinting, always perform distal neurovascular checks for circulation, sensory, and motor function. (PCPP 4–240 EPC 1004)

40.

A. To best maintain proper neurovascular function, you should immobilize an injured limb halfway between flexion and extension, also called the position of function. In this position, you place the least amount of stress on the joint ligaments and the muscles and tendons surrounding the injury. (PCPP 4–240   EPC 1004)

41.

C. The standard mnemonic for musculoskeletal injuries is RICE. This stands for **R**est, **I**ce, **C**ompression, and **E**levation. Heat may be applied 48 hours after the injury to promote healing and circulation. (PCPP 4–257   EPC 1021)

42.

A. Because reducing a dislocation is risky, you should attempt to reduce a dislocated joint in the field only if there is a significant neurovascular deficit, there is a prolonged extrication or transport time, there are no other associated serious injuries, and you are sure the injury is a dislocation. (PCPP 4–245 EPC 1009)

43.

D. Fractures to the pelvic ring are especially worrisome because of the danger of severe bleeding and associated injuries to the reproductive, digestive, and urinary organs. Management of a pelvic fracture includes immobilization of the pelvic ring with the pneumatic antishock garment, IV fluid replacement, and rapid transport to a trauma center. (PCPP 4–246   EPC 1010)

44.

A. The traction splint is the best device to splint the hemodynamically stable patient with an isolated femur fracture. (PCPP 4–247   EPC 1011)

45.

C. Commonly fractures will occur at the distal end of the radius, breaking it just above the articular surface. This is known as a Colles' fracture and presents with the wrist turned up at an unusual angle. (PCPP 4–249   EPC 1013)

46.

B. Fracture of the femur near the hip may be difficult to differentiate from an anterior hip dislocation. While you may expect a broken leg to be slightly shorter than the unbroken one, the difference may be slight and unnoticeable if the legs are not straight and parallel. (PCPP 4–247   EPC 1011)

47.

B. The foot turned outward and the head of the femur palpable in the inguinal region suggest an anterior hip dislocation. Management is aimed at immobilization on a spine board with lots of padding for comfort. Do not attempt to reduce an anterior hip dislocation. (PCPP 4–250   EPC 1014)

48.

D. As in any reduction of a dislocation, success is determined by the following criteria: hearing a "pop" as the bone ends realign, normal alignment of the joint is accomplished, a reduction in pain is de-

scribed, and an increase in mobility is seen. (PCPP 4–253   EPC 1017)

49.

D. Since nitrous oxide easily diffuses into air-filled spaces and can dramatically increase the pressure within these spaces, any patient with associated or preexisting problems (COPD, pneumothorax, bowel obstruction, middle ear obstruction) should not receive nitrous oxide. (PCPP 4–255   EPC 1019)

41

Head, Facial, and Neck Trauma

DIRECTIONS Each of the questions or incomplete statements below is followed by suggested answers or completions. Select the **one answer** that is best in each case.

1. Which of the following is NOT a component of the scalp?
   A. Skin
   B. Aponeurotica
   C. Cranium
   D. Periosteum

2. The irregular bone at the base of the skull is the
   A. falx cerebri
   B. central sulcus
   C. cribriform plate
   D. tentorium

3. The three meningeal layers of the brain from the inside out are the
   A. dura mater, pia mater, arachnoid membrane
   B. pia mater, dura mater, arachnoid membrane
   C. arachnoid membrane, pia mater, dura mater
   D. pia mater, arachnoid membrane, dura mater

4. Cerebrospinal fluid circulates through which meningeal layer?
   A. Epidural space
   B. Cerebellar space
   C. Subarachnoid space
   D. Intracerebral space

5. The area of the brain that is the center of conscious thought is the
   A. cerebrum
   B. cerebellum
   C. central sulcus
   D. falx cerebri

6. The cerebrum is separated from the cerebellum by the
   A. falx cerebri
   B. central sulcus
   C. cribriform plate
   D. tentorium

Match the following components of the brain with the functions they control:

7. ____ Frontal lobe
8. ____ Parietal lobe
9. ____ Temporal lobe
10. ____ Occipital lobe
11. ____ Cerebellum
12. ____ Hypothalamus
13. ____ Reticular activating system
14. ____ Medulla

   A. Fine motor coordination
   B. Sight
   C. Personality
   D. Endocrine function
   E. Cardiorespiratory centers
   F. Motor and sensory function
   G. Speech
   H. Consciousness

15. Cerebral perfusion pressure is the difference between the mean arterial pressure and the _____ pressure.
   A. mean venous
   B. capillary wedge
   C. pulse
   D. intracranial

16. The ascending reticular activating system is responsible for
    A. the sleep-wake cycle
    B. endocrine function
    C. voluntary muscle control
    D. maintenance of cerebral perfusion pressure

17. The prominent bone of the cheek is known as the
    A. mandible
    B. maxilla
    C. sphenoid
    D. zygoma

Match the following cranial nerves with their respective functions:

18. ____ Olfactory
19. ____ Optic
20. ____ Occulomotor
21. ____ Trochlear
22. ____ Trigeminal
23. ____ Abducens
24. ____ Facial
25. ____ Acoustic
26. ____ Glossopharyngeal
27. ____ Vagus
28. ____ Accessory
29. ____ Hypoglossal

A. The ability to smile
B. Chewing muscles
C. Pupil constriction
D. Parasympathetic tone
E. Balance
F. Tongue movement
G. Vision
H. Conjugate gaze
I. Neck muscles
J. Swallowing
K. Smell
L. Looking to the side

30. We hear because of the vibration of the
    A. tympanic membrane
    B. cochlea
    C. semicircular canals
    D. dens

31. Positional sense is regulated by our
    A. tympanic membrane
    B. cochlea
    C. semicircular canals
    D. dens

Match the following parts of the eye with their respective definitions:

32. ____ Vitreous humor
33. ____ Aqueous humor
34. ____ Pupil
35. ____ Iris
36. ____ Conjunctiva
37. ____ Lacrimal ducts
38. ____ Sclera

A. Provides nourishment and lubrication
B. Colored portion of the eye
C. White, vascular area of the eye
D. Gelatinous fluid found in eye globe
E. Thin, clear layer covering iris and cornea
F. Liquid found in anterior chamber of eye
G. Opening in the center of the iris

39. Which of the following statements is true regarding scalp lacerations?
    A. They tend to bleed profusely
    B. They result in severe bleeding that can lead to shock
    C. The blood vessels lack effective muscular control
    D. All of the above

40. Battle's sign and periorbital ecchymosis are classic signs of a/an
    A. intracerebral hemorrhage
    B. basilar skull fracture

C. depressed skull fracture

D. subdural hematoma

41. A brain injury occurring on the opposite side of the side of impact is known as a
    A. concussion
    B. contusion
    C. contrecoup
    D. cochlea

42. A patient who has sustained a closed head injury with a brief loss of consciousness but no tissue damage and who experiences a complete recovery of function has suffered a
    A. concussion
    B. contusion
    C. contrecoup
    D. cochlea

43. A patient who has sustained a closed head injury with resulting tissue damage has suffered a
    A. concussion
    B. contusion
    C. contrecoup
    D. cochlea

44. A person who cannot remember the events that occurred before the trauma that caused the condition is said to have _____ amnesia.
    A. anterograde
    B. retrograde
    C. post-traumatic
    D. concussive

45. Your patient presents with obvious fractures to both the maxilla and the nasal bones in which the midface and zygoma move concurrently. What LeFort classification level is this?
    A. I
    B. II
    C. III
    D. IV

46. A pool of blood in the anterior chamber of the eye is known as
    A. conjunctival hemorrhage
    B. retinal artery occlusion
    C. hyphema
    D. corneal abrasion

47. A patient who complains of sudden painless loss of vision in one eye has most likely suffered a
    A. retinal detachment
    B. retinal artery occlusion
    C. hyphema
    D. blowout fracture

48. Which of the following is a complication of jugular vein laceration?
    A. Pulmonary embolism
    B. Air embolism
    C. Hemorrhagic shock
    D. All of the above

49. Which of the following is NOT part of Cushing's response?
    A. Hypertension
    B. Bradycardia
    C. Altered respirations
    D. Hypothermia

50. A patient who responds only to deep pain by abnormally flexing the arms has a Glasgow Coma Score of
    A. 3
    B. 5
    C. 7
    D. 9

SCENARIO

Questions 51–60 refer to the following scenario.

Your patient is a 25-year-old boxer who was knocked out with a left hook to the side of the head and now lies in the dressing room fully awake. His initial vital signs are BP 130/80, pulse 80, respirations 18, and pupils equal and reactive to light. En route to the hospital, he begins to lose consciousness and complains of being sleepy. His breathing becomes erratic, his pulse slows to 60, and his blood pressure rises to 180/90. His left pupil is larger than the right and is slow to react to light.

51. This patient is probably suffering from a/an
    A. epidural hematoma
    B. subdural hematoma
    C. basilar skull fracture
    D. concussion

52. The rapid onset of signs and symptoms is most likely due to the
    A. fracture of the cribriform plate
    B. rupture of the middle meningeal artery
    C. leakage of CSF into soft tissues
    D. jarring of the reticular activating system

53. This patient also shows the classic signs and symptoms of
    A. increasing intracranial pressure
    B. decreasing cerebral blood volume
    C. basilar skull fracture
    D. contrecoup injury

54. These signs and symptoms are caused by
    A. brain shrinkage
    B. cerebral blood flow interruption
    C. brainstem herniation
    D. abnormally low carbon dioxide levels

55. His abnormal breathing pattern is caused by
    A. high levels of carbon dioxide
    B. pressure on the medulla
    C. the leakage of cerebrospinal fluid into the nasal cavity
    D. foramen magnum collapse

56. This patient may hyperventilate in an attempt to
    A. vasodilate the brain vasculature
    B. vasoconstrict the brain vasculature
    C. increase carbon dioxide levels
    D. cause a metabolic alkalosis

57. The larger left pupil is caused by compression of the
    A. third cranial nerve
    B. reticular activating system
    C. extraoccular muscles
    D. iris muscle

58. This patient may vomit without accompanying nausea due to
    A. high levels of carbon dioxide
    B. brain hypoxia
    C. Cushing's reflex
    D. pressure on the medulla

59. Prehospital management of this patient includes all of the following EXCEPT
    A. prophylactic hyperventilation with 100% oxygen
    B. maximizing oxygen concentration
    C. spinal immobilization
    D. all of the above

60. Pharmacological therapy for this patient may include
    A. furosemide
    B. diazepam
    C. succinylcholine
    D. all of the above

SCENARIO

Questions 61–63 refer to the following scenario.

Your patient is a 75-year-old nursing home resident who presents with a decreased level of response. The staff claims he began acting strangely hours before calling you. He has no history of diabetes or CNS disease. His only history is that of a minor fall he took one week ago. He presents with a slow bounding pulse; a systolic blood pressure of 170, which is high for him; an erratic breathing pattern; and a slightly larger right pupil. His blood sugar is 120, and there is no history or evidence of substance abuse.

61. This patient has probably suffered a/an
    A. epidural hematoma
    B. subdural hematoma

C. basilar skull fracture

D. concussion

62. The signs and symptoms of this type of injury often present themselves hours or days following the injury because
    A. significant brain swelling takes that long to develop
    B. the bleeding is from a small vein

C. the bleeding is from a large artery

D. there is no real tissue damage

63. High-risk factors for this type of injury include
    A. alcoholism
    B. the elderly
    C. recent head injuries
    D. all of the above

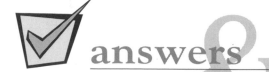

answers & rationales

1.

C. The scalp, which helps protect and insulate the skull and brain, is comprised of **S**kin, **C**onnective tissue, **A**poneurotica, **L**ayer of areolar tissue, and **P**eriosteum—SCALP. (PCPP 4–264   EPC 153)

2.

C. The cribriform plate is an irregular and bony plate at the base of the skull. It has surfaces against which the brain may abrade, lacerate, or contuse in severe deceleration injuries. This is the location of the common basilar skull fracture. (PCPP 4–265 EPC 154)

3.

D. The meninges are a group of three tissues between the skull and the brain and between the inside of the spinal foramen and the cord. The outermost layer is the dura mater. The layer closest to the brain and spinal cord is the pia mater, and separating the two layers is connective tissue called the arachnoid membrane. From the inside out, they form a "PAD" for the brain and spinal cord. (PCPP 4–265   EPC 154)

4.

C. Beneath the arachnoid membrane is the subarachnoid space, which is filled with cerebrospinal fluid. Cerebrospinal fluid is the medium that surrounds the central nervous system and acts to absorb the shock of minor deceleration. (PCPP 4–266   EPC 155)

5.

A. The cerebrum is the largest of the brain regions and occupies most of the cranial cavity. It is the center of conscious thought, personality, speech, motor control, and visual, auditory, and tactile perception. (PCPP 4–266   EPC 156)

6.

D. The tentorium is an extension of the dura mater separating the cerebrum from the cerebellum. It is a fibrous sheet and runs at right angles to the falx cerebri. (PCPP 4–267   EPC 156)

Matching   (PCPP 4–267   EPC 182)

7. C	Frontal lobe	**A.** Fine motor
8. F	Parietal lobe	coordination
9. G	Temporal lobe	**B.** Sight
10. B	Occipital lobe	**C.** Personality
11. A	Cerebellum	**D.** Endocrine function
12. D	Hypothalamus	**E.** Cardiorespiratory
13. H	Reticular	centers
	activating system	**F.** Motor and sensory
14. E	Medulla	function
		G. Speech
		H. Consciousness

15.

D. Cerebral perfusion pressure is the pressure moving blood through the brain. It is the difference between the mean arterial pressure and intracranial pressure. When brain swelling or bleeding increases intracranial pressure, the brain signals the cardiovascular system to raise the mean arterial pressure in order to perfuse the brain. (PCPP 4–269   EPC 157)

16.

A. The ascending reticular activating system is responsible for the sleep-wake cycle. It is our on-off switch for consciousness. (PCPP 4–269   EPC 157)

17.

D. The zygoma is the prominent bone of the cheek. It protects the eyes and the muscles controlling eye and jaw movement. (PCPP 4–271   EPC 153)

Matching   (PCPP 4–270   EPC 189)

18. K	Olfactory	A.	The ability to smile
19. G	Optic	B.	Chewing muscles
20. C	Occulomotor	C.	Pupil constriction
21. H	Trochlear	D.	Parasympathetic tone
22. B	Trigeminal	E.	Balance
23. L	Abducens	F.	Tongue movement
24. A	Facial	G.	Vision
25. E	Acoustic	H.	Conjugate gaze
26. J	Glossopharyngeal	I.	Neck muscles
27. D	Vagus	J.	Swallowing
28. I	Accessory	K.	Smell
29. F	Hypoglossal	L.	Looking to the side

30.

A. Hearing occurs when sound waves cause the tympanic membrane, or ear drum, to vibrate. The ear drum transmits the vibrations through three very small bones to the cochlea, the organ of hearing. These vibrations stimulate the auditory nerve, which, in turn, transmits the signal to the brain. (PCPP 4–273   EPC 161)

31.

C. The semicircular canals are three rings of the inner ear. They are responsible for sensing the motion of the head and providing positional sense for the body. This positional sense is present even when the eyes are closed. If injury or illness disturbs this center, excess signals are sent to the brain. Patients complain of a spinning feeling known as vertigo. (PCPP 4–273   EPC 161)

Matching   (PCPP 4–162)

32. D	Vitreous humor	A.	Provides nourishment and lubrication
33. F	Aqueous humor		
34. G	Pupil	B.	Colored portion of the eye
35. B	Iris		
36. E	Conjunctiva	C.	White, vascular area of the eye
37. A	Lacrimal ducts		
38. C	Sclera	D.	Gelatinous fluid found in eye globe
		E.	Thin, clear layer covering iris and cornea
		F.	Liquid found in anterior chamber of eye
		G.	Opening in the center of the iris

39.

D. The scalp is an area frequently subjected to soft tissue injury. Because this area is extremely vascular and because the scalp vessels are larger and not quite as muscular as other vessels, blood loss can be rapid and difficult to control. Severe and persistent bleeding from scalp lacerations can contribute to shock. (PCPP 4–278   EPC 1028)

40.

B. Battle's sign is a black-and-blue discoloration over the mastoid process just behind the ear. Bilateral periorbital ecchymosis is a black-and-blue discoloration of the area surrounding the eyes. Both of these signs are normally associated with a basilar skull fracture. (PCPP 4–280   EPC 1030)

41.

C. A contrecoup injury occurs on the opposite side of the side of impact. The brain impacts the interior of the skull on the opposite side, causing soft tissue injury such as contusions, lacerations, and hemorrhages. (PCPP 4–282   EPC 1032)

42.

A. A person who has sustained a closed head injury with a brief loss of consciousness but no tissue damage and who experiences a complete recovery of function, has suffered a concussion. (PCPP 4–284   EPC 1034)

43.

B. A contusion is a more significant jarring than a concussion and results in cell damage. It is a closed wound in which the skin is unbroken, although damage has occurred to the tissue beneath. If the loss of consciousness is longer than 5 minutes, the patient is usually admitted to the hospital. (PCPP 4–282   EPC 1032)

44.

B. A patient who cannot recall the events that occurred before the trauma that caused his condition is said to have retrograde amnesia. If he cannot recall the events that occurred after the trauma, he is said to have anterograde amnesia. Both are signs of brain injury. (PCPP 4–287 EPC 1037)

45.

B. The LeFort facial fracture classification system is as follows: (PCPP 4–290   EPC 1040)

I   Maxilla fracture only, slight instability, no displacement

II   Fracture of both maxilla and nasal bones

III Fracture involving entire face below brow ridge

46.

C. Hemorrhage into the anterior chamber of the eye will pool and display a level of blood in front of the pupil and iris. This condition is known as hyphema and is not emergent. It does, however, require evaluation by an ophthalmologist. (PCPP 4–293   EPC 1043)

47.

B. Retinal artery occlusion is a vascular emergency in which an embolus, or traveling clot, blocks the blood supply to the eye. The patient complains of sudden and painless loss of vision in one eye. (PCPP 4–294   EPC 1044)

48.

D. Jugular veins at times maintain a pressure less than atmospheric pressure. An open wound may draw air into a vessel, affecting the heart or pulmonary circulation. Jugular veins, although rather low-pressure vessels, still carry large volumes of blood and will bleed profusely. (PCPP 4–294   EPC 1044)

49.

D. In cases of increasing intracranial pressure, the brain displaces away from the side of the hematoma toward the foramen magnum. This movement pushes the medulla oblongata into the foramen magnum, producing changes in vital signs. The pulse rate slows, respirations become erratic, and the blood pressure rises. This collective change in vital signs is called Cushing's response. (PCPP 4–287   EPC 1037)

50.

B. The Glasgow Coma Scale objectively rates your patient in three categories: eye opening, best verbal response, and best motor response. Since this patient does not open his eyes, he gets a score of 1 in the first category. Since he does not respond to verbal commands, he gets a 1 in the second category. He flexes abnormally to pain, earning a score of 3 in the last category, making his total score 5. (PCPP 4–301   EPC 1051)

51.

A. An epidural hematoma is an accumulation of blood between the dura mater and the cranium. (PCPP 4–283   EPC 1033)

52.

B. The rapid onset of signs and symptoms following an epidural hematoma occurs because the bleeding involves arterial vessels, often the middle meningeal artery. The condition progresses rapidly while the patient moves quickly toward unconsciousness. Since the bleeding is arterial, intracranial pressure builds rapidly, compressing the cerebrum and increasing the pressure within the skull. (PCPP 4–283 EPC 1033)

53.

A. This patient shows the classic signs and symptoms of increasing intracranial pressure: an altered respiratory pattern, bradycardia, hypertension, unequal pupils, and a decreasing level of consciousness. (PCPP 4–287   EPC 1037)

54.

C. These signs and symptoms are caused by brainstem herniation. As the pressure in the cranium increases, the brain is pushed downward through the tentorium toward the brain stem. Because the brain stem houses our cardiac and respiratory centers, these vital signs are affected. (PCPP 4–287   EPC 1037)

55.

B. Pressure on the medulla oblongata causes alterations in respiratory control. Your patient may hyperventilate, exhibit Cheyne-Stokes respirations, and eventually stop breathing altogether. (PCPP 4–287   EPC 1037)

56.

B. High levels of carbon dioxide cause the brain vasculature to dilate. This results in increased blood volume, which, in turn, increases the pressure within the skull. In an attempt to vasoconstrict these vessels and reverse the process, the body may begin to hyperventilate. (PCPP 4–287   EPC 1037)

57.

A. Pressure on the third cranial nerve, the occulomotor nerve, causes the pupil on that side to dilate. An early indicator of increasing intracranial pressure is a slightly larger pupil that reacts slowly to light. As the pressure increases, the pupil will become fixed and totally dilated. (PCPP 4–287   EPC 1037)

58.

D. The vomit center is located in the medulla oblongata. Pressure on this center will cause immediate vomiting without accompanying nausea. The vomiting is usually forceful and known as "projectile vomiting." (PCPP 4–303   EPC 1053)

59.

B. Prehospital management of a patient with increasing intracranial pressure includes the following: spinal immobilization; elevation of the head of the stretcher to maximize venous drainage; aggressive airway management and intubation as soon as possible to protect the airway from the eventual vomiting; and high-flow O_2 to maximize brain oxygenation and prevent tissue swelling. Only in the event of severe deterioration from brain swelling should you perform hyperventilation. (PCPP 4–303   EPC 1053)

60.

D. Pharmacological therapy for this patient may include diuretics, such as furosemide or mannitol, to decrease intravascular blood volume; paralytics, such as succinylcholine or pancuronium, to facilitate intubation; and anticonvulsants, such as diazepam or midazolam, to control seizures and sedate your patient. (PCPP 4–311   EPC 1061)

61.

B. A subdural hematoma is a collection of blood directly beneath the dura mater. (PCPP 4–283 EPC 1033)

62.

B. The signs and symptoms following a subdural hematoma occur very slowly and are subtle in presentation because blood loss is usually due to rupture of a small venous vessel. (PCPP 4–283   EPC 1033)

63.

D. You will frequently encounter subdural hematomas in elderly patients or chronic alcoholics. Because the aging process and chronic alcoholism shrink the brain, both groups are prone to this condition following even seemingly minor head injuries. Your patient's altered behavior pattern may be caused by a subdural hematoma. (PCPP 4–284 EPC 1034)

42 Spinal Trauma

DIRECTIONS Each of the questions or incomplete statements below is followed by suggested answers or completions. Select the **one answer** that is best in each case.

1. Which mechanism of injury causes the majority of spinal cord injuries?
   A. Penetrating trauma
   B. Sports-related trauma
   C. Falls
   D. Motor vehicle crashes

2. Approximately how many spinal cord injuries result from improper handling after the incident?
   A. 5%
   B. 25%
   C. 50%
   D. 75%

3. The finger-like process of the second vertebra around which the first cervical vertebra rotates is the
   A. atlas
   B. axis
   C. odontoid
   D. mastoid

4. The opening on the vertebrae through which the spinal cord passes is the
   A. foramen magnum
   B. odontoid process
   C. spinal canal
   D. dura mater

5. Cerebrospinal fluid circulates through which meningeal layer?
   A. Epidural space
   B. Subdural space
   C. Subarachnoid space
   D. Intracerebral space

6. The first spinous process that you can palpate just above the shoulders is
   A. C-2
   B. C-4
   C. C-7
   D. T-1

7. Which section of the spinal canal has the largest foramen?
   A. Cervical
   B. Thoracic
   C. Sacral
   D. Lumbar

8. Bundles of nerves that transmit impulses from the body to the brain are known as
   A. descending tracts
   B. ascending tracts
   C. anterior medial fissures
   D. posterior medial sulci

9. The phrenic nerve is comprised of peripheral nerve roots
   A. C-1–C-8
   B. C-3–C-5
   C. T-1–T-3
   D. L-1 and below

10. Topographical regions of the body innervated by specific nerve roots are known as
    A. dermatomes
    B. cauda equina
    C. neurilemma
    D. axons

Match the following mechanisms of injury with their respective example (A term can be used more than once):

11. _____ Flexion
12. _____ Compression
13. _____ Hyperextension
14. _____ Distraction
15. _____ Rotation

A. Hanging
B. Axial loading
C. Whiplash
D. Left hook
E. In-line impacts

16. If your patient presents with loss of motor function and sensation to pain, light touch, and temperature below T-1, while retaining positional and vibration sense, he has most likely sustained a/an
    A. complete cord transection
    B. central cord syndrome
    C. Brown-Séquard's syndrome
    D. anterior cord syndrome

SCENARIO

Questions 17–21 refer to the following scenario.

Your patient is a 45-year-old male who was ejected from a vehicle in a one-car rollover accident. He presents on the ground complaining of the inability to move his arms and legs. His airway is clear, and his vital signs are respirations 18 with no chest rise, BP 70/30, pulse 50, and skin warm and dry. He also presents with priapism and the hands in the "hold-up" position.

17. Your field diagnosis of this patient should include
    A. neurogenic shock
    B. cervical spinal cord interruption
    C. bilateral paralysis
    D. all of the above

18. His unusual vital sign presentation is due to
    A. peripheral nerve interruption
    B. loss of sympathetic nervous system control
    C. loss of parasympathetic nervous system control
    D. blood loss below the injury

19. The priapism is caused by
    A. parasympathetic stimulation
    B. sympathetic stimulation
    C. total autonomic nervous system dysfunction
    D. none of the above

20. The absence of chest rise is due to
    A. intercostal muscle paralysis
    B. rupture of the diaphragm
    C. damage to the third cranial nerve
    D. Cushing's reflex

21. Prehospital management includes which of the following procedures?
    A. IV fluid replacement
    B. Atropine IV
    C. Spinal immobilization
    D. All of the above

✓ answers & rationales

1.

D. The majority of spinal cord injuries (48%) are the result of motor vehicle crashes, most commonly in young men ages 16–30. (PCPP 4–322   EPC 1069)

2.

B. As many as 25% of all spinal cord injuries result from improper handling of the spinal column (and the patient) after an injury. This is often caused by bystanders. (PCPP 4–323)

3.

C. The second cervical vertebra, the axis, has a small finger-like upper projection, called the odontoid process, which forms the pivot point around which the head rotates. The first cervical vertebra, the atlas, sits atop this protrusion. (PCPP 4–325   EPC 167)

4.

C. The spinal canal (or foramen) is the opening in the vertebrae through which the spinal cord passes. The cord travels from the skull to the second lumbar vertebra. This tube must remain aligned to prevent injury to the spinal cord. (PCPP 4–324 EPC 168)

5.

C. Beneath the arachnoid membrane is the subarachnoid space, which is filled with cerebrospinal fluid. Cerebrospinal fluid is the medium that surrounds the central nervous system and acts to absorb the shock of minor deceleration. (PCPP 4–328   EPC 172)

6.

C. The last cervical vertebra (C-7) is the first bony prominence you can feel just above the shoulders. It is an important landmark when counting vertebrae. (PCPP 4–326   EPC 169)

7.

D. The lumbar spine has the largest vertebral bodies, the thickest intervertebral disks, and the largest foramen (spinal canal). (PCPP 4–327   EPC 170)

8.

B. Bundles of axons that transmit sensory impulses from the body to the brain are known as the ascending tracts. These tracts are paired with the descending tracts (which carry motor impulses from the brain to the body) on each side of the spinal cord. Injury may affect one, some, or all of these tracts. (PCPP 4–329   EPC 185)

9.

B. The phrenic nerve is comprised of peripheral nerve roots C-3 through C-5. It innervates the diaphragm, the main muscle for breathing. (PCPP 4–330 EPC 185)

10.

A. Dermatomes are body regions corresponding to various nerve routes. As these peripheral routes branch off the spine, they perceive sensation lower and lower on the body. (PCPP 4–331   EPC 187)

Matching   (PCPP 4–334   EPC 1071)

11. **E**	Flexion	**A.**	Hanging
12. **B, E**	Compression	**B.**	Axial loading
13. **C**	Hyperextension	**C.**	Whiplash
14. **A**	Distraction	**D.**	Left hook
15. **D**	Rotation	**E.**	In-line impacts

16.

D. Anterior cord syndrome is caused by bony fragments or pressure compressing the arteries that perfuse the anterior cord. This causes a loss of motor function and sensation to pain, light touch, and temperature below the injured site. Potential for recovery is poor. (PCPP 4–338   EPC 1075)

17.

D. Your prehospital diagnosis of this patient should include cervical spinal cord interruption, bilateral paralysis, and neurogenic shock. (PCPP 4–338 EPC 1075)

18.

B. Patients in shock usually present with hypotension, tachycardia, and cool, clammy skin. These signs indicate that the sympathetic nervous system compensatory mechanism has been activated. Your patient's unusual vital sign presentation (i.e., hypotension, bradycardia, warm and dry skin) indicates the loss of sympathetic nervous system control. (PCPP 4–339 EPC 1076)

19.

A. Priapism is a painful penile erection. In this case, it is caused by the loss of sympathetic nervous system tone, allowing parasympathetic stimulation to dominate. (PCPP 4–339 EPC 1076)

20.

A. Interruption of the spinal cord in the cervical region will cause the intercostal muscles of the chest to become dysfunctional. Patients with this problem exhibit "belly breathing," characterized by movement of the diaphragm. (PCPP 4–330 EPC 185)

21.

D. Prehospital management of this patient includes spinal immobilization, IV fluid replacement with normal saline or lactated Ringer's, and atropine to raise the heart rate. Other interventions include a steroid, such as methylprednisolone or dexamethasone, to decrease cord swelling and dopamine to raise the blood pressure if atropine fails to improve cardiac output. (PCPP 4–360 EPC 1096)

43

Thoracic Trauma

DIRECTIONS Each of the questions or incomplete statements below is followed by suggested answers or completions. Select the **one answer** that is best in each case.

1. The uppermost part of the sternum is the
   A. mediastinum
   B. manubrium
   C. sternal body
   D. xiphoid process

2. The heart is suspended in the chest by the aortic arch and the ligamentum
   A. arteriosum
   B. cardiosum
   C. teres
   D. pericardium

3. Which of the following statements is true regarding multiple high rib fractures (1–3)?
   A. They are the most commonly fractured
   B. They are the least protected
   C. They have an associated mortality of <15%
   D. You should suspect severe intrathoracic injuries

SCENARIO

Questions 4–7 refer to the following scenario.

Your patient is a 15-year-old male who fell off his bicycle and hit the ground very hard. He presents with paradoxical chest movement on the right side, dyspnea, and guarded respirations. His vital signs are BP 140/80, pulse 100, respirations 30 and shallow, and diminished breath sounds on both sides.

4. Your field diagnosis is
   A. pneumothorax
   B. flail chest
   C. traumatic asphyxia
   D. hemothorax

5. The paradoxical movement is due to
   A. the instability of the chest wall

B. air in the pleural space
C. blood in the pleural space
D. paralysis of the respiratory muscles

6. The major complication from this injury is
   A. bleeding into the pericardial space
   B. air leaking into the subcutaneous tissues
   C. decreased tidal volumes
   D. rib displacement

7. Prehospital management of this patient includes
   A. positive pressure ventilation
   B. emergency chest decompression
   C. pericardiocentesis
   D. having the patient breathe into a paper bag

SCENARIO

Questions 8–10 refer to the following scenario.

Your patient is a 35-year-old female who was stabbed in the right chest after a quarrel with her girlfriend. You quickly discover a sucking wound in the right chest. She presents with diminished breath sounds on the right side, hyperresonance to percussion on the right side, ecchymosis from T-5 to T-8 on the right side, and dyspnea. BP is 120/70, pulse 90, and respirations 26 and shallow.

8. In addition to the sucking wound, your field diagnosis is
   A. massive hemothorax
   B. pneumothorax
   C. pericardial tamponade
   D. tension pneumothorax

9. Her condition is due to
   A. blood in the pleural space
   B. air in the pleural space
   C. blood in the pericardial sac
   D. air in the pericardial sac

10. Your initial management of this patient is to
    A. intubate the trachea
    B. ventilate with 100% oxygen
    C. seal the open wound with an occlusive dressing
    D. decompress the chest immediately

SCENARIO

Questions 11–13 refer to the following scenario.

Your patient is a 26-year-old who was shot with a small-caliber handgun in the right chest. She presents with dyspnea, distended neck veins, absent breath sounds on the right side, diminished breath sounds on the left side, hyperresonance on both sides, and tracheal deviation toward the left side. Her vital signs are BP 70/30, pulse 120 and weak, and respirations 30 and shallow.

11. Your field diagnosis is
    A. simple pneumothorax
    B. tension pneumothorax
    C. pericardial tamponade
    D. massive hemothorax

12. Her hypotension could be caused by
    A. decreased venous return
    B. tamponade effect on the heart
    C. blood loss
    D. all of the above

13. Emergency field management of this patient includes
    A. pneumatic antishock garment
    B. needle chest decompression
    C. pericardiocentesis
    D. none of the above

SCENARIO

Questions 14–15 refer to the following scenario.

Your patient is a 67-year-old female who was struck by a car and lies on the ground. She presents with dyspnea, pain to the right chest, dull percussion on the right side, and diminished breath sounds on the right side. Her vital signs are BP 80/60, pulse 110, respirations 30, skin cool and clammy, and flat neck veins.

14. Your field diagnosis is
    A. tension pneumothorax
    B. hemothorax
    C. pericardial tamponade
    D. traumatic asphyxia

15. Emergency field management of this patient includes
    A. rapid IV fluid replacement
    B. pericardiocentesis
    C. needle decompression
    D. pneumatic antishock garment

SCENARIO

Questions 16–18 refer to the following scenario.

Your patient is a 35-year-old unbelted male driver who hit the steering wheel and windshield in a one-car accident. He presents unconscious with the following vital signs: BP 110/90, pulse 120 and weak, respirations 28 and shallow, lungs equal and clear, distant heart sounds, skin cool and clammy, and distended neck veins. His only external sign of trauma is a midsternal bruise.

16. Your field diagnosis is
    A. tension pneumothorax
    B. massive hemothorax
    C. traumatic asphyxia
    D. pericardial tamponade

17. This patient's primary problem is
    A. air filling the pleural space
    B. fluid in the pericardial sac
    C. severe crushing injury to the chest
    D. blood in the pleural space

18. Emergency management of this patient includes
    A. needle decompression
    B. chest tube
    C. pneumatic antishock garment
    D. pericardiocentesis

SCENARIO

Questions 19–20 refer to the following scenario.

Your patient is a 45-year-old who presents with a bluish discoloration above the nipple line, absent vital signs, bloodshot eyes, and distended neck veins. He was pinned for a short time underneath his car following a rollover accident.

19. He is most likely suffering from
    A. tension pneumothorax
    B. traumatic asphyxia
    C. massive hemothorax
    D. pericardial tamponade

20. The bluish discoloration is caused by
    A. lack of oxygen in the tissues
    B. low PaO_2
    C. the bursting of capillaries
    D. high $PaCO_2$

answers

& rationales

1.

B. The sternum is divided into three parts. The uppermost part is a triangular-shaped bone called the manubrium. The manubrium is the attaching point for the clavicles and first ribs. (PCPP 4–368)

2.

A. The heart is suspended in the chest by the aortic arch and the ligamentum arteriosum. The ligamentum arteriosum is the remnant of the fetal vessel that connected the pulmonary artery to the aorta. At birth, this vessel closes to redirect blood flow to the lungs. (PCPP 4–379)

3.

D. It takes a tremendous force to fracture ribs 1–3 because they are well-protected by the shoulder girdle and heavy musculature of the upper chest. Their fracture is frequently associated with severe intrathoracic injuries, such as aortic rupture, tracheobronchial tears, and other vascular injuries. (PCPP 4–383)

4.

B. Paradoxical chest movement is a classic sign of a flail chest. Flail chest occurs when three or more ribs are fractured in multiple places, causing a floating segment and reducing the stability of the chest wall. (PCPP 4–386)

5.

A. The paradoxical movement is due to the instability of the chest wall. During inspiration, the negative pressures within the chest wall cause the flail segment to suck in. Upon exhalation, the positive intrathoracic pressures cause the flail segment to bow out. These movements are the opposite of how the the rest of the chest wall moves. (PCPP 4–386)

6.

C. Flail chest can result in severe respiratory compromise. The hypoventilation results in decreased air available for gas exchange, leading to hypoxia and hypercarbia. Broken rib pieces can also cause penetrating injuries to the lungs. (PCPP 4–386)

7.

A. Prehospital management of a patient suspected of having a flail chest includes positive pressure ventilation to ensure good ventilation and stabilizing the loose flail segment. (PCPP 4–386)

8.

B. This patient's presentation of diminished breath sounds on the right side with hyperresonance and ecchymosis indicates pneumothorax. (PCPP 4–388)

9.

B. A pneumothorax is caused by a tear in the pleura. Air enters the pleural space, collapsing the lung in that particular area. (PCPP 4–388)

10.

C. Initial management of this patient is aimed at sealing the wound with an occlusive dressing during exhalation. At the end of exhalation, cover the wound and tape it on three sides to prevent air from entering upon inhalation, but allowing air to escape during exhalation. (PCPP 4–389)

11.

B. This patient who presents with absent lung sounds on one side and decreased sounds on the other, with hyperresonance, jugular venous distention, and a deviated trachea, has a tension pneumothorax. (PCPP 4–389)

12.

D. Her hypotension could be the result of a combination of factors. The high intrathoracic pressures caused by the injury may decrease venous return. The tension could produce a tamponade effect on the heart, severely decreasing cardiac output. She may have blood loss from bleeding within the chest or other injuries. (PCPP 4–389)

13.

B. Emergency management of this patient includes immediate and rapid evacuation of the air trapped in the pleural space. Needle decompression is done by placing a large-bore IV catheter into the chest at the second intercostal space, midclavicular line. Then remove the needle and attach a one-way valve device, allowing air to escape, but not enter. (PCPP 4–390)

14.

B. This patient's presentation of dyspnea, pain to the right chest, diminished breath sounds on the right side, dull to percussion on the right side, and shock indicates hemothorax. A hemothorax is caused by bleeding into the pleural space. (PCPP 4–390)

15.

A. Emergency field management of this patient includes treating for shock by replacing blood fluid volume rapidly. (PCPP 4–391)

16.

D. This patient's presentation of distant heart sounds, distended neck veins, and a narrow pulse pressure indicates pericardial tamponade. This is the classic Beck's triad. (PCPP 4–394)

17.

B. Pericardial tamponade is the filling of the pericardial sac with fluid, which, in turn, limits the filling of the heart. (PCPP 4–394)

18.

D. Definitive emergency management of this patient includes pericardiocentesis. This procedure involves the insertion of a large-bore spinal needle into the pericardial sac and aspirating the excess blood. This procedure has many complications and is seldom performed by paramedics in the field. This patient requires rapid transport. (PCPP 4–395)

19.

B. Sudden compression of the chest from a crushing injury can lead to traumatic asphyxia. The compression severely limits chest excursion and results in hypoventilation. It may also cause a backup of venous blood within the head and neck, causing the classic bloodshot eyes, bulging blue tongue, distended neck veins, and cyanotic upper body, the classic "hood sign." (PCPP 4–398)

20.

C. Backflow of venous blood through the jugular veins into the head causes tremendous pressures in the capillaries, resulting in bursting. The result is petechiae, which gives the patient a purplish look above the nipples. (PCPP 4–398)

44 Abdominal Trauma

DIRECTIONS Each of the questions or incomplete statements below is followed by suggested answers or completions. Select the **one answer** that is best in each case.

1. The kidneys, spleen, and part of the pancreas are located within the _____ cavity.
   A. peritoneal
   B. retroperitoneal
   C. pleural
   D. pericardial

2. The sigmoid colon is located in the
   A. right upper quadrant
   B. left upper quadrant
   C. right lower quadrant
   D. left lower quadrant

3. The appendix is located in the
   A. right upper quadrant
   B. left upper quadrant
   C. right lower quadrant
   D. left lower quadrant

4. The gallbladder is located in the
   A. right upper quadrant
   B. left upper quadrant
   C. right lower quadrant
   D. left lower quadrant

5. The stomach is located in the
   A. right upper quadrant
   B. left upper quadrant
   C. right lower quadrant
   D. left lower quadrant

6. The continuous tube that extends from the esophagus to the rectum is the
   A. duodenal canal
   B. digestive tract
   C. parenteral canal
   D. peritoneal tract

7. The wave-like muscular motion of the intestines is known as
   A. alimentation
   B. peristalsis
   C. omentum
   D. mesentery action

8. Which of the following is a function of the liver?
   A. Detoxifying blood from the intestines
   B. Storing body energy reserves
   C. Producing plasma proteins
   D. All of the above

9. Bile is stored in the
   A. liver
   B. gallbladder
   C. pancreas
   D. spleen

10. The small bowel consists of which following three sections in order?
    A. Ileum, duodenum, jejunum
    B. Jejunum, omentum, duodenum
    C. Duodenum, jejunum, ileum
    D. Omentum, ileum, jejunum

11. The liver is suspended in the abdomen by the
    A. ligamentum teres
    B. bundle of Kent
    C. isle of Langerhans
    D. mesentery

12. Bile is produced in the
    A. stomach
    B. liver
    C. gallbladder
    D. pancreas

13. The pancreas
    A. produces glucagon and insulin
    B. secretes digestive enzymes
    C. is a solid, encapsulated organ
    D. all of the above

14. The most delicate and fragile abdominal organ is the
   A. pancreas
   B. spleen
   C. duodenum
   D. gallbladder

15. Pregnancy affects maternal circulation by
   A. decreasing blood volume
   B. decreasing heart rate
   C. increasing cardiac output
   D. increasing hematocrit

16. The abdominal aorta bifurcates into two _____ arteries.
   A. femoral
   B. iliac
   C. mesentery
   D. pelvic

17. The secondary circulatory system that transports intestinal blood to the liver for detoxification is known as the _____ system.
   A. mesentery
   B. omentum
   C. peritoneal
   D. portal

18. Which of the following organs is located in the retroperitoneal space?
   A. Small intestine
   B. Mesentery
   C. Pancreas
   D. Stomach

19. Your patient is a 24-year-old male who was stabbed in the left upper quadrant. He presents alert and oriented in moderate respiratory distress and with minor external blood loss. His airway is clear, but his breathing is shallow at a rate of 36/minute. He has good peripheral pulses, and his skin is warm and pink. He complains of pain upon inspiration in the left chest. Upon auscultation, you hear what sounds like bowel sounds in the left lower lobes. The right lungs are clear. Your likely field diagnosis is
   A. tension pneumothorax
   B. massive hemothorax
   C. cardiac tamponade
   D. diaphragmatic herniation

20. Which of the following is NOT a result of a hollow abdominal organ rupture?
   A. Hematochezia
   B. Hemoptysis
   C. Hematuria
   D. Hematemesis

21. Rebound tenderness is a classic sign that suggests
   A. diaphragmatic tear
   B. hypovolemic shock
   C. peritoneal irritation
   D. aortic aneurysm

22. Abdominal guarding usually indicates
   A. diaphragmatic tear
   B. hypovolemic shock
   C. peritoneal irritation
   D. aortic aneurysm

23. Which of the following conditions may occur during pregnancy if the mother sustains blunt trauma to the abdomen?
   A. Abruptio placenta
   B. Placenta previa
   C. Ruptured ectopic pregnancy
   D. Pregnancy-induced hypotension

SCENARIO

Questions 24–25 refer to the following scenario.

Your patient is a 57-year-old female who was a passenger in a two-car accident. She was ejected from the vehicle and lies on the ground next to the car. She presents unconscious with no obvious signs of trauma. Her vital signs are BP 50/30, pulse 120 and weak, respirations 38 and shallow, lungs equal and clear, and flat neck veins. Upon exam, you find discoloration around the umbilicus and abdominal guarding.

24. Your field diagnosis is
    A. tension pneumothorax
    B. pericardial tamponade
    C. intra-abdominal hemorrhage
    D. ruptured diaphragm

25. Field management of this patient includes
    A. pneumatic antishock garment
    B. IV fluid replacement
    C. rapid transport to a trauma center
    D. all of the above

answers & rationales

1.
B. The retroperitoneal space lies behind the layers of the peritoneum. The organs within this space include the kidneys, spleen, and part of the pancreas. (PCPP 4–415)

2.
D. The left lower quadrant houses the sigmoid colon as well as portions of the small and large intestines. (PCPP 4–415)

3.
C. The right lower quadrant contains the appendix. (PCPP 4–415)

4.
A. The right upper quadrant contains the liver, right kidney, gallbladder, duodenum, and part of the pancreas. (PCPP 4–415)

5.
B. The left upper quadrant includes the stomach, left kidney, spleen, and most of the pancreas. (PCPP 4–416)

6.
B. The digestive tract (alimentary canal) is a continuous tube that begins with the esophagus and ends with the rectum. In this canal, food goes through the digestive process. (PCPP 4–416)

7.
B. Peristalsis is the wave-like muscular motion of the esophagus and bowel, moving food through the digestive system. (PCPP 4–416)

8.
D. The liver occupies the area below and under the rib cage in the right upper quadrant. A large and vascular organ, it detoxifies the blood coming from the digestive field, stores body energy reserves, produces plasma proteins, and performs many other important functions. (PCPP 4–418)

9.
B. Beneath and behind the liver is the gallbladder, a storehouse for bile. Bile is a product of the liver that helps in the digestion of fat. (PCPP 4–418)

10.
C. The small intestine consists of three sections. The first section is called the duodenum. The second section is called the jejunum, and the third section is the ileum. (PCPP 4–418)

11.
A. The ligamentum teres suspends the liver. In deceleration, the ligament may slice the liver as cheese is sliced by a wire cutter. This laceration is severe, often resulting in rapid hemorrhage. (PCPP 4–418)

12.
B. Bile, produced in the liver and stored in the gallbladder, helps the body by emulsifying ingested fats that would otherwise remain in clumps during the digestive process. (PCPP 4–418)

13.
D. The pancreas, a solid, encapsulated organ, secretes hormones that regulate blood sugar (insulin and glucagon) and powerful digestive enzymes. (PCPP 4–419)

14.
B. The spleen, part of the immune system, is the most delicate abdominal organ. Since it is engorged with blood, it has the potential for life-threatening hemorrhage when injured. Luckily, it is well-protected by the ribs, spine, and flank and back muscles. (PCPP 4–419)

15.

C. During pregnancy, maternal physiology undergoes significant changes in circulation. By the third trimester, circulating volume increases by 45% with no increase in red blood cell production. The heart rate increases by 15 beats per minute, and cardiac output increases by up to 40%. (PCPP 4–422)

16.

B. The abdominal aorta bifurcates into two iliac arteries. When these arteries pass through the pelvis at the inguinal ligament, they eventually become the femoral arteries. (PCPP 4–423)

17.

D. The portal system transports venous blood from the intestines to the liver. Here the liver detoxifies the fluid, stores excess nutrients, adds nutrients when they are deficient, and then sends the blood into the inferior vena cava for a return to the general circulation. When a drug is given orally, it makes this "first pass" through the liver and may lose some of its potency through this detoxifying process. (PCPP 4–423)

18.

C. The retroperitoneal space lies behind the peritoneum. Organs within this space include the kidneys, pancreas, posterior portions of the ascending and descending colon, rectum, duodenum, and urinary bladder. (PCPP 4–424)

19.

D. Bowel sounds in the chest following penetrating trauma to either the lower chest or the upper abdomen usually indicate a ruptured diaphragm. Upon inspiration, the negative pressure in the chest draws the intestines through the hole in the diaphragm into the chest, resulting in bowel sounds in the lower lobes. This commonly occurs on the left side, as the right side of the diaphragm is well-protected by the massive liver. (PCPP 4–427)

20.

B. Hematochezia (frank blood in the stool), hematuria (blood in the urine), and hematemesis (blood in emesis) are all classic signs of a ruptured abdominal organ. Hemoptysis is the presence of blood in sputum (lungs). (PCPP 4–428)

21.

C. Rebound tenderness is pain upon the release of your hand during deep palpation, allowing the patient's abdominal wall to return to its normal position. It is a classic sign of peritoneal irritation and suggests a bacterial or chemical irritation caused by intra-abdominal bleeding or hollow organ rupture. (PCPP 4–430)

22.

C. The peritoneum can become irritated by the presence of blood. The patient with peritoneal irritation often presents with guarding because it hurts to move. (PCPP 4–430)

23.

A. Blunt trauma to the uterus may cause the placenta to detach from the uterine wall. This condition is known as abruptio placenta and presents a life-threatening risk to both the mother and the baby. (PCPP 4–432)

24.

C. Any patient who presents with signs and symptoms of shock and discoloration around the umbilicus, also known as Cullen's sign, should be suspected of having an intra-abdominal hemorrhage. (PCPP 4–437)

25.

D. Field management of this patient includes the pneumatic antishock garment, IV fluid replacement, and rapid transport to a trauma center. (PCPP 4–439)

45

Shock Trauma
Resuscitation

DIRECTIONS Each of the questions or incomplete statements below is followed by suggested answers or completions. Select the **one answer** that is best in each case.

SCENARIO

Questions 1–12 refer to the following scenario.

You are awakened in the middle of the night for a call on a quiet country road. Your patient was the unrestrained driver in a one-car high-speed auto accident involving frontal impact with a telephone pole. He is a 19-year-old male who presents unconscious and partially trapped in the severely deformed vehicle. According to witnesses, he was driving at a high rate of speed. Upon initial examination, you immediately hear gurgling respirations. Vital signs are weak carotid pulse of 120; BP 70/40; respirations 36 and shallow; skin cool, pale, and clammy; and capillary refill time 4 seconds. Pulse oximetry reads 70%. Upon physical exam, you discover a bruise to the front chest wall with a loose flail segment and some abdominal guarding. Lung sounds are diminished on the right side with some hyperresonance in that area.

1. Which of the following programs is aimed at preventing such an incident?
   A. Fire department explorer program
   B. "Just say no"
   C. OSHA night driving course
   D. "Let's not meet by accident"

2. Your initial management of this patient should be to
   A. perform immediate nasotracheal intubation
   B. start two large-bore IVs
   C. manually stabilize his head and neck
   D. place an oxygen mask on him

3. The gurgling noise that accompanies his breathing calls for immediate
   A. suctioning
   B. intubation
   C. head-tilt/chin-lift procedure
   D. chest decompression

4. You are concerned about the right-sided flail segment because
   A. it indicates lung tissue damage beneath the injury
   B. it severely inhibits ventilation and oxygenation
   C. it is usually accompanied by pericardial tamponade
   D. underlying damage to the heart is expected

5. His respiratory situation indicates the need for immediate
   A. chest decompression
   B. Trendelenburg positioning
   C. intubation
   D. positive pressure ventilation

6. Your patient's pulse and blood pressure indicate which stage of shock?
   A. Compensated
   B. Irreversible
   C. Decompensated
   D. None of the above

7. The most likely cause of your patient's shock is
   A. loss of alveolar function
   B. internal blood loss
   C. massive vasodilation
   D. acute myocardial infarction

8. Peripheral vascular resistance is regulated in which blood vessels?
   A. Veins
   B. Venules
   C. Arteries
   D. Arterioles

9. Which of the following statements is TRUE regarding this patient?
   A. Anaerobic metabolism is occurring
   B. Resuscitation is still possible
   C. Irreversible shock will ensue if left untreated
   D. All of the above

10. This patient responds to pain stimuli by moaning. He earns a _____ on the AVPU scale.
    A. A
    B. V
    C. P
    D. U

11. Prehospital fluid resuscitation of this patient should include
    A. lactated Ringer's
    B. 0.45% sodium chloride
    C. 5% dextrose and water
    D. any of the above

12. Which of the following IV equipment would best help this patient?
    A. 20 gauge, 2 inch catheter, 60 drop/ml tubing

B. 14 gauge, 1 inch catheter, 10 drop/ml tubing
C. 16 gauge, 3 inch catheter, 60 drop/ml tubing
D. 22 gauge, 1/2 inch catheter, 10 drop/ml tubing

13. In general, fluid resuscitation in the field should be limited to
    A. 1 liter
    B. 2 liters
    C. 3 liters
    D. none of the above

14. During a hot load, you should always
    A. approach the helicopter from the rear
    B. stay clear of the tail rotor
    C. direct lights directly at the pilot
    D. use flares instead of flashlights

15. The appropriate helicopter landing zone for a large aircraft is at least
    A. 60 × 60 feet
    B. 75 × 75 feet
    C. 120 × 120 feet
    D. 200 × 200 feet

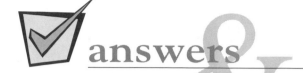

answers & rationales

1.

D. "Let's not meet by accident" is a program developed by a trauma system and prehospital care providers. It is designed to acquaint high school students with EMS and to alert them to the trauma hazards in our society. (PCPP 4–449)

2.

C. Always stabilize a cervical spine if the mechanism of injury strongly suggests an injury in this area. Assign one of your crew to stabilize the head manually while you continue your primary assessment. Release manual stabilization only after you secure the head to a long spine board. (PCPP 4–455)

3.

A. Always ensure a patent airway immediately. Examine it for fluids, obstruction, or signs of trauma and apply suction as necessary. A noisy airway is an obstructive airway. (PCPP 4–458)

4.

B. Always be concerned about a flail segment because it may severely inhibit ventilation and oxygenation. Your patient may become hypoxic and hypercarbic. (PCPP 4–463)

5.

D. This patient's respiratory situation indicates the need for positive pressure ventilation with a bag-valve-mask and supplemental oxygen. (PCPP 4–458)

6.

C. Your patient's blood pressure and pulse indicate that he is in decompensated shock. It is during this stage that the body's normal defense mechanisms are failing. (PCPP 4–459)

7.

B. The most probable cause of this patient's shock is internal blood loss, probably in the abdomen. (PCPP 4–460)

8.

D. Peripheral vascular resistance is regulated in the arterioles. Arterioles have the ability to affect blood pressure and direct blood flow from the heart to various organs. They can open and close with a valve-like function and can vary their inner diameter by as much as a factor of 5. (PCPP 4–459, 4–102)

9.

D. In decompensated shock, anaerobic metabolism occurs. Anaerobic metabolism occurs when there is insufficient oxygen for the cell to function. As a result of this inefficient process, acids accumulate. Resuscitation at this point is still possible, but irreversible shock will ensue if this patient is left untreated. (PCPP 4–469, 4–109)

10.

C. Since this patient responds only to pain stimuli, he earns a P on the AVPU scale. (PCPP 4–457)

11.

A. Prehospital fluid resuscitation is accomplished using normal saline or lactated Ringer's. These isotonic solutions are ideal for fluid resuscitation because they tend to remain in the intravascular space for a period of time. (PCPP 4–469)

12.

B. In order to maximize fluid flow, use an IV catheter with the largest gauge and shortest length, and 10 drop per milliliter IV tubing. (PCPP 4–469)

13.

C. Fluid resuscitation in the field is very controversial. In general, it should be limited to three liters of crystalloid solution. Reasons for the controversy include the loss of two-thirds of the fluid from the vascular space within one hour, its inability to transport oxygen to the tissues, and its possible interference with normal clotting. (PCPP 4–469)

14.

B. Hot loading refers to loading a patient into a helicopter while the rotors continue to turn. If you are asked to help load the patient, stay close to the flight crew, and avoid the area of the tail rotor. The tail rotor spins at speeds in excess of 2000 rpm and is almost invisible. (PCPP 4–484)

15.

C. A landing zone should be a minimum of 60×60 feet for small helicopters, 75×75 feet for medium ones, and 120×120 feet for large ones. (PCPP 4–483)

46

Neonatology

1. Which of the following is considered an antepartum risk factor for possible complications in newborns?
   A. More than one fetus
   B. Mother's age is >35
   C. Post-term gestation
   D. All of the above

Match the following congenital anomalies with their respective descriptions:

2. ____ Meningomyelocele
3. ____ Omphalocele
4. ____ Choanal atresia
5. ____ Cleft palate
6. ____ Pierre Robin syndrome

A. Spinal cord herniation
B. Small jaw/large tongue/no gag
C. Nasopharyngeal blockage
D. Fissure in roof of mouth
E. Umbilical herniation

7. Which of the following is recommended immediately following delivery of the infant?
   A. Position the baby, head down, at the level of the vagina
   B. Suction the mouth and then the nose
   C. Dry the baby off
   D. All of the above

8. Which of the following is recommended practice regarding the umbilical cord?
   A. Milk the cord toward the baby
   B. Milk the cord toward the mother
   C. Clamp and cut the cord shortly after delivery
   D. Disregard the cord until the placenta delivers

9. The normal respiratory rate of the neonate should be _____ breaths per minute.
   A. 10–20
   B. 20–40
   C. 40–60
   D. 60–100

10. A pulse rate of less than 100 beats per minute in the newborn infant
    A. is normal after 2–3 minutes postpartum
    B. indicates an infant in distress
    C. requires immediate atropine administration
    D. requires aggressive fluid therapy

11. Which of the following statements is true regarding the APGAR score?
    A. It should be calculated at 1 and 5 minutes after delivery
    B. An infant with a score of 3 requires immediate resuscitation
    C. Scores in the 7–10 range indicate a normal infant
    D. All of the above

12. The presence of meconium at birth requires immediate
    A. bag-valve-mask ventilation
    B. suctioning of the trachea
    C. stimulation of the baby to breathe
    D. cardiopulmonary resuscitation

13. Which of the following statements is true regarding neonatal suctioning?
    A. Normal suctioning should be performed by bulb syringe or Delee trap
    B. Suctioning should last no longer than 10 seconds
    C. Meconium should be suctioned through an endotracheal tube
    D. All of the above

14. Which of the following is **NOT** part of the first step of the inverted pyramid?
    A. Oxygen administration
    B. Tactile stimulation
    C. Drying and warming
    D. Positioning

15. An infant's best indicator of distress is the
    A. respiratory effort
    B. heart rate
    C. cardiac rhythm
    D. blood pressure

16. If the infant presents with cyanosis after performing step 1 of the inverted pyramid, you should
    A. administer blow-by oxygen
    B. perform bag-valve-mask ventilation
    C. begin CPR
    D. insert an endotracheal tube

17. If the heart rate is less than 100 or the infant is still cyanotic after performing step 2, you should
    A. administer blow-by oxygen
    B. perform bag-valve-mask ventilation
    C. begin CPR
    D. insert an endotracheal tube

18. If the infant's heart rate is less than 80 after performing steps 1–3, you should
    A. administer atropine
    B. perform chest compression
    C. insert an endotracheal tube
    D. administer epinephrine

19. The infant's heart rate can best be checked by
    A. auscultating the heart at the apex
    B. feeling the umbilical cord
    C. palpating the brachial pulse
    D. all of the above

20. Which of the following is true regarding neonatal resuscitation?
    A. Pop-off valves on bag-valve devices should be disengaged
    B. Cuffed ET tubes should be used on all neonates
    C. Chest compression should be performed on the midsternum
    D. All of the above

21. The umbilicus contains
    A. two arteries and two veins
    B. two arteries and one vein
    C. one artery and two veins
    D. one artery and one vein

22. Mothers taking narcotics have been known to produce infants with
    A. low birth weight
    B. withdrawal symptoms and tremors
    C. respiratory depression
    D. all of the above

SCENARIO

Questions 23–26 refer to the following scenario.

Your newborn infant presents with respiratory distress and cyanosis; unresponsiveness to ventilations; a small, flat abdomen; heart sounds displaced to the right; and bowel sounds in the chest.

23. Your suspected field diagnosis is
    A. spontaneous pneumothorax
    B. herniated diaphragm
    C. pericardial tamponade
    D. phrenic nerve paralysis

24. Proper positioning of this patient is
    A. Trendelenburg
    B. left lateral recumbent
    C. supine with head and chest elevated
    D. prone

25. Which of the following treatments is CONTRA-INDICATED for this patient?
    A. Oxygen administration
    B. Bag-valve-mask ventilation
    C. Orogastric tube insertion and gastric suctioning
    D. Endotracheal intubation

26. Bradycardia in the newborn is most often caused by
    A. hyperthyroidism
    B. alkalosis
    C. dehydration
    D. hypoxia

SCENARIO

Questions 27–28 refer to the following scenario.

Your newborn presents with pale, cool skin; diminished peripheral pulses; capillary refill time of 6 seconds; and oliguria.

27. Your field diagnosis is
    A. hypoglycemia
    B. hypovolemic shock
    C. increasing intracranial pressure
    D. severe hypoxia

28. Proper field management includes
    A. epinephrine 0.01mg/kg IV
    B. 10 mL/kg normal saline IV
    C. 20 mL/kg lactated Ringer's IV
    D. 10% dextrose solution IV

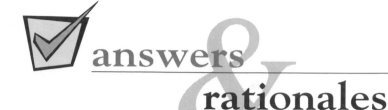

answers & rationales

1.

D. Approximately 6% of field deliveries require neonatal life support. Antepartum (before birth) risk factors that indicate the possibility of complications in newborns include multiple gestation, inadequate prenatal care, mother younger than 16 or older than 35, history of perinatal morbidity or mortality, post-term gestation (baby overdue), drugs or medications, and toxemia/hypertension/diabetes during pregnancy. (PCPP 5–5 EPC 1682)

Matching (PCPP 5–8 EPC 1685)

2. A Meningomyelocele
3. E Omphalocele
4. C Choanal atresia
5. D Cleft palate
6. B Pierre Robin syndrome

A. Spinal cord herniation
B. Small jaw/large tongue/no gag
C. Nasopharyngeal blockage
D. Fissure in roof of mouth
E. Umbilical herniation

7.

D. Routine care of the newborn infant is the first step of the inverted pyramid. This step includes drying and warming the baby; positioning the baby, head down, at the level of the vagina; suctioning the mouth and then the nose; and performing tactile stimulation if necessary. (PCPP 5–9 EPC 1686)

8.

C. After you have stabilized the neonate's airway and prevented heat loss, clamp and cut the umbilical cord. Apply the umbilical clamps within 30–45 seconds after birth. Place the first clamp approximately 10 cm from the neonate; place the second clamp approximately 5 cm distal from the first clamp; then cut the cord between the two clamps. After the cord is cut, inspect it periodically to make sure there is no additional bleeding. (PCPP 5–12 EPC 1688)

9.

C. The normal respiratory rate of the neonate should be 40–60 breaths per minute. (PCPP 5–8 EPC 1685)

10.

B. The heart rate is the critical component of neonatal resuscitation. A pulse rate of less than 100 beats per minute in the newborn indicates an infant in distress. (PCPP 5–8 EPC 1685)

11.

D. As soon as possible assign the neonate an APGAR score. Do this at 1 and 5 minutes after birth. A score of 7–10 indicates an active and vigorous neonate that requires only routine care. Neonates with APGAR scores of less than 4 are severely distressed and require immediate resuscitation. (PCPP 5–8 EPC 1685)

12.

B. The presence of fetal meconium at birth indicates the possibility of fetal respiratory distress. Aspiration of meconium can cause severe lung inflammation and pneumonia in the neonate. If you spot meconium during delivery, do not induce respiratory effort until you have removed the meconium from the trachea by suctioning under direct visualization with the laryngoscope. This is a true emergency. (PCPP 5–13 EPC 1688)

13.

D. Normal suctioning of the neonate should be performed by bulb syringe or Delee trap and should last no longer than 10 seconds. Meconium should be suctioned through an endotracheal tube. (PCPP 5–10   EPC 1686)

14.
A. As stated in question 1, the first step of the inverted pyramid includes drying and warming the infant; positioning the baby, head down, at the level of the vagina; suctioning the mouth and nose; and providing tactile stimulation when necessary. (PCPP 5–15   EPC 1690)

15.
B. An infant's best indicator of stress is the heart rate. If the heart rate is greater than 100 beats per minute and spontaneous respirations are present, continue assessing the baby. If the heart rate is less than 100 beats per minute, begin positive pressure ventilation immediately. If the heart rate is less than 60 beats per minute, or between 60 and 80 beats per minute after 30 seconds of positive pressure ventilation and supplemental oxygen, begin chest compression. (PCPP 5–19   EPC 1693)

16.
A. If the infant presents with cyanosis after performing step 1 of the inverted pyramid, you should then move to step 2 and administer blow-by oxygen. (PCPP 5–19   EPC 1695)

17.
B. If the heart rate is less than 100 or the infant is still cyanotic after performing step 2, immediately move to step 3 and perform bag-valve-mask ventilation. (PCPP 5–20   EPC 1695)

18.
B. If the infant's heart rate is less than 80 after performing steps 1, 2, and 3, move to step 4 and perform chest compression. Encircle the neonate's chest and place both of your fingers on the lower third of the sternum. Compress the sternum 1/3 to 1/2 of the chest's total height at a rate of at least 100/min. (PCPP 5–21   EPC 1696)

19.
D. The infant's heart rate can best be checked by auscultating the heart at the apex, feeling for pulsation at the umbilical cord, or palpating the brachial pulse. (PCPP 5–19   EPC 1693)

20.
A. When performing bag-valve-mask ventilation on the neonate, the pop-off valve, if present, should be disengaged. This will prevent underinflation of the infant's lungs. (PCPP 5–20   EPC 1696)

21.
B. The umbilicus contains three vessels—two arteries and one vein. The vein is easy to locate as it is larger and has a thinner wall. Accessing the umbilical vein for resuscitation is a relatively easy process. (PCPP 5–22   EPC 1698)

22.
D. Maternal abuse of narcotics can produce infants with low birth weight, withdrawal symptoms and tremors, and respiratory depression. Unless the mother is a narcotic addict, administer naloxone to reverse any respiratory depression if the mother used within fours of delivery. For the child of a narcotic addict, provide ventilation instead to avoid infant narcotic withdrawal. (PCPP 5–23   EPC 1700)

23.
B. Diaphragmatic hernias occur very rarely, in approximately 1 in 2,200 births. When they do occur, the mortality is 50% for an infant presenting with respiratory distress in the first 18 to 24 hours. Signs and symptoms include respiratory distress and cyanosis unresponsive to ventilations; a small, flat abdomen; heart sounds displaced to the right; and bowel sounds in the chest. (PCPP 5–27   EPC 1702)

24.
C. Proper positioning of an infant with a herniated diaphragm is supine with the head and chest higher than the abdomen. (PCPP 5–28   EPC 1703)

25.
B. Do not use bag-valve-mask ventilation with an infant suspected of having a herniated diaphragm, as it may worsen the condition by causing gastric distention. If necessary, deliver positive pressure ventilation directly to the lungs through an endotracheal tube. (PCPP 5–28   EPC 1703)

26.
D. Bradycardia in the newborn is most often caused by hypoxia. For this reason, treat bradycardia with airway management, ventilation, and oxygenation. If your patient's condition does not improve, then

consider medications such as epinephrine. (PCPP 5–29   EPC 1704)

27.

B. Hypovolemia is the leading cause of shock in newborns. It may result from dehydration, hemorrhage, or third-spacing of fluids. (PCPP 5–30   EPC 1705)

28.

B. Field management of hypovolemic shock includes airway management, oxygenation, and IV fluid replacement with normal saline or Ringer's lactate at 10mL/kg. Some newborns may require 40 to 60 mL/kg. (PCPP 5–31   EPC 1706)

47 Pediatrics

DIRECTIONS Each of the questions or incomplete statements below is followed by suggested answers or completions. Select the **one answer** that is best in each case.

1. The leading cause of death between the ages of 1 and 15 years is
   A. accidents
   B. respiratory illness
   C. SIDS
   D. congenital problems

2. Children between the ages of _____ years are most obsessed with monsters and mutilation.
   A. 1 and 3
   B. 3 and 5
   C. 5 and 12
   D. 12 and 15

3. A sunken anterior fontanel may indicate
   A. increased intracranial pressure
   B. meningitis
   C. epidural hematoma
   D. dehydration

4. Your 2-year-old patient requires head and neck immobilization on a backboard. Which of the following techniques will most likely maintain the child's head in the neutral position?
   A. Padding underneath the head
   B. Padding underneath the back and shoulders
   C. No padding
   D. Padding underneath the head, back, and shoulders

5. As a rule, as a child gets older
   A. the BP falls and the pulse rate rises
   B. the BP rises and the pulse rate falls
   C. the BP and pulse rate fall
   D. the BP and pulse rate rise

6. In young children, the narrowest part of the upper airway is the
   A. glottis
   B. vocal cords
   C. cricoid ring
   D. thyroid cartilage

7. Which of the following statements is true regarding the skin and body surface area of children as compared to adults?
   A. The skin of a child is thicker
   B. Children have more subcutaneous fat
   C. Children have a larger body surface-to-weight ratio
   D. All of the above

8. The three components of the pediatric assessment triangle are
   A. airway, breathing, circulation
   B. airway, pulses, neuro
   C. appearance, vital signs, neuro
   D. appearance, breathing, circulation

9. The most common cause of cardiac arrest in infants and young children is
   A. respiratory arrest
   B. circulatory collapse
   C. cardiac dysrhythmia
   D. drug overdose

10. Usually the first sign of respiratory distress in infants is
   A. bradycardia
   B. tachycardia
   C. bradypnea
   D. tachypnea

11. Bradycardia in a distressed infant or young child is usually
    A. an ominous sign of cardiac arrest
    B. transient
    C. a normal response to effective treatment
    D. the first sign of circulatory collapse

12. Which of the following signs may signify impending cardiac arrest in a child?
    A. Respiratory rate over 60
    B. Pulse rate 170
    C. Pulse rate 70 in a 5-year-old
    D. None of the above

13. Your patient is a 6-month-old girl who appears to have a complete upper airway obstruction. Which of the following foreign body removal techniques is recommended?
    A. Abdominal thrusts
    B. Heimlich maneuver
    C. Back blows
    D. Blind finger sweeps

14. Which of the following complications may occur as a result of performing oropharyngeal suctioning with a rigid-tip catheter?
    A. Bradycardia
    B. Vagal stimulation
    C. Hypoxia
    D. All of the above

15. Which of the following airways is approved and recommended for pediatric use?
    A. Esophageal obturator airway (EOA)
    B. Oropharyngeal airways
    C. Pharyngotracheal lumen airway (PTL)
    D. None of the above

16. Pop-off valves should be functional when ventilating the pediatric patient
    A. to avoid overinflation of the lungs
    B. to avoid causing a pneumothorax
    C. to avoid barotrauma to the lungs
    D. none of the above

17. Which of the following is an approved method for estimating the correct ET tube size in an infant or young child?
    A. Diameter of the patient's ring finger
    B. Diameter of the patient's nasal opening
    C. Patient's age in years $\times 4 + 16$
    D. All of the above

18. The commonly accepted age limit for attempting an intraosseous infusion is
    A. 3 years old
    B. 6 years old
    C. 8 years old
    D. none of the above

19. Verifying proper placement of an intraosseous needle includes
    A. noting a lack of resistance
    B. observing the needle standing upright
    C. achieving free flow of the infusion without infiltration
    D. all of the above

20. The initial dose for defibrillation in the pediatric patient is
    A. 1 j/kg
    B. 2 j/kg
    C. 4 j/kg
    D. 200 j

21. A 3-year-old child who burns both legs and arms has burned approximately _____% of his entire body surface area.
    A. 54
    B. 46
    C. 72
    D. 36

22. Which of the following children may be at a higher risk for child abuse?
    A. Child with disabilities
    B. Twin child
    C. Premature child
    D. All of the above

23. Which of the following is a classic characteristic of a child abuser?
    A. Parent who spends majority of time with child
    B. Parent who was abused as child
    C. Parent who is experiencing financial or marital stress
    D. All of the above

24. Prehospital management of the abused child includes all of the following EXCEPT
    A. treating all injuries
    B. eliciting a complete history from child and parents
    C. allowing parent to drive child to hospital
    D. reporting your findings to the emergency department staff

25. Which of the following statements regarding febrile seizures is true?
    A. They usually occur between the ages of 6 months and 1 year
    B. They are caused by extremely high temperatures
    C. They are caused by a sudden increase in temperature
    D. The patient usually does not need to be transported

26. Which of the following statements is true regarding SIDS?
    A. It usually occurs between the ages of 1 and 3 years
    B. Death usually occurs during sleep

C. It is usually caused by external suffocation
D. All children are at equal risk

SCENARIO

Questions 27–29 refer to the following scenario.

Your patient is a 2-month-old who presents lethargic and febrile. His mother says that he has been ill with upper respiratory congestion for 2 days. He has not eaten well, and he generally appears to be very ill. His anterior fontanels are sunken; he is tachycardic and tachypneic, with a 4 second capillary refill.

27. You should suspect _____ until proven otherwise.
    A. Reye's syndrome
    B. Down's syndrome
    C. meningitis
    D. bronchiolitis

28. His vital signs indicate that this patient
    A. is in respiratory failure
    B. is in shock
    C. has increased intracranial pressure
    D. none of the above

29. Prehospital management should include oxygen and
    A. IV mannitol
    B. 20 mL/kg IV fluid challenge
    C. IV antibiotics
    D. the pneumatic antishock garment

SCENARIO

Questions 30–32 refer to the following scenario.

Your patient is a 3-year-old who presents with a sudden onset of severe difficulty in breathing. She has not been ill and had been playing with friends at the time of onset. She presents afebrile with inspiratory stridor, a weak cough, and ashen skin.

30. You should suspect
    A. foreign body obstruction
    B. croup
    C. epiglottitis
    D. asthma

31. Initial prehospital management of this patient includes
    A. back blows
    B. abdominal thrusts
    C. leaving the patient alone
    D. encouraging the patient to cough

32. Further management of this patient may include
    A. direct laryngoscopy
    B. removal with Magill forceps
    C. cricothyrotomy
    D. all of the above

SCENARIO

Questions 33–35 refer to the following scenario.

Your patient is a 5-year-old who presents sitting forward using all accessory muscles to breathe. He has inspiratory stridor, retractions, and a sore throat, and he drools. He is febrile and has been ill for almost a week prior to this incident.

33. In this patient, you should suspect
    A. foreign body obstruction
    B. croup
    C. epiglottitis
    D. asthma

34. Initial prehospital management of this patient includes
    A. racemic epinephrine
    B. direct laryngoscopy
    C. Heimlich maneuver
    D. none of the above

35. If the patient totally occludes his airway, you should immediately
    A. deliver five abdominal thrusts
    B. perform bag-valve-mask ventilation
    C. inject 0.03 mg/kg epinephrine 1:1000 SC
    D. none of the above

SCENARIO

Questions 36–38 refer to the following scenario.

Your patient is an 8-month-old child who presents with difficulty in breathing. She has diffuse expiratory wheezing and retractions and uses accessory muscles to move air. She is tachypneic and tachycardic. She is warm and has been ill since yesterday.

36. In this patient, you should suspect
    A. asthma
    B. bronchitis
    C. bronchiolitis
    D. croup

37. Signs that this patient is in imminent respiratory arrest include
    A. slowing of the respiratory rate
    B. decrease in the respiratory effort
    C. decrease in breath sounds
    D. all of the above

38. Prehospital management of this patient should include
    A. administering oxygen
    B. administering albuterol via nebulizer
    C. sitting the child upright
    D. all of the above

SCENARIO

Questions 39–40 refer to the following scenario.

Your patient is a 4-year-old who presents listless and appears very ill. She has a decreased level of consciousness and responds only to loud voices. Her mother says she has had diarrhea for 2 days and has not been able to keep food or drink down. She has tenting, dry mucous membranes, tachycardia, and delayed capillary refill.

39. From this patient's presentation, you should suspect
    A. respiratory failure
    B. severe dehydration
    C. pulmonary edema
    D. respiratory infection

40. Prehospital management should include oxygen and
    A. 20 mL/kg IV fluid challenge
    B. 40 mg furosemide IV
    C. IV antibiotics
    D. albuterol via nebulizer

SCENARIO

Questions 41–42 refer to the following scenario.

Your patient is a 6-year-old boy who presents with a rapid heart rate (260 beats per minute) and complains of palpitations. He is alert and oriented, his skin is warm and dry, he has no respiratory distress, and his blood pressure is 106/88. The ECG shows a narrow-complex tachycardia.

41. You suspect his problem is caused by
    A. dehydration
    B. airway compromise
    C. cardiac dysrhythmia
    D. any of the above

42. Proper initial field management of this patient includes all of the following EXCEPT
    A. oxygen administration
    B. adenosine administration
    C. synchronized cardioversion
    D. fluid challenge

43. Which of the following analgesics is NOT recommended for children?
    A. Morphine
    B. Fentanyl
    C. Meperidine
    D. Nalbuphine

44. The leading cause of poisoning in toddlers and preschoolers is
    A. cardiac medications
    B. cleaning supplies
    C. iron-containing vitamins
    D. aspirin

45. The most common type of burn injury suffered in the home by children is
    A. electrical
    B. chemical
    C. scald
    D. direct fire

46. Prehospital fluid resuscitation of children should be accomplished with
    A. 10 mL/kg IV colloid
    B. 10 mL/kg IV crystalloid
    C. 20 mL/kg IV 0.45% sodium chloride
    D. 20 mL/kg IV lactated Ringer's

47. Which of the following is the correct initial dose of epinephrine for a child in asystolic cardiac arrest?
    A. 0.1 mg/kg IV of 1:1000
    B. 0.01 mg/kg IV of 1:1000
    C. 0.1 mg/kg ET of 1:10,000
    D. 0.01 mg/kg IO of 1:10,000

48. Which of the following prehospital treatments is NOT indicated for a patient with croup?
    A. Administering cool mist oxygen
    B. Administering racemic epinephrine
    C. Starting an IV
    D. Sitting on mother's lap during transport

49. Epiglottitis has become a rare childhood disease due to
    A. better parental care at home
    B. the *H. flu* vaccine
    C. the advent of non-aspirin-containing analgesics
    D. more tonsillectomies being performed

50. A paramedic should never attempt to visualize the oropharynx of a child suspected of having
    A. croup
    B. epiglottitis
    C. laryngotracheobronchitis
    D. all of the above

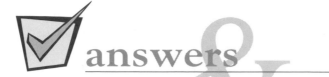

answers & rationales

1.

A. Accidents of all types are the leading cause of death between the ages of 1 and 15 years. (PCPP 5–47   EPC 1719)

2.

B. Children in the 3–5 age group have vivid imaginations and may see monsters as part of their world. During this stage of development, children have a fear of mutilation and may view treatment procedures as hostile. (PCPP 5–47   EPC 1719)

3.

D. The anterior fontanel should be inspected in all infants. It should be level with the surface of the skull or slightly sunken, and it may pulsate. With dehydration, the anterior fontanel may often fall below the level of the skull and appear sunken. (PCPP 5–51   EPC 1722)

4.

B. As a rule, for children under the age of 3, padding underneath the back and shoulders will be necessary to maintain a neutral position due to the large occiput. (PCPP 5–51   EPC 1722)

5.

B. As a rule, as a child gets older, the blood pressure rises and the pulse rate falls. (PCPP 5–61   EPC 1730)

6.

C. In young children, the narrowest part of the upper airway is at the cricoid ring. It acts as an anatomical cuff, which holds an endotracheal tube in place. This is why for children under the age of 8 we use uncuffed tubes. (PCPP 5–52   EPC 1723)

7.

C. There are three distinguishing features of a child's skin and body surface area-to-weight ratio. Their skin is thinner than that of adults, they have less subcutaneous fat, and they have a larger body surface-to-weight ratio. (PCPP 5–53   EPC 1724)

8.

D. The new pediatric assessment triangle includes three components: general appearance, work of breathing, and circulation. (PCPP 5–57   EPC 1727)

9.

A. The most common causes of cardiac arrest in infants and young children are airway and respiratory problems. (PCPP 5–58   EPC 1727)

10.

D. In general, the first manifestation of respiratory distress in infants and young children is tachypnea. (PCPP 5–60   EPC 1729)

11.

A. Bradycardia in a distressed infant or young child is an ominous sign of impending cardiac arrest. Bradycardia is age dependent, so it is important to know the normal heart rate for each age group. (PCPP 5–62   EPC 1730)

12.

A. Recognizing and preventing cardiac arrest in the pediatric patient is the key. Vital signs that place a pediatric patient at risk for cardiopulmonary arrest include a respiratory rate >60, heart rate >180, and heart rate <80 (under 5 years) and <60 (over 5 years). (PCPP 5–62   EPC 1731)

13.

C. For children less than 1 year old, back blows and chest thrusts are the only techniques recommended for removal of a foreign body. (PCPP 5–69   EPC 1737)

14.

D. Even when performing oropharyngeal suctioning properly, complications may occur in the infant and small child. These include vagal stimulation and the resulting bradycardia, and hypoxia. To reduce the possibility of these complications, limit suctioning to less than 10 seconds, reduce the suction pressure to less than 100 mm/Hg, and frequently monitor your patient for signs of hypoxia and bradycardia. (PCPP 5–71   EPC 1737)

15.

B. Certain airways in pediatrics are contraindicated because of variations in airway size in children. Avoid esophageal obturator airways, pharyngotracheal lumen airways, and esophageal combitubes. (PCPP 5–72   EPC 1739)

16.

D. Pediatric bag-valve-masks should not contain pressure pop-off valves. If one exists, it should be disengaged. The reason is that higher pressures may be needed to ventilate the pediatric patient. (PCPP 5–75   EPC 1741)

17.

B. Approved techniques for estimating the correct ET tube size for infants and young children include the diameter of the patient's little finger, the diameter of the nasal opening, and the patient's age in years + 16 divided by 4. Of course, you can always refer to a chart for the recommended size for your patient's age and size. (PCPP 5–77   EPC 1743)

18.

B. Indications for intraosseous infusion include an unresponsive child less than 6 years of age in shock or cardiac arrest, after unsuccessful attempts at peripheral IV insertion. In children over the age of 6, the bones become more solid. (PCPP 5–83 EPC 1749)

19.

D. Placement of the needle into the marrow cavity can be determined by noting a lack of resistance if the needle passes through the bony cortex. Other indications include the needle standing upright without support, the ability to aspirate bone marrow into a syringe, and the free flow of the infusion without infiltration into the subcutaneous tissues. (PCPP 5–84   EPC 1750)

20.

B. The initial dose for defibrillation in pediatric patients is 2 joules per kilogram. Perform all subsequent defibrillation attempts at 4 joules per kilogram. (PCPP 5–86   EPC 1752)

21.

B. Estimation of the burn surface is slightly different for children. When using the rule of nines to calculate the percentage of burns in infants and small children, each leg is worth 14%, while the head is worth 18%. For this patient who burned both legs and arms, the body surface area adds up to 46%. (PCPP 5–126   EPC 1789)

22.

D. There are several characteristics common to abused children. Often they are seen as special and different from others. Also, premature infants or twins, children less than 5 years of age, children with disabilities, uncommunicative children, boys, and children of the wrong sex are at higher risk. (PCPP 5–127   EPC 1790)

23.

D. The child abuser can come from any geographic, religious, ethnic, occupational, educational, or socioeconomic group. However, people who abuse children tend to share certain characteristics. The abuser is usually a parent or someone in the role of a parent. When the mother spends most time with the child, she is the parent most frequently identified as the abuser. Most child abusers were abused as children. Common crises (financial stress, marital or relationship stress, and physical illness in a parent or child) may precipitate abuse. (PCPP 5–127   EPC 1791)

24.

C. The prehospital management of the abused child includes appropriately treating the injuries, protecting the child from further abuse, notifying the proper authorities, obtaining as much information as possible in a nonjudgmental manner, and documenting all findings or statements in the patient report. (PCPP 5–130   EPC 1793)

25.

C. Febrile seizures occur as a result of a sudden increase in body temperature. They seem related to the rate at which the body temperature increases, not to the degree of fever. (PCPP 5–109   EPC 1773)

26.

B. Sudden infant death syndrome (SIDS) usually occurs in children between the ages of 1 month and 1 year during sleep. It is not caused by any type of external suffocation. Certain children (males, infants with a low birth weight, children of young mothers, and infants from lower socioeconomic groups) are predisposed to SIDS. (PCPP 5–126 EPC 1789)

27.

C. Documented fever in a child less than 3 months of age is considered meningitis until proven otherwise. (PCPP 5–110   EPC 1774)

28.

B. The patient's vital signs, sunken anterior fontanels, tachycardia, tachypnea, and delayed capillary refill all indicate shock. (PCPP 5–102   EPC 1766)

29.

B. Prehospital management of this patient should include oxygen and a fluid challenge of 20 milliliters per kilogram of IV crystalloid (normal saline, lactated Ringer's). (PCPP 5–110   EPC 1774)

30.

A. Any afebrile child who presents with a sudden onset of stridor without previous history of illness should be suspected as having a foreign body obstruction. (PCPP 5–96   EPC 1760)

31.

B. Initial prehospital management of this patient includes delivering five abdominal thrusts. (PCPP 5–96   EPC 1760)

32.

D. Further management of this patient may include direct laryngoscopy and removal of the foreign body with Magill forceps and, as a last resort, needle cricothyrotomy. (PCPP 5–96   EPC 1760)

33.

C. Your 5-year-old patient who sits forward, drooling and presenting with stridor, fever, and illness, should be suspected of having epiglottitis. (PCPP 5–94   EPC 1758)

34.

D. Initial prehospital management of this patient includes placing the child in a position of comfort and administering humidified oxygen by face mask or blow-by. Direct visualization of the larynx may cause laryngospasm and is contraindicated. (PCPP 5–94   EPC 1759)

35.

B. If the patient totally closes his airway (usually from laryngospasm), immediately perform bag-valve-mask ventilation. (PCPP 5–95   EPC 1759)

36.

C. In this patient, who is less than 1 year old, presenting with wheezing and difficulty breathing, you should suspect bronchiolitis. (PCPP 5–98 EPC 1762)

37.

D. Signs that a pediatric patient is in imminent respiratory arrest include a slowing of the respiratory rate, a decrease in the respiratory effort, and a decrease in breath sounds. (PCPP 5–91   EPC 1755)

38.

D. Prehospital management of this patient should include oxygen administration, sitting the child upright, and administering albuterol via nebulizer. (PCPP 5–98   EPC 1762)

39.

B. This child who presents with dry mucous membranes, poor skin turgor, tachycardia, and delayed capillary refill is suspected of having severe dehydration. (PCPP 5–102   EPC 1765)

40.

A. Prehospital management of this patient should include oxygen and 20 milliliters per kilogram of IV crystalloid (normal saline, lactated Ringer's). (PCPP 5–102   EPC 1766)

41.

C. A heart rate of 260 indicates a cardiac dysrhythmia, rather than any other cause such as dehydration or hypoxia. The narrow complex suggests supraventricular tachycardia. (PCPP 5–102   EPC 1769)

42.

C. For this stable patient in probable supraventricular tachycardia, proper field management includes oxygen therapy, IV–KVO, and adenosine administration (0.1–0.2 mg/kg IV) to convert the rhythm. If the patient becomes unstable, deliver synchronized cardioversion (0.5–1 joule/kg). (PCPP 5–105 EPC 1769)

43.

D. Unless there is a contraindication, children should receive pain management. Natural analgesics, such as morphine, meperidine, and fentanyl, are effective. Synthetic analgesics, such as nalbuphine and butorphanol, should be avoided because their effects on children are unpredictable. (PCPP 5–122 EPC 1785)

44.

C. Iron-containing vitamin supplements are the leading cause of poisoning in the toddler and preschool age groups. (PCPP 5–114   EPC 1788)

45.

C. The most common type of burn injury suffered by children in the home is a scald injury, usually by pulling hot liquids off a table or stove. In cases of abuse, hot water immersion is the typical cause. (PCPP 5–125   EPC 1783)

46.

D. Prehospital fluid therapy for a child is accomplished with an isotonic solution, such as normal saline (0.9% sodium chloride) or lactated Ringer's, at 20 mL/kg initial bolus. (PCPP 5–84   EPC 1750)

47.

D. The initial dose of epinephrine for a child in asystolic cardiac arrest is 0.01 mg/kg of 1:10,000 IV/IO or 0.1 mg/kg of 1:1000 ET. (PCPP 5–85 EPC 1751)

48.

C. Prehospital management of a child with croup includes administering cool mist oxygen by face mask or blow-by, administering racemic epinephrine or albuterol via nebulizer if the attack is severe, and avoiding anything that will agitate the child, such as starting an IV. (PCPP 5–93 EPC 1757)

49.

B. Epiglottitis is caused by a bacterial infection—usually the Hemophilus influenza type B. With the advent of the *H. flu* vaccine, epiglottitis has become a rare pediatric disease. (PCPP 5–94   EPC 1758)

50.

D. If you suspect your pediatric patient may have croup (laryngotracheobronchitis) or epiglottitis, never put anything into their mouths. This may worsen the tissue swelling, cause further upper airway obstruction, and even result in a complete obstruction and apnea. (PCPP 5–95   EPC 1759)

48

Geriatric Emergencies

DIRECTIONS Each of the questions or incomplete statements below is followed by suggested answers or completions. Select the **one answer** that is best in each case.

1. The fastest-growing segment of our population is the elderly because of
   A. a declining birth rate
   B. an absence of major wars and catastrophies
   C. an improved health care system
   D. all of the above

2. Which of the following best describes changes in the respiratory system of elderly patients?
   A. Lung elasticity decreases
   B. Vital capacity decreases
   C. Respiratory muscle strength decreases
   D. All of the above

3. Which of the following best describes changes in the cardiovascular system of elderly patients?
   A. Left ventricular hypertrophy
   B. Conduction system degeneration
   C. Decreased cardiac output
   D. All of the above

4. Osteoporosis, kyphosis, and spondylolysis are the result of
   A. the demineralizing of bone
   B. fibrosis
   C. decreased nerve conduction velocity
   D. the reduced number of nephrons

5. Which of the following tends to complicate the assessment of the elderly?
   A. The elderly often suffer more than one disease at a time
   B. The primary problem often is different from the chief complaint
   C. The patient's perception of pain may be diminished or absent
   D. All of the above

6. Assessing an elderly patient who presents with poor peripheral pulses, rales, and dependent edema may be difficult because
   A. his presentation is consistent with congestive heart failure
   B. his signs and symptoms may be caused by the aging process
   C. it is often difficult to distinguish acute from chronic problems
   D. all of the above

7. Your patient who complains that the room is spinning and who is nauseated, pale, and sweating may be suffering from
   A. dementia
   B. delirium
   C. Alzheimer's
   D. vertigo

Match the following causes of syncope with their respective descriptions:

8. ____ Vasodepressor
9. ____ Orthostatic
10. ____ Vasovagal
11. ____ Cardiac
12. ____ TIA

   A. Temporary stroke
   B. Stokes-Adams syndrome
   C. Rising from a seated or supine position
   D. The common faint
   E. Valsalva maneuver

13. Chronic global mental impairment is known as
   A. organic brain syndrome
   B. senile dementia
   C. senility
   D. all of the above

14. Which of the following renders the elderly susceptible to making medication errors?
    A. Forgetfulness
    B. Limited income
    C. Vision impairment
    D. All of the above

SCENARIO

Questions 15–16 refer to the following scenario.

Your patient is an 89-year-old female who presents with multiple bruises. She lives with her son, who says she is always falling down and is just generally clumsy. She appears somewhat undernourished and frightened. She cowers when you approach her and reluctantly allows you to inspect her bruises. Her son behaves very strangely toward you and your partner and nervously attempts to explain each bruise. She is incontinent of urine and appears not to have been washed in days. You suspect elderly abuse.

15. In which socioeconomic class is this problem most prevalent?
    A. Lower
    B. Middle class
    C. Wealthy
    D. All classes

16. In this case, the paramedic should do all of the following EXCEPT
    A. obtain a complete patient and family history
    B. report any suspicions to the ED staff
    C. be honest with her son about your concerns
    D. watch for inconsistencies in stories

SCENARIO

Questions 17–19 refer to the following scenario.

Your patient is an 82-year-old woman who presents with some vague complaints about feeling weak and fatigued. She denies any chest pain. She has a long history of cardiac, respiratory, and diabetic problems. She takes a host of medications for each but cannot remember what she took today. In your exam, you notice her swollen ankles and weak peripheral pulses, and you auscultate some fine bibasilar rales. You suspect she is having a cardiac episode and begin appropriate prehospital management.

17. Which of the following is true regarding this elderly patient?
    A. Absence of chest pain does not rule out myocardial infarction
    B. Her peripheral edema and rales may be normal findings
    C. The first 2 hours after the onset of symptoms are critical
    D. All of the above

18. Atypical presentations of myocardial infarction include
    A. dental pain
    B. syncope
    C. dyspnea
    D. all of the above

19. All of the following statements are true regarding the management of the elderly cardiac patient EXCEPT
    A. they are treated much the same as the younger patient
    B. medication orders may be modified
    C. oxygen administration must be carefully monitored
    D. fluid administration may be decreased

answers & rationales

1.

D. The fastest-growing segment of our population is the elderly due to a declining birth rate, the absence of major wars and catastrophies, and an improved health care system since World War II. (PCPP 5–140 EPC 1800)

2.

D. The effects of aging on the respiratory system include increased chest wall stiffness, loss of lung elasticity, increased air trapping, and reduced strength and endurance of the respiratory muscles, all decreasing vital capacity, maximum breathing capacity, and maximum oxygen uptake. (PCPP 5–161 EPC 1813)

3.

D. Changes in the cardiovascular system include left ventricular hypertrophy, fibrosis in the heart and peripheral vascular system, conductive system degeneration, and decreased cardiac output. (PCPP 5–162 EPC 1814)

4.

A. Osteoporosis, kyphosis, and spondylolysis are the result of the demineralizing of bone. This results in the softening of bone tissue. (PCPP 5–165 EPC 1817)

5.

D. It is difficult to assess the elderly because they often suffer more than one disease at a time. Their primary problem is often different from the chief complaint, and their perception of pain may be diminished or absent. (PCPP 5–149 EPC 1803)

6.

D. Assessing elderly patients who present with poor peripheral pulses, rales, and edema may be difficult because their presentation is consistent with congestive heart failure, and yet their signs and symptoms may be caused simply by the aging process. It is often difficult to distinguish the acute from the chronic problem. (PCPP 5–149 EPC 1803)

7.

D. Vertigo is a specific sensation of motion perceived by the patient as spinning or whirling. It is often accompanied by sweating, pallor, nausea, and vomiting. (PCPP 5 –176 EPC 1828)

Matching (PCPP 5–174 EPC 1826)

8. D Vasodepressor
9. C Orthostatic
10. E Vasovagal
11. B Cardiac
12. A TIA
A. Temporary stroke
B. Stokes-Adams syndrome
C. Rising from a seated or supine position
D. The common faint
E. Valsalva maneuver

13.

D. Dementia, a chronic, global mental impairment, is often progressive or irreversible and usually is due to underlying neurological disease. This mental deterioration is often called organic brain syndrome, senile dementia, or senility. (PCPP 5–177 EPC 1830)

14.

D. Underdosing and overdosing of medication are very common in the elderly. This may be due to confusion, vision impairment, forgetfulness, or limited income. (PCPP 5–150 EPC 1803)

15.

D. Abuse of the elderly knows no socioeconomic bounds. It occurs in all classes of our society and is a major health and social problem. (PCPP 5–197 EPC 1846)

16.

C. In cases where you suspect geriatric abuse, you should obtain a complete patient and family history and watch for inconsistencies in the stories. You should report any suspicions to the ED staff and always avoid confrontations with the family. (PCPP 5–198 EPC 1847)

17.

D. In this case, the absence of chest pain does not rule out myocardial infarction because many elderly patients suffer silent myocardial infarctions. Her peripheral edema and rales may be normal findings of the aging process, and as in all cardiac patients, the first 2 hours after the onset of symptoms are the most critical. (PCPP 5–171 EPC 1823)

18.

D. Atypical presentations of myocardial infarction include dental pain, syncope, dyspnea, confusion, neck pain, epigastric pain, and fatigue. (PCPP 5–171 EPC 1823)

19.

C. Managing the elderly cardiac patient is somewhat the same as managing the younger cardiac patient, with a few differences. Medication orders may be modified and fluid administration may be decreased based on the presence of congestive heart failure, liver disease, and other metabolic problems. (PCPP 5–172 EPC 1824)

49 Abuse and Assault

DIRECTIONS

Each of the questions or incomplete statements below is followed by suggested answers or completions. Select the **one answer** that is best in each case.

1. Reasons for not reporting an abusive partner include
   A. fear of reprisal
   B. humiliation
   C. denial
   D. all of the above

2. Which of the following is one of the ten generic risk factors identified in domestic abuse?
   A. The male is a white-collar worker
   B. The partners are married
   C. The male is between 18 and 30 years old
   D. All of the above

3. When interviewing a battered partner, which of the following phrases represents an appropriate response?
   A. "Why don't you leave?"
   B. "How awful."
   C. "I hear what you are telling me."
   D. "You are so nice and that guy is a real jerk."

4. Which of the following statements is believed to be true regarding domestic elder abuse?
   A. The elders are usually in good health
   B. The abusers are usually well-adjusted with few problems of their own
   C. There is seldom a family history of elder abuse
   D. None of the above

5. The main perpetrators of elder abuse are
   A. grandchildren
   B. adult children
   C. spouses
   D. brothers and sisters

6. Which of the following is a characteristic of child abusers?
   A. They rarely feel guilt or remorse
   B. They usually identify with the child's pain and suffering
   C. Alcohol or drug abuse is uncommon
   D. They usually want the child's injuries treated

SCENARIO

Questions 7–8 refer to the following scenario.

Your patient is a 9-year-old boy who has suffered a possible fractured clavicle while tree climbing in the backyard with his friends. You notice he has multiple bruises on his legs and arms in various stages of healing. He acts normally and relates the story to you without hesitation. The story matches the one told by his father, who appears very concerned for his child's welfare and wants transportation to the "best" hospital.

7. You suspect his bruises were caused by
   A. obvious child abuse from the father
   B. normal play and "roughhousing"

8. Which of the following statements is true regarding child abuse injuries?
   A. Splash burns indicate child abuse
   B. Rib fractures in young children suggest child abuse
   C. Shaken baby syndrome never causes death of the infant
   D. Head injuries are usually the first sign in child abuse

9. What differentiates sexual assault from rape?
   A. Intent of the perpetrator
   B. Consent of the victim
   C. Use of a condom
   D. Vaginal or rectal penetration

10. Which of the following statements is true regarding sexual assault and rape?

    A. Most victims are older than 18

    B. Most crimes occur in the afternoon

    C. Most women are raped by someone they know

    D. Most rapists use weapons

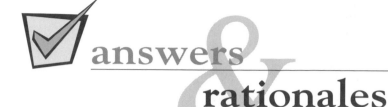

answers & rationales

1.

D. So why don't these people just report the abuse? Reasons for not reporting partner abuse include fear of reprisal, fear of humiliation, denial, lack of knowledge, and lack of financial resources. That's why. (PCPP 5–207   EPC 1854)

2.

C. The generic risk factors include the following: The male is unemployed or is a blue-collar worker, uses illegal drugs at least once a year, did not graduate from high school, is between 18 and 30 years old, and watched his father abuse his mother. The partners are unmarried, they have different religious backgrounds, their family income is below the poverty level, and either partner is violent toward children at home. (PCPP 5–207   EPC 1854)

3.

C. When interviewing a suspected battered partner, avoid judgmental questions or statements. Just use common active listening techniques that let the patient know that you are listening and interested. (PCPP 5–209   EPC 1856)

4.

D. There are four main theories concerning elder abuse. Caregivers are stressed themselves and ill-equipped to care for their elder family members. The elders are usually in poor physical or mental health and cannot report the abuse. There is a family history of elder abuse or a cycle of violence. Finally, the abuse increases with the personal problems of the caregivers. (PCPP 5–211   EPC 1856)

5.

B. The main perpetrators of elder abuse are adult children, by far. Also, they often exhibit alcoholic be-havior, drug addiction, or some mental impair-ment. (PCPP 5–212   EPC 1857)

6.

A. Child abusers usually demonstrate no regard for the child's welfare, no concern for the injuries inflicted or the pain suffered, and no remorse or guilt for what has happened. Drug and alcohol use or abuse is common. (PCPP 5–213   EPC 1859)

7.

B. Differentiating signs of child abuse from the normal injury patterns of an active child is a challenging task. In this scenario, there are a number of important clues that this is not child abuse. The stories from the child and father are identical and match the injury pattern. The child does not hesitate to tell the story, and the father makes no attempt to cover up the truth. The father is obviously concerned with his son's welfare. Finally, any active 9-year-old gets bruises from playing with his friends. The evidence presented in this case should lead you not to suspect child abuse. (PCPP 5–214   EPC 1859)

8.

B. Splash burns usually indicate that a child accidentally got into hot water. Shaken baby syndrome can indeed cause death of the infant. Over time, injuries from abuse tend to progress from the extremities and trunk to the head. Rib fractures in young children suggest child abuse because of the tremendous force necessary to fracture them. (PCPP 5–214   EPC 1860)

9.

D. Sexual assault is unwanted oral, genital, rectal, or manual sexual contact. Rape is penile penetration of the genitalia or rectum without the consent of the victim. (PCPP 5–217   EPC 1863)

10.

C. Most victims are adolescent females under the age of 18. Most sexual crimes occur between 6 P.M. and 6 A.M. in a place familiar to the victim. Most women are raped by someone they know. Only 30% of rapists use weapons. (PCPP 5–217   EPC 1863)

50 The Challenged Patient

DIRECTIONS

Each of the questions or incomplete statements below is followed by suggested answers or completions. Select the **one answer** that is best in each case.

1. The curable type of deafness is known as
   A. sensorineural
   B. labyrinthitis
   C. conductive
   D. presbycusis

2. Which of the following techniques will aid you in communicating with a hearing-impaired patient?
   A. Speak in high-pitched tones
   B. Speak from behind the patient
   C. Yell and use exaggerated gestures
   D. Use a low-pitched voice

3. Glaucoma is caused by
   A. other eye diseases
   B. diabetic retinopathy
   C. unknown causes
   D. all of the above

4. Which of the following should you NOT do if your patient has a seeing eye dog and it is in its harness?
   A. Pet it
   B. Grab the harness
   C. Grab the patient's arm
   D. All of the above

5. The type of aphasia that occurs when your patient can understand you but cannot speak is known as _____ aphasia.
   A. motor
   B. global
   C. sensory
   D. articulatory

6. Down's syndrome is caused by
   A. a viral infection
   B. an extra chromosome
   C. congenital hypoxia
   D. fetal alcohol syndrome

7. Patients on chemotherapy may develop
   A. neutropenia
   B. sarcoma
   C. angiocarcinoma
   D. all of the above

8. The most common type of cerebral palsy, characterized by a state of permanent stiffness and contracture, is known as _____ cerebral palsy.
   A. athetoid
   B. spastic
   C. diplegic
   D. quadriplegic

9. An inherited disorder that involves the exocrine glands producing heavy mucous obstruction in the lungs and in the pancreas is known as
   A. multiple sclerosis
   B. muscular dystrophy
   C. cystic fibrosis
   D. hypermucosis

Match the following neurological system disorders with their respective characteristics:

10. ____ Multiple sclerosis
11. ____ Muscular dystrophy
12. ____ Poliomyelitis
13. ____ Spina bifida
14. ____ Myasthenia gravis
15. ____ Cerebral palsy

A. Blocked neurotransmitters
B. Damage to the cerebrum in utero
C. Genetic degeneration of muscle fibers
D. Inflammation of myelin sheath
E. Viral attack on gray matter
F. Open defect in spinal canal and backbone

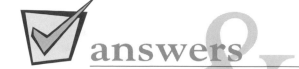

answers & rationales

1.

C. Conductive deafness is curable. It is caused when there is a blocking of the transmission of sound waves through the external ear canal to the middle or inner ear. Otitis media is a common cause of conductive deafness in infants. (PCPP 5–225 EPC 1868)

2.

D. When talking with a hearing-impaired patient, use a low-pitched voice, eliminate background noise if possible, speak directly in front of his or her face, and never yell or use exaggerated gestures. (PCPP 5–227 EPC 1869)

3.

D. Glaucoma, a group of eye diseases that result in increased intraocular pressure on the optic nerve and can lead to blindness, can be caused by diabetic retinopathy and by other eye diseases. It can also be of unknown origin. (PCPP 5–228 EPC 1870)

4.

D. If your patient has a seeing eye dog and it is in its harness, this means it is working. In this scenario, do not touch the dog, grab its leash or the harness, or grab the patient's arm without permission. (PCPP 5–228 EPC 1871)

5.

A. The type of aphasia that occurs when your patient can understand you but cannot speak is known as motor aphasia. It is important to allow your patient to express himself in whatever way he can. (PCPP 5–230 EPC 1871)

6.

B. Down's syndrome, named after Dr. J. Langdon Down, results from an extra chromosome. Instead of the usual 46, the Down's child has 47. (PCPP 5–234 EPC 1875)

7.

A. Patients on chemotherapy may develop neutropenia, a condition that results from an abnormally low neutrophil count in the blood. This increases the patient's risk for infection. (PCPP 5–236 EPC 1878)

8.

B. Spastic cerebral palsy is the most common form of cerebral palsy. It is characterized by a state of permanent stiffness and contracture. When both legs are affected, the knees turn inward, causing the characteristic "scissor gait." (PCPP 5–237 EPC 1879)

9.

C. Cystic fibrosis is an inherited disorder that involves the exocrine (mucus-producing) glands in the lungs and the pancreas. This results in thick mucous obstruction in the lungs and pancreatic duct blockage. Because of the poor prognosis, the majority of cystic fibrosis patients you see will be children and adolescents. (PCPP 5–237 EPC 1879) (PCPP 5–238 to 5–240 EPC 1802)

Matching (PCPP 5–238 to 5–240 EPC 1802)

10. **D** Multiple sclerosis
11. **C** Muscular dystrophy
12. **E** Poliomyelitis
13. **F** Spina bifida
14. **A** Myasthenia gravis
15. **B** Cerebral palsy

A. Blocked neurotransmitters
B. Damage to the cerebrum in utero
C. Genetic degeneration of muscle fibers
D. Inflammation of myelin sheath
E. Viral attack on gray matter
F. Open defect in spinal canal and backbone

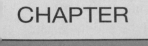

51

Acute Interventions for the Chronic-Care Patient

DIRECTIONS Each of the questions or incomplete statements below is followed by suggested answers or completions. Select the **one answer** that is best in each case.

1. Which of the following techniques is used with an endotracheal tube?
   A. BPAP
   B. PEEP
   C. CPAP
   D. All of the above

2. Which of the following drugs is **NOT** administered via a nebulizer?
   A. Metaproterenol
   B. Methylprednisolone
   C. Albuterol
   D. Ipratropium

3. A patient with cystic fibrosis will likely require emergency care for which of the following problems?
   A. Pulmonary hemorrhage
   B. Pneumothorax
   C. Hemoptysis
   D. All of the above

4. Your patient is an infant being treated for bronchopulmonary dysplasia. He is being weaned off his respirator by a process called intermittent mandatory ventilation. When you arrive, you find the infant obviously hypoxic and sick-looking. Which of the following treatments is indicated?
   A. Oxygen administration
   B. Ventilatory support
   C. Prompt transport to a neonatal center
   D. All of the above

5. Which of the following is **NOT** a treatment for sleep apnea?
   A. Alcohol nightcap
   B. CPAP
   C. Weight loss
   D. Surgical alteration of the airway

6. Your patient has a tracheostomy and is on a ventilator. He presents in acute respiratory distress. You assess his trach tube and it appears clear, but there is something wrong with the ventilator. You do not notice any loose fittings or disconnected tubes. The airway is clear and he is sitting upright. What is your next step?
   A. Call the manufacturer's service hotline
   B. Try to further troubleshoot the ventilator
   C. Disconnect the patient and ventilate him with a bag-valve device
   D. Connect your oxygen tank directly to the tracheostomy tube

7. The poncho wrap, cuirass, and iron lung all work on the principle of
   A. positive pressure ventilation
   B. negative pressure ventilation
   C. osmosis and diffusion
   D. active transport

8. Patients with _____ are at high risk for developing ulcers, especially on the feet.
   A. atherosclerosis
   B. cystic fibrosis
   C. diabetes mellitus
   D. COPD

9. Postpartum depression occurs in roughly _____ of mothers.
   A. one-half
   B. one-third
   C. two-thirds
   D. three-fourths

10. Which of the following surgically implanted medication delivery devices requires a special-shaped needle for access?
    A. Hickman catheter
    B. PICC line
    C. Port-A-Cath
    D. Groshong

answers & rationales

1.

B. Positive end expiratory pressure (PEEP) is provided through an endotracheal tube. Continuous positive airway pressure (CPAP) and bilevel positive airway pressure (BiPAP) are provided with a tight-fitting mask. (PCPP 5–264   EPC 1898)

2.

B. Often home-care patients are prescribed medications administered via a nebulizer. These include sympathomimetic bronchodilators, such as albuterol and metaproterenol, and anticholinergics, such as ipratropium. Methylprednisolone is a corticosteroid administered intravenously or orally. (PCPP 5–264   EPC 1898)

3.

D. Patients with cystic fibrosis suffer severe coughing spells in an attempt to clear the airways of mucus. From these coughing spells, hemoptysis, pneumothorax, severe pulmonary hemorrhage, and pulmonary hypertension can occur. (PCPP 5–265   EPC 1899)

4.

D. Patients with bronchopulmonary dysplasia have been treated for respiratory distress and have not been completely weaned from the ventilator. They are sent home and treated with intermittent mandatory ventilation systems that are set at increasingly lower settings until the weaning is complete. If your patient presents hypoxic, treat him for hypoxia—oxygen administration, ventilation as needed, and prompt transport to a neonatal center. (PCPP 5–266 EPC 1900)

5.

A. Treatment for sleep apnea includes surgery, medications, weight loss, avoidance of alcohol or any CNS depressant, and use of a CPAP ventilator. (PCPP 5–266   EPC 1900)

6.

C. If the problem is not immediately apparent, do not waste time troubleshooting the machine. Disconnect the machine, attach your bag-valve device to the trach tube, and provide ventilation. (PCPP 5–270   EPC 1904)

7.

B. The poncho wrap, cuirass, and iron lung all work on the principle of negative pressure ventilation. They expand, pulling on the chest, causing it to expand also, and allowing air to flow into the lungs. (PCPP 5–272   EPC 1905)

8.

C. Patients with diabetes have alterations in peripheral circulation that result in poor perfusion to the extremities, especially the feet. These patients are at high risk for unhealing wounds and ulcers. (PCPP 5–251   EPC 1887)

9.

D. Postpartum depression occurs in 70–80% of mothers. In these cases, women have difficulty caring for their babies and themselves. In extreme cases, babies have been neglected or even harmed. (PCPP 5–281   EPC 1915)

10.

C. Surgically implanted medication delivery devices that can be accessed with a regular needle include the Hickman, Groshong, Broviac, and PICC lines. The Port-A-Cath and Medi-Port devices are disc-shaped and have a diaphragm that requires a specially shaped needle. (PCPP 5–274   EPC 1908)

52 Assessment-Based Management

1. Most of the time for a patient with a medical condition you will formulate your field diagnosis based on the
   A. history
   B. physical exam
   C. vital signs
   D. monitor strip

2. Pattern recognition is based on experience and
   A. circumstances
   B. knowledge
   C. vital signs
   D. protocols

3. Which of the following statements is true regarding the use of protocols?
   A. Deviation from protocol is prohibited
   B. Standing orders replace a paramedic's judgment
   C. Exercising judgment is a dangerous proposition
   D. Protocols are guidelines that require judicious application

4. Which of the following circumstances can affect your on-scene decision-making capabilities?
   A. Extreme environmental temperatures
   B. A loud, abusive patient
   C. Gory injuries
   D. All of the above

5. In a two-paramedic ambulance crew, which of the following tasks is performed by the team leader?
   A. Gathering scene information
   B. Interrogating the patient
   C. Starting the IV
   D. Obtaining vital signs

6. Your patient presents with chest pain, normal mental status, and normal vital signs. The correct approach would be the _____ approach.
   A. contemplative
   B. resuscitative
   C. immediate evacuation
   D. none of the above

7. Which of the following patients requires a complete head-to-toe physical exam?
   A. Patient with an isolated ankle sprain
   B. Responsive patient with suspected AMI
   C. Unresponsive stroke patient
   D. Alert and oriented 14-year-old with moderate asthma attack

8. Your patient is unstable. You should perform an ongoing assessment every _____ minutes.
   A. 5
   B. 10
   C. 15
   D. 20

9. The "A" in SOAP stands for
   A. allergies
   B. actions
   C. acute
   D. none of the above

10. An effective oral presentation should last no more than _____.
    A. 15 seconds
    B. 1 minute
    C. 2 minutes
    D. 5 minutes

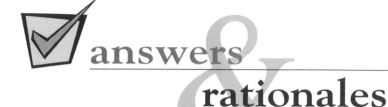

answers & rationales

1.

A. Doctors will base 80% of their diagnosis on the history. Your ability to elicit a good history will determine your success in formulating an accurate field diagnosis. (PCPP 5–293   EPC 1923)

2.

B. Pattern recognition is based on your experience and knowledge base. The greater both are, the more likely you are to recognize patterns. This is why the perfect team is a seasoned paramedic (experienced, street savvy) and a new graduate (recent knowledge, enthusiasm). (PCPP 5–294 EPC 1924)

3.

D. Protocols and standing orders are guidelines only. You must add your clinical judgment when deciding to use or not use them. Of course, clinical judgment comes from experience. Experience comes from having had bad judgment. (PCPP 5–294 EPC 1924)

4.

D. A number of factors can affect your ability to make an on-scene decision. These include your personal attitude, your patient's attitude, distracting injuries, and environmental factors. Understanding this, try to maintain focus on the problem and disregard the distractions. (PCPP 5–294 EPC 1924)

5.

B. In a typical two-paramedic crew, the duties are sometimes divided into the team leader and patient care provider roles. The team leader obtains the history, performs the physical exam, presents the patient, and handles documentation. The patient care provider surveys the scene, obtains vital signs, and performs interventions. In a multiple-casualty inci-

dent, the team leader assumes EMS command, while his or her partner begins triage. (PCPP 5–297 EPC 1927)

6.

A. Use the contemplative approach when your patient does not require immediate intervention. In this case, a good history and physical exam are worth some added on-scene time because they will yield vital information. (PCPP 5–300   EPC 1930)

7.

C. A complete head-to-toe exam consists of a rapid trauma assessment for the trauma patient or a rapid medical assessment for the medical patient. These exams are performed on medical patients who are unresponsive and on trauma patients with significant mechanisms of injury or altered mental status. Responsive medical patients and patients with isolated injuries receive physical exams directed at the body systems involved. (PCPP 5–301   EPC 1931)

8.

A. The ongoing assessment must be performed on all patients to monitor for trends and changes in the patient's condition—every 5 minutes for an unstable patient, every 15 minutes for stable patients. The ongoing assessment includes reassessing the initial assessment and focused exam, and reevaluating transport priorities and vital signs, as well as the effectiveness of interventions and management plans. (PCPP 5–301   EPC 1931)

9.

D. SOAP is the universal format for presenting a patient to another health care professional. The mnemonic stands for **S**ubjective, **O**bjective, **A**ssessment, and **P**lan. You should always use SOAP or some variation of it when presenting your patient on the radio or in person at the ED. (PCPP 5–303   EPC 1933)

10.

B. An effective patient report, either on the radio or in person, should last no longer than 1 minute. Other health care providers, especially busy emergency department personnel, have little interest or time to listen to unimportant details. Use the SOAP format and get to the point quickly. (PCPP 5–303 EPC 1933)

53 Ambulance Operations

DIRECTIONS
Each of the questions or incomplete statements below is followed by suggested answers or completions. Select the **one answer** that is best in each case.

1. Which of the following agencies has established standards for ambulance design and EMS operations?
   A. USDOT
   B. OSHA
   C. NIOSH
   D. All of the above

2. A computerized personnel and ambulance deployment system is known as
   A. peak loading reinforcement
   B. demographic deployment
   C. system status management
   D. tiered response

3. A study of emergency ambulance collisions demonstrated that the majority of collisions occurred
   A. at intersections
   B. at night
   C. during inclement weather
   D. during turning

4. Inexperienced drivers tend to _____ when they hear a siren approaching.
   A. pull to the right
   B. stop
   C. speed up
   D. pull to the left

5. In general, it is a good practice to use a police escort when responding to a scene.
   A. True
   B. False

6. If you arrive first on the scene of an automobile collision and there is no sign of fire or escaping liquids or fumes, you should park your vehicle
   A. 100 feet beyond the crash
   B. 50 feet beyond the crash
   C. 100 feet in front of the crash
   D. 50 feet in front of the crash

7. Fixed-wing aircraft usually are used when transporting patients over distances of more than _____ miles.
   A. 250
   B. 500
   C. 100
   D. 50

8. The first use of helicopters to evacuate patients occurred during the _____ War.
   A. Second World
   B. Korean
   C. Vietnam
   D. Gulf

9. A standard helicopter landing zone should be
   A. a 25 ft × 25 ft triangle
   B. a 100 ft × 100 ft square
   C. a 50 ft × 50 ft rectangle × square
   D. none of the above

10. Which of the following statements is true regarding helicopter transport?
    A. Most treatment should be done prior to loading the patient
    B. Helicopter transport is relatively inexpensive
    C. Patient care is seldom affected during the flight
    D. Pressure changes do not affect equipment such as PASG, ET tubes, etc.

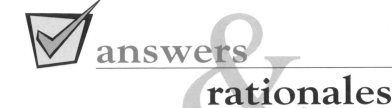

answers & rationales

1.

D. A number of government and private agencies have established mandatory and voluntary standards for ambulance design, safety, and EMS operations. These include the United States Department of Transportation (USDOT), the National Institute for Occupational Safety and Health (NIOSH), the Occupational Safety and Health Administration (OSHA), the National Flight Paramedics Association (NFPA), the Federal Communications Commission (FCC), the National Flight Nurses Association (NFNA), the National Fire Protection Association (NFPA), the Commission on Accreditation of Ambulance Services (CAAS), and the American College of Surgeons (ACS), just to name a few. (PCPP 5–318 EPC 1941)

2.

C. System status management, developed by EMS system designer Jack Stout, is a computerized personnel and ambulance deployment strategy designed to meet service demands with fewer resources and to ensure appropriate response time and vehicle location. (PCPP 5–322 EPC 1943)

3.

A. New York State studied emergency ambulance collisions that occurred from 1974 to 1996. The data collected demonstrated that the majority of collisions occurred on clear days, during daylight hours, and on dry roads while the vehicle was "blowing through" an intersection. (PCPP 5–324 EPC 1944)

4.

C. Inexperienced drivers tend to increase their driving speed by 10–15 mph when they hear an approaching siren. When you use lights and siren, you are held to a higher standard than the normal driver. Use extreme caution when you drive "code red." (PCPP 5–327 EPC 1947)

5.

B. In general, it is not good practice to use a police escort when responding to an emergency scene for a number of reasons. The two vehicles have different acceleration speeds and braking distances, and other motorists become confused because they expect only one responding vehicle coming through an intersection. Use this responding technique sparingly. (PCPP 5–328 EPC 1947)

6.

D. If you arrive first on the scene, you should park your ambulance 50 feet (100 feet if you suspect impending fire or explosion) in front of the crash scene to warn approaching motorists. (PCPP 5–328 EPC 1948)

7.

C. Normally, fixed-wing aircraft (airplanes) are used to transport patients distances over 100 miles. These types of transports are common in remote areas of Canada and Alaska. (PCPP 5–331 EPC 1949)

8.

B. In Korea, helicopters rescued downed soldiers at the front and evacuated them to aid stations. If you answered "D" (Gulf War), you are not old enough to be a paramedic. (PCPP 5–331 EPC 1949)

9.

B. A standard helicopter landing zone is a 100 ft × 100 ft square on flat terrain. Always approach the ship from the front or side in a crouch. Always be mindful of the tail rotor. (PCPP 5–334 EPC 1952)

10.

A. Helicopter transport is challenging and controversial. While there are many advantages to rapid transport, there are also many disadvantages. Most patient care will be done prior to transport due to confining space in the ship; patient care during transport is often affected due to lighting, confined space, personnel, and flight safety; and pressure changes at certain altitudes can affect therapies such as PASG, ET tubes, Foley catheters, and air-splints. Finally, air medical transport is never inexpensive. (PCPP 5–334   EPC 1949)

54 Medical Incident Command

DIRECTIONS Each of the questions or incomplete statements below is followed by suggested answers or completions. Select the **one answer** that is best in each case.

1. National consensus standards for managing mass-casualty incidents were developed by
   A. FEMA
   B. NFPA
   C. OSHA
   D. DOT

2. All of the following are components of an incident management system **EXCEPT**
   A. command
   B. finance/administration
   C. logistics
   D. triage

3. Incident command should be established
   A. when top-ranking officers arrive
   B. when the fire department arrives
   C. when law enforcement arrives
   D. when the first unit arrives

4. Which of the following would be described as a "closed" incident?
   A. Multivehicle collision
   B. Office building fire with people trapped
   C. Train crash with explosion capabilities
   D. Ammonia leak

5. In order to avoid congestion at the scene, it is useful to
   A. stage vehicles at a central location until needed at the scene
   B. request only the number of vehicles you absolutely need
   C. limit responding units to a minimum
   D. have responding units park away from the scene and only send personnel in

6. The incident commander should radio brief progress reports approximately every _____ minutes until the incident has been resolved.

   A. 5
   B. 10
   C. 15
   D. 20

7. An orderly transfer-of-command process includes
   A. face-to-face communication
   B. a radio announcement
   C. a formal briefing
   D. all of the above

Match the following MCI roles with their respective functions:

8. _____ Safety officer
9. _____ Liaison officer
10. _____ Public information officer
11. _____ CISM team
12. _____ Finance/administration
13. _____ Logistics
14. _____ Operations
15. _____ Planning

A. Carries out tactical objectives
B. Provides past, present, and future information about incident
C. Coordinates outside agencies
D. Procures and distributes medical resources
E. Keeps records of incident
F. Monitors for potential hazards
G. Relays information to press
H. Monitors emotional status of responders

16. The sector normally assigned to work in the hazard zone is
    A. triage
    B. treatment
    C. extrication
    D. supply

17. Locating and removing victims from the hazard zone is the responsibility of the _____ sector.
    A. extrication
    B. treatment
    C. triage
    D. transportation

18. Providing a safe area to collect patients once removed from the hazard zone is the responsibility of the _____ sector.
    A. extrication
    B. treatment
    C. triage
    D. staging

19. Establishing an ambulance loading zone is the responsibility of the _____ sector.
    A. staging
    B. treatment
    C. triage
    D. transportation

20. As you encounter walking wounded, you should
    A. move them to the treatment area
    B. ignore them
    C. move them to an area other than the treatment area
    D. transport them immediately

Indicate whether you would categorize the following patients as Immediate or Delayed:

21. _____ 56-year-old male bleeding from a scalp laceration, respirations 26, radial pulse, confused and disoriented.

22. _____ 23-year-old female with abdominal pain, respirations 20, radial pulse, alert and oriented.

23. _____ 25-year-old male with abdominal pain and guarding, respirations 28, no radial pulse, disoriented.

24. _____ 35-year-old female with unstable flail chest, respirations 36, radial pulse, alert.

25. _____ 78-year-old male with fractured humerus, respirations 20, radial pulse, alert.

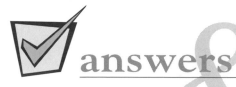

answers & rationales

1.

B. National consensus standards, or widely agreed upon guidelines, for managing a mass-casualty incident were developed by the National Fire Protection Association (NFPA). The national curriculum for implementing the incident management system is taught by the National Fire Academy at Emmitsburg, Maryland. (PCPP 5–343   EPC 1954)

2.

D. C–FLOP is a mnemonic used to describe the components of an incident management system. It stands for **C**ommand—**F**inance, **L**ogistics, **O**perations, **P**lanning. (PCPP 5–343   EPC 1954)

3.

D. The basic principle of the incident command system is that overall incident command responsibilities are fixed on one person. This system further requires that a strong, direct, and visible command mode be established as early as possible during the operation, preferably by the first arriving unit. (PCPP 5–345   EPC 1954)

4.

A. In a "closed" incident, the injuries have already occurred by the time you arrive at the scene. In an "open" incident, such as a fire or hazardous materials leak, the potential for more patients is apparent. (PCPP 5–346   EPC 1956)

5.

A. Staging describes the collecting of vehicles at a central location for distribution as needed at a major incident scene. It is used to avoid scene congestion. Primary staging occurs close to the scene, while secondary staging occurs in another location and acts as a contingency. (PCPP 5–346   EPC 1957)

6.

B. The incident commander should radio brief progress reports approximately every 10 minutes until the incident has been resolved. These reports should restate goals and objectives, tactics, and resources needed to manage the incident. (PCPP 5–347   EPC 1958)

7.

D. An orderly transfer-of-command process includes face-to-face communication with a formal briefing and/or a radio announcement. (PCPP 5–349   EPC 1958)

Matching (PCPP 5–350   EPC 1959)

8. F   Safety officer
9. C   Liaison officer
10. G   Public information officer
11. H   CISM team
12. E   Finance/administration
13. D   Logistics
14. A   Operations
15. B   Planning

A. Carries out tactical objectives
B. Provides past, present, and future information about incident
C. Coordinates outside agencies
D. Procures and distributes medical resources
E. Keeps records of incident
F. Monitors for potential hazards
G. Relays information to press
H. Monitors emotional status of responders

16.

C. The first sector usually established by the incident commander is the extrication sector. The extrication sector operates within the hazard zone. (PCPP 5–360 EPC 1968)

17.

A. Locating and removing victims from the hazard zone is a responsibility of the extrication sector. This sector is usually the responsibility of the fire department. (PCPP 5–360 EPC 1968)

18.

B. Providing a safe area to collect patients once removed from the hazard zone is the responsibility of the treatment sector. (PCPP 5–358 EPC 1966)

19.

D. Establishing an ambulance loading zone is the responsibility of the transportation sector. (PCPP 5–359 EPC 1967)

20.

C. The first on-scene rescuers clear the site of any walking wounded by verbally telling them to walk to a designated location. This location should be different from the treatment area and staffed with personnel to process them appropriately. (PCPP 5–354 EPC 1963)

Triage Exercise (PCPP 5–354 EPC 1963)

21.

This patient's confusion and decreased mental status make him Immediate.

22.

This patient has no major respiratory, circulatory, or neurological deficits and is Delayed.

23.

This patient's absence of radial pulse and decreased mental status make him Immediate.

24.

This patient's respiratory rate of 36 makes her Immediate.

25.

This patient has no major respiratory, circulatory, or neurological deficits and is Delayed.

55 Rescue Awareness and Operations

DIRECTIONS Each of the questions or incomplete statements below is followed by suggested answers or completions. Select the **one answer** that is best in each case.

1. The highest priority in any rescue situation is
   A. patient care
   B. rescuer safety
   C. time management
   D. extrication

2. The paramedic's responsibilities in a rescue operation include
   A. assessing the patient as soon as possible
   B. maintaining patient care throughout disentanglement
   C. accompanying the patient during removal and transport
   D. all of the above

3. The decision whether to attempt or not to attempt a dangerous rescue should be made by the
   A. rescue captain
   B. fire chief
   C. safety officer
   D. paramedic in charge

4. Which of the following is included in the screening criteria for rescue personnel?
   A. Psychological testing
   B. Physical capabilities
   C. Phobia testing
   D. All of the above

5. Which of the following foods are recommended for extended rescue operations?
   A. Complex carbohydrates and water
   B. Cookies and milk
   C. Coffee and doughnuts
   D. Soda and pretzels

6. Which of the following is included in the rescue assessment?
   A. Nature of the situation

B. Number of victims
C. Scene hazards
D. All of the above

7. Which of the following may be helpful during a rescue operation?
   A. Search dogs
   B. Electronic detection devices
   C. Experienced search managers
   D. All of the above

8. Guidelines for managing patients with prolonged exposure to the elements are published by the
   A. Wilderness Medical Society
   B. Wilderness EMT Course
   C. National Association for Search and Rescue
   D. all of the above

9. Which of the following would be helpful in providing psychological support for a victim?
   A. Avoid using his name
   B. Do not introduce yourself
   C. Explain all delays in the rescue operation
   D. Never describe the technical aspects of the operation

10. Water causes heat loss _____ times faster than air.
    A. 10
    B. 15
    C. 20
    D. 25

11. The HELP system was designed to
    A. activate the dive team
    B. eliminate the need for a personal floatation device

C. reduce the likelihood of laryngospasm

D. reduce body heat loss

12. The water rescue model is
    A. Throw—Reach—Go—Row
    B. Reach—Throw—Row—Go
    C. Row—Go—Reach—Throw
    D. Go—Throw—Row—Reach

13. If you find yourself in swift-moving water, you should
    A. try to stand up
    B. stay to the outside of a curve
    C. look for eddies
    D. float on your back, head first

14. The mammalian diving reflex is a protective mechanism designed to reduce body heat loss. Its effects include
    A. tachycardia and vasoconstriction
    B. bradycardia and vasodilation
    C. tachycardia and vasodilation
    D. bradycardia and vasoconstriction

15. According to NIOSH, the majority of confined-space fatalities are due to
    A. alcohol intoxication
    B. recreational activities
    C. rescue attempts
    D. secondary collapse

16. The largest single hazard associated with EMS highway operations is

A. explosion

B. traffic flow

C. power lines

D. sharp objects

17. The safest way to extinguish a road flare is to
    A. let it burn out
    B. pick it up and snuff it out with a gloved hand
    C. douse it with a fire hose
    D. pick it up and rub it onto the ground

18. Windshields are made of
    A. tempered glass
    B. reinforced glass
    C. plexi glass
    D. safety glass

19. Low-angle rescues can be safely attempted when the slope is less than _____ degrees.
    A. 10
    B. 20
    C. 30
    D. 40

20. A helicopter extrication technique in which a person is attached to a rope that is attached to a helicopter is known as a
    A. short haul
    B. leapfrog
    C. tip line
    D. scrambling line

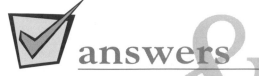

answers & rationales

1.

B. Your own personal safety is your first and major concern in any rescue situation. (PCPP 5–372 EPC 1973)

2.

D. In a rescue situation, the paramedic has three major responsibilities: initiating patient assessment and care as soon as possible, maintaining patient care procedures throughout disentanglement, and accompanying the patient during removal and transport. (PCPP 5–372   EPC 1973)

3.

C. The safety officer is the person with the knowledge and authority to intervene in an unsafe rescue situation. This person should make all go/no-go decisions for every rescue operation. (PCPP 5–376 EPC 1976)

4.

D. Search-and-rescue teams often use personnel screening to determine who may participate in a rescue process. Programs are available that identify physical capabilities of crew members. In addition, psychological testing and phobia screening may be desirable. (PCPP 5–376   EPC 1976)

5.

A. Predetermined policies regarding food and hydration are an important part of the rescue preplan. To maintain maximum personnel performance, rescuers should eat frequently but in small amounts. The diet should be high in complex carbohydrates and low in sugars and fats. Liquid replacement should consist of plain water or relatively dilute electrolyte solutions. (PCPP 5–377   EPC 1977)

6.

D. The rescue assessment begins with the dispatcher's call and your subsequent arrival at the scene. It is necessary to evaluate the nature of the situation, any on-scene hazards, specific patient location, and number of victims involved. (PCPP 5–378 EPC 1977)

7.

D. On rare occasions, you will come across rescue situations that hide patients. If possible, ask your dispatcher to send an on-scene specialist to meet the crew. Search dogs, electronic detection devices, or experienced search managers may also be required. (PCPP 5–378   EPC 1977)

8.

D. Position papers of the Wilderness Medical Society and the Wilderness EMT Course, sponsored by the National Association for Search and Rescue, can serve as guidelines for protocols that anticipate prolonged patient care situations. (PCPP 5–407 EPC 1999)

9.

C. In order to provide more in-depth psychological support for rescue patients in a prolonged extrication operation, you should do the following:

- Learn and use the patient's name.
- Be sure the patient knows your name and that you will not abandon him or her.
- Be sure that other team members know and use the patient's correct name.
- Avoid negative comments regarding the operation or the patient's condition within earshot of the patient.
- Explain all delays to the patient and reassure him or her if problems arise.
- Ask special rescue teams to explain technical aspects of the operation that could directly impact the patient's condition. Translate these operations into clear, simple terms for the patient. (PCPP 5–382   EPC 1979)

10.

D. Water causes heat loss 25 times faster than air. A person submerged in water just above freezing will survive only 15–20 minutes. (PCPP 5–385 EPC 1982)

11.

D. The heat escape lessening position (HELP) system was designed for persons submerged in cold water. To reduce body heat loss, place the body in a fetal tuck with the head above water and floating until help arrives. (PCPP 5–385 EPC 1982)

12.

B. The water rescue model is Reach (with a pole or long rescue device), Throw (a floatation device), Row (a rescue boat if available), and Go (into the water). (PCPP 5–386 EPC 1982)

13.

C. If you find yourself in swift-running water, you should float on your back and travel feet-first, steering with your feet. Try and steer toward the shore or toward an eddy, which can sweep you toward shore. Never attempt to stand up. (PCPP 5–388 EPC 1985)

14.

D. The mammalian diving reflex occurs when the face of a mammal is plunged into water less than 68°F. The heart rate decreases, the blood pressure drops, and the blood vessels constrict—all to preserve body heat. (PCPP 5–390 EPC 1986)

15.

C. According to NIOSH, nearly 60% of confined-space fatalities are people attempting to rescue a victim. Make sure your enthusiasm for rescuing your patient does not place you and your crew in harm's way. (PCPP 5–392 EPC 1987)

16.

B. The largest single hazard associated with EMS operations on a highway is traffic flow. Work closely with law enforcement to ensure a safe working environment for you and your crew. (PCPP 5–397 EPC 1990)

17.

A. Let a road flare burn out by itself. Any other method of trying to extinguish it is an unsafe practice that could cause you or a crew member harm. (PCPP 5–397 EPC 1991)

18.

D. Windshields are made from three layers of fused materials: glass/plasticlaminate/glass. This is known as safety glass. It is designed to stay intact when shattered or broken. The side and rear windows are made from tempered glass, which crumbles into small beads when broken. (PCPP 5–400 EPC 1993)

19.

D. Low-angle rescues can be safely attempted when the slope is less than 40° unless the surface is extremely smooth. Then a high-angle rescue team should be called. (PCPP 5–404 EPC 1996)

20.

A. Short hauling is a helicopter extrication technique in which a person is attached to a rope that is attached to a helicopter. The aircraft lifts off with the person attached to it. This means of extrication requires highly specialized skills. (PCPP 5–407 EPC 1998)

56 Hazardous Materials Incidents

DIRECTIONS
Each of the questions or incomplete statements below is followed by suggested answers or completions. Select the **one answer** that is best in each case.

1. Which of the following is NOT traditionally a responsibility of a paramedic on the scene of a hazardous materials incident?
   A. Scene size-up
   B. Containment and control
   C. Assessment of the toxicological risk
   D. Activation of the incident management system

2. All of the following agencies have published standards or regulations for dealing with hazardous materials incidents EXCEPT
   A. OSHA
   B. EPA
   C. NFPA
   D. NAEMT

3. The absence of a warning placard on a vehicle rules out the possibility of a hazardous material onboard.
   A. True
   B. False

Match the following symbols to their respective hazard types:

4. ____ Flame
5. ____ Ball on fire
6. ____ Propeller
7. ____ Skull and crossbones

   A. Poison
   B. Flammable
   C. Oxidizer
   D. Radioactive

8. Which of the following is an on-scene source of information for EMS personnel during a haz-mat incident?
   A. CHEMTREC
   B. CAMEO
   C. Poison control center
   D. North American Emergency Response Guidebook
   E. CHEMTEL
   F. All of the above

9. The type of radiation that requires lead shielding for your protection is
   A. alpha
   B. beta
   C. delta
   D. gamma

10. You have just come in contact with a person who inhaled a poisonous gas. What are your risks of secondary contamination from the victim through normal caregiver/patient contact?
   A. Low risk
   B. Medium risk
   C. High risk

11. Which of the following treatments is NOT recommended following a hazardous materials exposure?
   A. Tetracaine for eye irritation
   B. Tincture of green soap for skin decontamination
   C. Atropine for SLUDGE symptoms
   D. Induced vomiting for chemical ingestion
   E. Amyl nitrite for cyanide inhalation
   F. Hyperbaric therapy for CO poisoning
   G. Diazepam for seizures
   H. Furosemide for pulmonary edema

12. Which of the following methods of decontamination is not usually a prehospital activity?
   A. Dilution
   B. Absorption
   C. Neutralization
   D. Isolation

13. The four most common decontamination solvents are

A. water, tincture of green soap, isopropyl alcohol, hypochlorite solution

B. water, isopropyl alcohol, tincture of green soap, vegetable oil

C. water, tincture of green soap, hypochlorite solution, vegetable oil

D. water, isopropyl alcohol, vegetable oil, hypochlorite solution

14. A stretcher decon pool is used to

A. decontaminate ambulance personnel prior to transport

B. select which ambulance transports the next patient

C. neutralize certain contaminated substances

D. protect ambulance personnel during transport

15. Which of the following statements is true regarding hazardous materials incidents?

A. A field decontamination is a true decontamination

B. Never transport a semidecontaminated patient to the hospital

C. If the situation is emergent, use as much protection as possible, even if less than ideal

D. Heat stress is not a concern when wearing type A suits due to ventilation mesh

answers & rationales

1.

B. On the scene of a hazardous materials incident, paramedics traditionally will perform scene size-up, assess the toxicological risks, and activate the incident management system. Containment and control are traditional functions of a haz-mat team. (PCPP 5–416   EPC 2001)

2.

D. Standards or regulations for dealing with hazardous materials incidents have been published by the Occupational Safety and Health Administration (OSHA), the Environmental Protection Agency (EPA), and the National Fire Protection Administration (NFPA). (PCPP 5–416   EPC 2001)

3.

B. Regulations depend on the type of substance and/or the amount of substance in transit. If the vehicle is carrying 1 gallon less than the minimum amount needed to use a placard, a placard is not legally necessary. (PCPP 5–420   EPC 2005)

Matching   (PCPP 5–421   EPC 2005)

4. B	Flame	**A.**	Poison
5. C	Ball on fire	**B.**	Flammable
6. D	Propeller	**C.**	Oxidizer
7. A	Skull and crossbones	**D.**	Radioactive

8.

F. As an emergency responder to a hazardous materials incident, you have a wealth of information at your fingertips. These include CHEMTREC and CHEMTEL (two emergency hotlines), CAMEO (a computerized database and internet website), your regional poison control center, and the North American Emergency Response Guidebook. (PCPP 5–425   EPC 2007)

9.

D. Alpha radiation is stopped by clothing, paper, and intact skin. Beta radiation will penetrate a few millimeters of skin. Gamma rays require lead shielding for protection. (PCPP 5–428   EPC 2010)

10.

A. Gas exposure rarely results in secondary contamination. The substance enters the lungs and is dispersed and absorbed into the bloodstream with little or no external residue. Normal patient contact, along with universal precautions, should afford you solid protection and minimal risk. (PCPP 5–429   EPC 2011)

11.

D. Never induce vomiting in anyone who has ingested a corrosive chemical. Strong acids and alkalis will cause severe damage to the esophagus and oral mucosa if reintroduced during vomiting. (PCPP 5–431   EPC 2012)

12.

C. Dilution (applying large amounts of water), absorption (blotting up the material from the skin), and isolation (separating the victim from the substance) are all normal prehospital management stragies. Neutralization (adding a substance that reduces or eliminates the toxicity of the substance) is almost never used by EMS personnel. (PCPP 5–434   EPC 2014)

13.

B. Water (the universal decon agent), vegetable oil (for water-reactive substances), isopropyl alcohol (for some isocyanates), and tincture of green soap (used with the universal decon agent) can be used as decontamination solvents. (PCPP 5–436   EPC 2016)

14.

D. A decon pool is used in the back of the ambulance to protect the crew from secondary contamination during transport by isolating potentially contaminated body fluids. (PCPP 5–437   EPC 2017)

15.

C. A field decontamination is not considered a true decontamination. Patients may still have to undergo an invasive decontamination process at the medical facility. However, it is always better to transport a semidecontaminated live patient to the hospital than a perfectly decontaminated corpse. When wearing a type A suit, heat stress is always a concern due to the airtightness of the suit. If the situation is emergent, use as much protection as possible, even if less than ideal. (PCPP 5–439 EPC 2017)

57 Crime Scene Awareness

DIRECTIONS Each of the questions or incomplete statements below is followed by suggested answers or completions. Select the **one answer** that is best in each case.

1. Which of the following is an appropriate way to respond to a potentially violent crime scene?
   A. Always use lights and siren
   B. Follow police units to the scene
   C. Do not approach the scene until secured by police
   D. All of the above

2. When approaching a dark house, how should you hold your flashlight?
   A. Over your head
   B. To the side
   C. In front of you
   D. Behind you

3. Before you have completed assessing your patient, bystanders become unruly and threaten your life. Your stretcher is still in the ambulance. You feel in imminent danger. What is your most appropriate action?
   A. Continue assessing your patient
   B. Hold your ground and radio for immediate assistance
   C. Try and drag your patient down the stairs and into the ambulance
   D. Retreat without your patient and call for help

4. Which of the following statements is true with regard to approaching a vehicle at a roadside emergency?
   A. Approach from the passenger's side
   B. The driver should remain in the ambulance
   C. Don't walk between the ambulance and the vehicle
   D. All of the above

5. Violent crime most often takes place in
   A. the street
   B. the home

   C. a bar
   D. none of the above

6. You respond to a possible injury at a home in the seedy part of town. Police are on the scene of what they describe as a clandestine drug lab. Possible hazards at a scene such as this include
   A. toxic fumes
   B. booby traps
   C. volatile chemicals
   D. all of the above

7. The contact-and-cover technique is used to
   A. interview a victim on the street
   B. escape from immediate danger
   C. signal incoming agencies of potential danger
   D. retreat and return to the scene

8. Which of the following weapons will penetrate the typical body armor?
   A. Ice pick
   B. High-velocity rifle
   C. Dual-edged knife
   D. All of the above

9. Crime scene evidence containing body fluids is best preserved in a/n
   A. plastic bag
   B. brown paper bag
   C. ice chest
   D. sterile, airtight container

10. Which of the following is an acceptable way for a paramedic to avoid contaminating crime scene evidence?
    A. Move a gun by placing a pen into the barrel
    B. Place bloody clothes into one pile
    C. Use gloves
    D. All of the above

answers & rationales

1.

C. When responding to a potentially violent crime scene, avoid using lights and siren, and wait for law enforcement to secure the scene. (PCPP 5–445 EPC 2020)

2.

B. When approaching a dark house at night, hold your flashlight to the side rather than in front of you. If someone fires a gun, he or she usually aims at the light. (PCPP 5–446 EPC 2021)

3.

D. You may find yourself in a situation in which you must decide whether you can quickly package your patient and leave the scene or retreat without him. Abandoning your patient is a risky proposition but your safety is more important. Get out! (PCPP 5–448 EPC 2022)

4.

D. When approaching a vehicle at a roadside emergency, you should approach from the passenger's side and use the one-person approach. The driver should remain in the ambulance. Also, don't walk between the ambulance and the vehicle because then you are backlighted and make an easy target. (PCPP 5–449 EPC 448)

5.

A. According to statistics from the U.S. Department of Justice, most violent crime occurs on the streets, often within 5 miles of the victim's home. (PCPP 5–449 EPC 2024)

6.

D. When entering a "drug lab," always be aware of potential hazards that may have been meant to harm police. These include toxic fumes, volatile chemicals, and booby traps. The job of raiding and securing this type of scene belongs to specialized personnel—not EMS. (PCPP 5–452 EPC 2026)

7.

A. The contact-and-cover technique was developed by the San Diego police department after several officers were killed or injured while interviewing suspects. To use this procedure, one crew member interviews the victim while the other surveys the scene for potential danger. (PCPP 5–455 EPC 2028)

8.

D. Body armor is worn by an increasing number of EMS field personnel. It offers reasonable protection from many handguns, most knives, and blunt trauma. However, high-velocity rifle bullets, dual-edged knives, and even an ice pick can penetrate its fibers. (PCPP 5–456 EPC 2029)

9.

B. Crime scene evidence containing body fluids, such as blood-soaked clothing, should be preserved in a brown paper bag that allows for evaporation and prevents mold from forming. (PCPP 5–459 EPC 2032)

10.

C. To avoid contaminating crime scene evidence, the paramedic should wear gloves at all times and avoid touching anything unnecessarily. (PCPP 5–460 EPC 2032)

Appendix D.O.T. Objectives

UNIT TERMINAL OBJECTIVE

1–1   At the completion of this unit, the paramedic student will understand his or her roles and responsibilities within an EMS system, and how these roles and responsibilities differ from other levels of providers.

COGNITIVE OBJECTIVES

At the completion of this unit, the paramedic student will be able to:

1–1.1   Define the following terms: (C-1)
   a.   EMS systems
   b.   Licensure
   c.   Certification
   d.   Registration
   e.   Profession
   f.   Professionalism
   g.   Health care professional
   h.   Ethics
   i.   Peer review
   j.   Medical direction
   k.   Protocols

1–1.2   Describe key historical events that influenced the development of national Emergency Medical Services (EMS) systems. (C-1)

1–1.3   Identify national groups important to the development, education, and implementation of EMS. (C-1)

1–1.4   Differentiate among the four nationally recognized levels of EMS training/education, leading to licensure/certification/registration. (C-1)

1–1.5   Describe the attributes of a paramedic as a health care professional. (C-1)

1–1.6   Describe the recognized levels of EMS training/education, leading to licensure/certification in his or her state. (C-1)

1–1.7   Explain paramedic licensure/certification, recertification, and reciprocity requirements in his or her state. (C-1)

1–1.8   Evaluate the importance of maintaining one's paramedic license/certification. (C-3)

1–1.9   Describe the benefits of paramedic continuing education. (C-1)

1–1.10   List current state requirements for paramedic education in his/her state. (C-1)

1–1.11   Discuss the role of national associations and of a national registry agency. (C-1)

1–1.12   Discuss current issues in his/her state impacting EMS. (C-1)

1–1.13   Discuss the roles of various EMS standard setting agencies. (C-1)

1–1.14   Identify the standards (components) of an EMS system as defined by the National Highway Traffic Safety Administration. (C-1)

1–1.15   Describe how professionalism applies to the paramedic while on and off duty. (C-1)

1–1.16   Describe examples of professional behaviors in the following areas: integrity, empathy, self-motivation, appearance and personal hygiene, self-confidence, communications, time management, teamwork and diplomacy, respect, patient advocacy, and careful delivery of service. (C-1)

1–1.17   Provide examples of activities that constitute appropriate professional behavior for a paramedic. (C-2)

1–1.18   Describe the importance of quality EMS research to the future of EMS. (C-3)

1–1.19   Identify the benefits of paramedics teaching in their community. (C-1)

1–1.20   Describe what is meant by "citizen involvement in the EMS system." (C-1)

1–1.21   Analyze how the paramedic can benefit the health care system by supporting primary care to patients in the out-of-hospital setting. (C-3)

1–1.22   List the primary and additional responsibilities of paramedics. (C-1)

1–1.23   Describe the role of the EMS physician in providing medical direction. (C-1)

1–1.24   Describe the benefits of medical direction, both on-line and off-line. (C-1)

1–1.25   Describe the process for the development of local policies and protocols. (C-2)

1–1.26   Provide examples of local protocols. (C-1)

1–1.27   Discuss prehospital and out-of-hospital care as an extension of the physician. (C-1)

1–1.28   Describe the relationship between a physician on the scene, the paramedic on the scene, and the EMS physician providing on-line medical direction. (C-1)

1–1.29 Describe the components of continuous quality improvement. (C-1)

1–1.30 Analyze the role of continuous quality improvement with respect to continuing medical education and research. (C-3)

1–1.31 Define the role of the paramedic relative to the safety of the crew, the patient, and bystanders. (C-1)

1–1.32 Identify local health care agencies and transportation resources for patients with special needs. (C-1)

1–1.33 Describe the role of the paramedic in health education activities related to illness and injury prevention. (C-1)

1–1.34 Describe the importance and benefits of research. (C-2)

1–1.35 Explain the EMS provider's role in data collection. (C-1)

1–1.36 Explain the basic principles of research. (C-1)

1–1.37 Describe a process of evaluating and interpreting research. (C-3)

AFFECTIVE OBJECTIVES

At the completion of this unit, the paramedic student will be able to:

1–1.38 Assess personal practices relative to the responsibility for personal safety, the safety of the crew, the patient, and bystanders. (A-3)

1–1.39 Serve as a role model for others relative to professionalism in EMS. (A-3)

1–1.40 Value the need to serve as the patient advocate inclusive of those with special needs, alternate lifestyles, and cultural diversity. (A-3)

1–1.41 Defend the importance of continuing medical education and skills retention. (A-3)

1–1.42 Advocate the need for supporting and participating in research efforts aimed at improving EMS systems. (A-3)

1–1.43 Assess personal attitudes and demeanor that may distract from professionalism. (A-3)

1–1.44 Value the role that family dynamics plays in the total care of patients. (A-3)

1–1.45 Advocate the need for injury prevention, including abusive situations. (A-1)

1–1.46 Exhibit professional behaviors in the following areas: integrity, empathy, self-motivation, appearance and personal hygiene, self-confidence, communications, time management, teamwork and diplomacy, respect, patient advocacy, and careful delivery of service. (A-2)

PSYCHOMOTOR OBJECTIVES

None identified for this unit.

UNIT TERMINAL OBJECTIVE

1–2 At the completion of this unit, the paramedic student will understand and value the importance of personal wellness in EMS and serve as a healthy role model for peers.

COGNITIVE OBJECTIVES

At the completion of this unit, the paramedic student will be able to:

1–2.1 Discuss the concept of wellness and its benefits. (C-1)

1–2.2 Define the components of wellness. (C-1)

1–2.3 Describe the role of the paramedic in promoting wellness. (C-1)

1–2.4 Discuss the components of wellness associated with proper nutrition. (C-1)

1–2.5 List principles of weight control. (C-1)

1–2.6 Discuss how cardiovascular endurance, muscle strength, and flexibility contribute to physical fitness. (C-2)

1–2.7 Describe the impact of shift work on circadian rhythms. (C-1)

1–2.8 Discuss how periodic risk assessments and knowledge of warning signs contribute to cancer and cardiovascular disease prevention. (C-1)

1–2.9 Differentiate proper from improper body mechanics for lifting and moving patients in emergency and non-emergency situations. (C-3)

1–2.10 Describe the problems that a paramedic might encounter in a hostile situation and the techniques used to manage the situation. (C-1)

1–2.11 Given a scenario involving arrival at the scene of a motor vehicle collision, assess the safety of the scene and propose ways to make the scene safer. (C-3)

1–2.12 List factors that contribute to safe vehicle operations. (C-1)

1–2.13 Describe the considerations that should be given to: (C-1)
a. Using escorts
b. Adverse environmental conditions
c. Using lights and siren
d. Proceeding through intersections
e. Parking at an emergency scene

1–2.14 Discuss the concept of "due regard for the safety of all others" while operating an emergency vehicle. (C-1)

1–2.15 Describe the equipment available for self-protection when confronted with a variety of adverse situations. (C-1)

1–2.16 Describe the benefits and methods of smoking cessation. (C-1)

1–2.17 Describe the three phases of the stress response. (C-1)

1–2.18 List factors that trigger the stress response. (C-1)

1–2.19 Differentiate between normal/healthy and detrimental reactions to anxiety and stress. (C-3)

1–2.20 Describe the common physiological and psychological effects of stress. (C-1)

1–2.21 Identify causes of stress in EMS. (C-1)

1–2.22 Describe behavior that is a manifestation of stress in patients and those close to them and how these relate to paramedic stress. (C-1)

1–2.23 Identify and describe the defense mechanisms and management techniques commonly used to deal with stress. (C-1)

1–2.24 Describe the components of critical incident stress management (CISM). (C-1)

1–2.25 Provide examples of situations in which CISM would likely be beneficial to paramedics. (C-1)

1–2.26 Given a scenario involving a stressful situation, formulate a strategy to help cope with the stress. (C-3)

1–2.27 Describe the stages of the grieving process (Kubler-Ross). (C-1)

1–2.28 Describe the needs of the paramedic when dealing with death and dying. (C-1)

1–2.29 Describe the unique challenges for paramedics in dealing with the needs of children and other special populations related to their understanding or experience of death and dying. (C-1)

1–2.30 Discuss the importance of universal precautions and body substance isolation practices. (C-1)

1–2.31 Describe the steps to take for personal protection from airborne and bloodborne pathogens. (C-1)

1–2.32 Given a scenario in which equipment and supplies have been exposed to body substances, plan for the proper cleaning, disinfection, and disposal of the items. (C-3)

1–2.33 Explain what is meant by an exposure and describe principles for management. (C-1)

AFFECTIVE OBJECTIVES

At the completion of this unit, the paramedic student will be able to:

1–2.34 Advocate the benefits of working toward the goal of total personal wellness. (A-2)

1–2.35 Serve as a role model for other EMS providers in regard to a total wellness lifestyle. (A-3)

1–2.36 Value the need to assess his/her own lifestyle. (A-2)

1–2.37 Challenge him/herself to each wellness concept in his/her role as a paramedic. (A-3)

1–2.38 Defend the need to treat each patient as an individual, with respect and dignity. (A-2)

1–2.39 Assess his/her own prejudices related to the various aspects of cultural diversity. (A-3)

1–2.40 Improve personal physical well-being through achieving and maintaining proper body weight, regular exercise, and proper nutrition. (A-3)

1–2.41 Promote and practice stress management techniques. (A-3)

1–2.42 Defend the need to respect the emotional needs of dying patients and their families. (A-3)

1–2.43 Advocate and practice the use of personal safety precautions in all scene situations. (A-3)

1–2.44 Advocate and serve as a role model for other EMS providers relative to body substance isolation practices. (A-3)

PSYCHOMOTOR OBJECTIVES

At the completion of this unit, the paramedic student will be able to:

1–2.45 Demonstrate safe methods for lifting and moving patients in emergency and non-emergency situations. (P-2)

1–2.46 Demonstrate the proper procedures to take for personal protection from disease. (P-2)

UNIT TERMINAL OBJECTIVE

1–3 At the completion of this unit, the paramedic student will be able to integrate the implementation of primary injury prevention activities as an effective way to reduce death, disabilities, and health care costs.

COGNITIVE OBJECTIVES

At the completion of this unit, the paramedic student will be able to:

1.3–1 Describe the incidence, morbidity, and mortality of unintentional and alleged unintentional events. (C-1)

1.3–2 Identify the human, environmental, and socioeconomic impact of unintentional and alleged unintentional events. (C-1)

1.3–3 Identify health hazards and potential crime areas within the community. (C-1)

1.3–4 Identify local municipal and community resources available for physical, socioeconomic crises. (C-1)

1.3–5 List the general and specific environmental parameters that should be inspected to assess a patient's need for preventative information and direction. (C-1)

1.3–6 Identify the role of EMS in local municipal and community prevention programs. (C-1)

1.3–7 Identify the local prevention programs that promote safety for all age populations. (C-2)

1.3–8 Identify patient situations where the paramedic can intervene in a preventative manner. (C-1)

1.3–9 Document primary and secondary injury prevention data. (C-1)

AFFECTIVE OBJECTIVES

At the completion of this unit, the paramedic student will be able to:

1.3–10 Value and defend tenets of prevention in terms of personal safety and wellness. (A-3)

1.3–11 Value and defend tenets of prevention for patients and communities being served. (A-3)

1.3–12 Value the contribution of effective documentation as one justification for funding of prevention programs. (A-3)

1.3–13 Value personal commitment to success of prevention programs. (A-3)

PSYCHOMOTOR OBJECTIVES

At the completion of this unit, the paramedic student will be able to:

1.3–14 Demonstrate the use of protective equipment appropriate to the environment and scene. (P-3)

UNIT TERMINAL OBJECTIVE

1–4 At the completion of this unit, the paramedic student will understand the legal issues that impact decisions made in the out-of-hospital environment.

COGNITIVE OBJECTIVES

At the completion of this unit, the paramedic student will be able to:

1–4.1 Differentiate between legal and ethical responsibilities. (C-2)

1–4.2 Describe the basic structure of the legal system in the United States. (C-1)

1–4.3 Differentiate between civil and criminal law as it pertains to the paramedic. (C-1)

1–4.4 Identify and explain the importance of laws pertinent to the paramedic. (C-1)

1–4.5 Differentiate between licensure and certification as they apply to the paramedic. (C-1)

1–4.6 List the specific problems or conditions encountered while providing care that a paramedic is required to report, and identify in each instance to whom the report is to be made. (C-1)

1–4.7 Define the following terms: (C-1)
a. Abandonment
b. Advance directives
c. Assault
d. Battery
e. Breach of duty
f. Confidentiality

g. Consent (expressed, implied, informed, involuntary)
h. Do not resuscitate (DNR) orders
i. Duty to act
j. Emancipated minor
k. False imprisonment
l. Immunity
m. Liability
n. Libel
o. Minor
p. Negligence
q. Proximate cause
r. Scope of practice
s. Slander
t. Standard of care
u. Tort

1–4.8   Differentiate between the scope of practice and the standard of care for paramedic practice. (C-3)

1–4.9   Discuss the concept of medical direction, including off-line medical direction and on-line medical direction, and its relationship to the standard of care of a paramedic. (C-1)

1–4.10   Describe the four elements that must be present in order to prove negligence. (C-1)

1–4.11   Given a scenario in which a patient is injured while a paramedic is providing care, determine whether the four components of negligence are present. (C-2)

1–4.12   Given a scenario, demonstrate patient care behaviors that would protect the paramedic from claims of negligence. (C-3)

1–4.13   Explain the concept of liability as it might apply to paramedic practice, including physicians providing medical direction and paramedic supervision of other care providers. (C-2)

1–4.14   Discuss the legal concept of immunity, including Good Samaritan statutes and governmental immunity, as it applies to the paramedic. (C-1)

1–4.15   Explain the importance and necessity of patient confidentiality and the standards for maintaining patient confidentiality that apply to the paramedic. (C-1)

1–4.16   Differentiate among expressed, informed, implied, and involuntary consent. (C-2)

1–4.17   Given a scenario in which a paramedic is presented with a conscious patient in need of care, describe the process used to obtain consent. (C-2)

1–4.18   Identify the steps to take if a patient refuses care. (C-1)

1–4.19   Given a scenario, demonstrate appropriate patient management and care techniques in a refusal of care situation. (C-3)

1–4.20   Describe what constitutes abandonment. (C-1)

1–4.21   Identify the legal issues involved in the decision not to transport a patient, or to reduce the level of care being provided during transportation. (C-1)

1–4.22   Describe how hospitals are selected to receive patients based on patient need and hospital capability and the role of the paramedic in such selection. (C-1)

1–4.23   Differentiate between assault and battery and describe how to avoid each. (C-2)

1–4.24   Describe the conditions under which the use of force, including restraint, is acceptable. (C-1)

1–4.25   Explain the purpose of advance directives relative to patient care and how the paramedic should care for a patient who is covered by an advance directive. (C-1)

1–4.26   Discuss the responsibilities of the paramedic relative to resuscitation efforts for patients who are potential organ donors. (C-1)

1–4.27   Describe the actions that the paramedic should take to preserve evidence at a crime or accident scene. (C-1)

1–4.28   Describe the importance of providing accurate documentation (oral and written) in substantiating an incident. (C-1)

1–4.29   Describe the characteristics of a patient care report required to make it an effective legal document. (C-1)

1–4.30   Given a scenario, prepare a patient care report, including an appropriately detailed narrative. (C-2)

AFFECTIVE OBJECTIVES

At the completion of this unit, the paramedic student will be able to:

1–4.31   Advocate the need to show respect for the rights and feelings of patients. (A-3)

1–4.32   Assess his/her personal commitment to protecting patient confidentiality. (A-3)

1–4.33   Given a scenario involving a new employee, explain the importance of obtaining consent for adults and minors. (A-2)

1–4.34   Defend personal beliefs about withholding or stopping patient care. (A-3)

1–4.35   Defend the value of advance medical directives. (A-3)

PSYCHOMOTOR OBJECTIVES

None identified for this unit.

UNIT TERMINAL OBJECTIVE

1–5   At the completion of this unit, the paramedic student will understand the role that ethics plays in decision making in the out-of-hospital environment.

COGNITIVE OBJECTIVES

At the completion of this unit, the paramedic student will be able to:

1–5.1   Define ethics. (C-1)

1–5.2   Distinguish between ethical and moral decisions. (C-3)

1–5.3   Identify the premise that should underlie the paramedic's ethical decisions in out-of hospital care. (C-1)

1–5.4   Analyze the relationship between the law and ethics in EMS. (C-3)

1–5.5   Compare and contrast the criteria that may be used in allocating scarce EMS resources. (C-3)

1–5.6   Identify the issues surrounding the use of advance directives, in making a prehospital resuscitation decision. (C-1)

1–5.7   Describe the criteria necessary to honor an advance directive in your state. (C-1)

AFFECTIVE OBJECTIVES

At the completion of this unit, the paramedic student will be able to:

1–5.8   Value the patient's autonomy in the decision-making process. (A-2)

1–5.9   Defend the following ethical positions: (A-3)
a. The paramedic is accountable to the patient.
b. The paramedic is accountable to the medical director.
c. The paramedic is accountable to the EMS system.

    d. The paramedic is accountable for fulfilling the standard of care.

1–5.10 Given a scenario, defend or challenge a paramedic's actions concerning a patient who is treated against his/her wishes. (A-3)

1–5.11 Given a scenario, defend a paramedic's actions in a situation where a physician orders therapy the paramedic feels to be detrimental to the patient's best interests. (A-3)

PSYCHOMOTOR OBJECTIVES

None identified for this unit.

UNIT TERMINAL OBJECTIVE

1–6 At the completion of this unit, the paramedic student will be able to apply the general concepts of pathophysiology for the assessment and management of emergency patients.

COGNITIVE OBJECTIVES

At the completion of this unit, the paramedic student will be able to:

1–6.1 Discuss cellular adaptation. (C-1)

1–6.2 Describe cellular injury and cellular death. (C-1)

1–6.3 Describe the factors that precipitate disease in the human body. (C-1)

1–6.4 Describe the cellular environment. (C-1)

1–6.5 Discuss analyzing disease risk. (C-1)

1–6.6 Describe environmental risk factors. (C-1)

1–6.7 Discuss combined effects and interaction among risk factors. (C-1)

1–6.8 Describe aging as a risk factor for disease. (C-1)

1–6.9 Discuss familial diseases and associated risk factors. (C-1)

1–6.10 Discuss hypoperfusion. (C-1)

1–6.11 Define cardiogenic, hypovolemic, neurogenic, anaphylactic, and septic shock. (C-1)

1–6.12 Describe multiple organ dysfunction syndrome. (C-1)

1–6.13 Define the characteristics of the immune response. (C-1)

1–6.14 Discuss induction of the immune system. (C-1)

1–6.15 Discuss fetal and neonatal immune function. (C-1)

1–6.16 Discuss aging and the immune function in the elderly. (C-1)

1–6.17 Describe the inflammation response. (C-1)

1–6.18 Discuss the role of mast cells as part of the inflammation response. (C-1)

1–6.19 Describe the plasma protein system. (C-1)

1–6.20 Discuss the cellular components of inflammation. (C-1)

1–6.21 Describe the systemic manifestations of the inflammation response. (C-1)

1–6.22 Describe the resolution and repair from inflammation. (C-1)

1–6.23 Discuss the effect of aging on the mechanisms of self-defense. (C-1)

1–6.24 Discuss hypersensitivity. (C-1)

1–6.25 Describe deficiencies in immunity and inflammation. (C-1)

1–6.26 Describe homeostasis as a dynamic steady state. (C-1)

1–6.27 List types of tissue. (C-1)

1–6.28 Describe the systemic manifestations that result from cellular injury. (C-1)

1–6.29 Describe neuroendocrine regulation. (C-1)

1–6.30 Discuss the interrelationships between stress, coping, and illness. (C-1)

AFFECTIVE OBJECTIVES

At the completion of this unit, the paramedic student will be able to:

1–6.31 Advocate the need to understand and apply the knowledge of pathophysiology to patient assessment and treatment. (A-2)

PSYCHOMOTOR OBJECTIVES

None identified for this unit.

UNIT TERMINAL OBJECTIVE

1–7 At the completion of this unit, the paramedic student will be able to integrate pathophysiological principles of pharmacology and the assessment findings to formulate a field impression and implement a pharmacologic management plan.

COGNITIVE OBJECTIVES

At the completion of this unit, the paramedic student will be able to:

1–7.1 Describe historical trends in pharmacology. (C-1)

1–7.2 Differentiate among the chemical, generic (nonproprietary), and trade (proprietary) names of a drug. (C-3)

1–7.3 List the four main sources of drug products. (C-1)

1–7.4 Describe how drugs are classified. (C-1)

1–7.5 List the authoritative sources for drug information. (C-1)

1–7.6 List legislative acts controlling drug use and abuse in the United States. (C-1)

1–7.7 Differentiate among Schedule I, II, III, IV, and V substances. (C-3)

1–7.8 List examples of substances in each schedule. (C-1)

1–7.9 Discuss standardization of drugs. (C-1)

1–7.10 Discuss investigational drugs, including the Food and Drug Administration (FDA) approval process and the FDA classifications for newly approved drugs. (C-1)

1–7.11 Discuss special consideration in drug treatment with regard to pregnant, pediatric, and geriatric patients. (C-1)

1–7.12 Discuss the paramedic's responsibilities and scope of management pertinent to the administration of medications. (C-1)

1–7.13 Review the specific anatomy and physiology pertinent to pharmacology with additional attention to autonomic pharmacology. (C-1)

1–7.14 List and describe general properties of drugs. (C-1)

1–7.15 List and describe liquid and solid drug forms. (C-1)

1–7.16 List and differentiate routes of drug administration. (C-3)

1–7.17 Differentiate between enteral and parenteral routes of drug administration. (C-3)

1–7.18 Describe mechanisms of drug action. (C-1)

1–7.19 List and differentiate the phases of drug activity, including the pharmaceutical, pharmacokinetic, and pharmacodynamic phases. (C-3)

1–7.20 Describe the process called pharmacokinetics, pharmcodynamics, including theories of drug action, drug-response relationship, factors altering drug responses, predictable drug responses, Iatrogenic drug responses, and unpredictable adverse drug responses. (C-1)

1–7.21 Differentiate among drug interactions. (C-3)

1–7.22 Discuss considerations for storing and securing medications. (C-1)

1–7.23 List the components of a drug profile by classification. (C-1)

1–7.24 List and describe drugs that the paramedic may administer according to local protocol. (C-1)

1–7.25 Integrate pathophysiological principles of pharmacology with patient assessment. (C-3)

1–7.26 Synthesize patient history information and assessment findings to form a field impression. (C-3)

1–7.27 Synthesize a field impression to implement a pharmacologic management plan. (C-3)

1–7.28 Assess the pathophysiology of a patient's condition by identifying classifications of drugs. (C-3)

AFFECTIVE OBJECTIVES

At the completion of this unit, the paramedic student will be able to:

1–7.29 Serve as a model for obtaining a history by identifying classifications of drugs. (A-3)

1–7.30 Defend the administration of drugs by a paramedic to affect positive therapeutic affect. (A-3)

1–7.31 Advocate drug education through identification of drug classifications. (A-3)

PSYCHOMOTOR OBJECTIVES

None identified for this unit.

UNIT TERMINAL OBJECTIVE

1–8 At the completion of this unit, the paramedic student will be able to safely and precisely access the venous circulation and administer medications.

COGNITIVE OBJECTIVES

At the completion of this unit, the paramedic student will be able to:

1–8.1 Review the specific anatomy and physiology pertinent to medication administration. (C-1)

1–8.2 Review mathematical principles. (C-1)

1–8.3 Review mathematical equivalents. (C-1)

1–8.4 Differentiate temperature readings between the Centigrade and Fahrenheit scales. (C-3)

1–8.5 Discuss formulas as a basis for performing drug calculations. (C-1)

1–8.6 Discuss applying basic principles of mathematics to the calculation of problems associated with medication dosages. (C-1)

1–8.7 Describe how to perform mathematical conversions from the household system to the metric system. (C-1)

1–8.8 Describe the indications, equipment needed, technique used, precautions, and general principles of peripheral venous or external jugular cannulation. (C-1)

1–8.9 Describe the indications, equipment needed, technique used, precautions, and general principles of intraosseous needle placement and infusion. (C-1)

1–8.10 Discuss legal aspects affecting medication administration. (C-1)

1–8.11 Discuss the "six rights" of drug administration and correlate these with the principles of medication administration. (C-1)

1–8.12 Discuss medical asepsis and the differences between clean and sterile techniques. (C-1)

1–8.13 Describe use of antiseptics and disinfectants. (C-1)

1–8.14 Describe the use of universal precautions and body substance isolation (BSI) procedures when administering a medication. (C-1)

1–8.15 Differentiate among the different dosage forms of oral medications. (C-3)

1–8.16 Describe the equipment needed and general principles of administering oral medications. (C-3)

1–8.17 Describe the indications, equipment needed, techniques used, precautions, and general principles of administering medications by the inhalation route. (C-3)

1–8.18 Describe the indications, equipment needed, techniques used, precautions, and general principles of administering medications by the gastric tube. (C-3)

1–8.19 Describe the indications, equipment needed, techniques used, precautions, and general principles of rectal medication administration. (C-3)

1–8.20 Differentiate among the different parenteral routes of medication administration. (C-3)

1–8.21 Describe the equipment needed, techniques used, complications, and general principles for the preparation and administration of parenteral medications. (C-1)

1–8.22 Differentiate among the different percutaneous routes of medication administration. (C-3)

1–8.23 Describe the purpose, equipment needed, techniques used, complications, and general principles for obtaining a blood sample. (C-1)

1–8.24 Describe disposal of contaminated items and sharps. (C-1)

1–8.25 Synthesize a pharmacologic management plan including medication administration. (C-3)

1–8.26 Integrate pathophysiological principles of medication administration with patient management. (C-3)

AFFECTIVE OBJECTIVES

At the completion of this unit, the paramedic student will be able to:

1–8.27 Comply with paramedic standards of medication administration. (A-1)

1–8.28 Comply with universal precautions and body substance isolation (BSI). (A-1)

1–8.29 Defend a pharmacologic management plan for medication administration. (A-3)

1–8.30 Serve as a model for medical asepsis. (A-3)

1–8.31 Serve as a model for advocacy while performing medication administration. (A-3)

1–8.32 Serve as a model for disposing of contaminated items and sharps. (A-3)

PSYCHOMOTOR OBJECTIVES

At the completion of this unit, the paramedic student will be able to:

1–8.33 Use universal precautions and body substance isolation (BSI) procedures during medication administration. (P-2)

1–8.34 Demonstrate cannulation of peripheral or external jugular veins. (P-2)

1–8.35 Demonstrate intraosseous needle placement and infusion. (P-2)

1–8.36 Demonstrate clean technique during medication administration. (P-3)

1–8.37 Demonstrate administration of oral medications. (P-2)

1–8.38 Demonstrate administration of medications by the inhalation route. (P-2)

1–8.39 Demonstrate administration of medications by the gastric tube. (P-2)

1–8.40 Demonstrate rectal administration of medications. (P-2)

1–8.41 Demonstrate preparation and administration of parenteral medications. (P-2)

1–8.42 Demonstrate preparation and techniques for obtaining a blood sample. (P-2)

1–8.43 Perfect disposal of contaminated items and sharps. (P-3)

UNIT TERMINAL OBJECTIVE

1–9 At the completion of this unit, the paramedic student will be able to integrate the principles of therapeutic communication to effectively communicate with any patient while providing care.

COGNITIVE OBJECTIVES

At the completion of this unit, the paramedic student will be able to:

1–9.1 Define communication. (C-1)

1–9.2 Identify internal and external factors that affect a patient/bystander interview conducted by a paramedic. (C-1)

1–9.3 Restate the strategies for developing patient rapport. (C-1)

1–9.4 Provide examples of open-ended and closed or direct questions. (C-1)

1–9.5 Discuss common errors made by paramedics when interviewing patients. (C-1)

1–9.6 Identify the nonverbal skills that are used in patient interviewing. (C-1)

1–9.7 Restate the strategies to obtain information from the patient. (C-1)

1–9.8 Summarize the methods to assess mental status based on interview techniques. (C-1)

1–9.9 Discuss the strategies for interviewing a patient who is unmotivated to talk. (C-1)

1–9.10 Differentiate the strategies a paramedic uses when interviewing a patient who is hostile compared to one who is cooperative. (C-3)

1–9.11 Summarize developmental considerations of various age groups that influence patient interviewing. (C-1)

1–9.12 Restate unique interviewing techniques necessary to employ with patients who have special needs. (C-1)

1–9.13 Discuss interviewing considerations used by paramedics in cross-cultural communications. (C-1)

AFFECTIVE OBJECTIVES

At the completion of this unit, the paramedic student will be able to:

1–9.14 Serve as a model for an effective communication process. (A-3)

1–9.15 Advocate the importance of external factors of communication. (A-2)

1–9.16 Promote proper responses to patient communication. (A-2)

1–9.17 Exhibit professional nonverbal behaviors. (A-2)

1–9.18 Advocate development of proper patient rapport. (A-2)

1–9.19 Value strategies to obtain patient information. (A-2)

1–9.20 Exhibit professional behaviors in communicating with patients in special situations. (A-3)

1–9.21 Exhibit professional behaviors in communicating with patients from different cultures. (A-3)

PSYCHOMOTOR OBJECTIVES

None identified for this unit.

UNIT TERMINAL OBJECTIVE

1–10 At the completion of this unit, the paramedic student will be able to integrate the physiological, psychological, and sociological changes throughout human development with assessment and communication strategies for patients of all ages.

COGNITIVE OBJECTIVES

At the completion of this unit, the paramedic student will be able to:

1–10.1 Compare the physiological and psychosocial characteristics of an infant with those of an early adult. (C-3)

1–10.2 Compare the physiological and psychosocial characteristics of a toddler with those of an early adult. (C-3)

1–10.3 Compare the physiological and psychosocial characteristics of a preschool child with those of an early adult. (C-3)

1–10.4 Compare the physiological and psychosocial characteristics of a school-aged child with those of an early adult. (C-3)

1–10.5 Compare the physiological and psychosocial characteristics of an adolescent with those of an early adult. (C-3)

1–10.6 Summarize the physiological and psychosocial characteristics of an early adult. (C-3)

1–10.7 Compare the physiological and psychosocial characteristics of a middle-aged adult with those of an early adult. (C-3)

1–10.8 Compare the physiological and psychosocial characteristics of a person in late adulthood with those of an early adult. (C-3)

AFFECTIVE OBJECTIVES

At the completion of this unit, the paramedic student will be able:

1–10.9 Value the uniqueness of infant, toddler, preschool, school-aged, adolescent, early adulthood, middle-aged, and late adulthood physiological and psychosocial characteristics. (A-3)

PSYCHOMOTOR OBJECTIVES

None identified for this unit.

UNIT TERMINAL OBJECTIVE

2–1 At the completion of this unit, the paramedic student will be able to establish and/or maintain a patent airway, and oxygenate and ventilate a patient.

COGNITIVE OBJECTIVES

At the completion of this unit, the paramedic student will be able to:

2–1.1 Explain the primary objective of airway maintenance. (C-1)

2–1.2 Identify commonly neglected prehospital skills related to airway. (C-1)

2–1.3 Identify the anatomy of the upper and lower airway. (C-1)

2–1.4 Describe the functions of the upper and lower airway. (C-1)

2–1.5 Explain the differences between adult and pediatric airway anatomy. (C-1)

2–1.6 Define gag reflex. (C-1)

2–1.7 Explain the relationship between pulmonary circulation and respiration. (C-3)

2–1.8 List the concentration of gases that comprise atmospheric air. (C-1)

2–1.9 Describe the measurement of oxygen in the blood. (C-1)

2–1.10 Describe the measurement of carbon dioxide in the blood. (C-1)

2–1.11 Describe peak expiratory flow. (C-1)

2–1.12 List factors that cause decreased oxygen concentrations in the blood. (C-1)

2–1.13 List the factors that increase and decrease carbon dioxide production in the body. (C-1)

2–1.14 Define atelectasis. (C-1)

2–1.15 Define FiO_2. (C-1)

2–1.16 Define and differentiate between hypoxia and hypoxemia. (C-1)

2–1.17 Describe the voluntary and involuntary regulation of respiration. (C-1)

2–1.18 Describe the modified forms of respiration. (C-1)

2–1.19 Define normal respiratory rates and tidal volumes for the adult, child, and infant. (C-1)

2–1.20 List the factors that affect respiratory rate and depth. (C-1)

2–1.21 Explain the risk of infection to EMS providers associated with ventilation. (C-3)

2–1.22 Define pulsus paradoxes. (C-1)

2–1.23 Define and explain the implications of partial airway obstruction with good and poor air exchange. (C-1)

2–1.24 Define complete airway obstruction. (C-1)

2–1.25 Describe causes of upper airway obstruction. (C-1)

2–1.26 Describe causes of respiratory distress. (C-1)

2–1.27 Describe manual airway maneuvers. (C-1)

2–1.28 Describe the Sellick (cricoid pressure) maneuver. (C-1)

2–1.29 Describe complete airway obstruction maneuvers. (C-1)

2–1.30 Explain the purpose for suctioning the upper airway. (C-1)

2–1.31 Identify types of suction equipment. (C-1)

2–1.32 Describe the indications for suctioning the upper airway. (C-3)

2–1.33 Identify types of suction catheters, including hard or rigid catheters and soft catheters. (C-1)

2–1.34 Identify techniques of suctioning the upper airway. (C-1)

2–1.35 Identify special considerations of suctioning the upper airway. (C-1)

2–1.36 Describe the indications, contraindications, advantages, disadvantages, complications, equipment, and technique of tracheobronchial suctioning in the intubated patient. (C-3)

2–1.37 Describe the use of an oral and nasal airway. (C-1)

2–1.38 Identify special considerations of tracheobronchial suctioning in the intubated patient. (C-1)

2–1.39 Define gastric distention. (C-1)

2–1.40 Describe the indications, contraindications, advantages, disadvantages, complications, equipment, and technique for inserting a nasogastric tube and orogastric tube. (C-1)

2–1.41 Identify special considerations of gastric decompression. (C-1)

2–1.42 Describe the indications, contraindications, advantages, disadvantages, complications, and technique for inserting an oropharyngeal and nasopharyngeal airway. (C-1)

2–1.43 Describe the indications, contraindications, advantages, disadvantages, complications, and technique for ventilating a patient by: (C-1)
   a. Mouth-to-mouth
   b. Mouth-to-nose
   c. Mouth-to-mask
   d. One person bag-valve-mask
   e. Two person bag-valve-mask
   f. Three person bag-valve-mask
   g. Flow-restricted, oxygen-powered ventilation device

2–1.44 Explain the advantage of the two person method when ventilating with the bag-valve-mask. (C-1)

2–1.45 Compare the ventilation techniques used for an adult patient to those used for pediatric patients. (C-3)

2–1.46 Describe indications, contraindications, advantages, disadvantages, complications, and technique for ventilating a patient with an automatic transport ventilator (ATV). (C-1)

2–1.47 Explain safety considerations of oxygen storage and delivery. (C-1)

2–1.48 Identify types of oxygen cylinders and pressure regulators (including a high-pressure regulator and a therapy regulator). (C-1)

2–1.49 List the steps for delivering oxygen from a cylinder and regulator. (C-1)

2–1.50 Describe the use, advantages, and disadvantages of an oxygen humidifier. (C-1)

2–1.51 Describe the indications, contraindications, advantages, disadvantages, complications, liter flow range, and concentration of delivered oxygen for supplemental oxygen delivery devices. (C-3)

2–1.52 Define, identify, and describe a tracheostomy, stoma, and tracheostomy tube. (C-1)

2–1.53 Define, identify, and describe a laryngectomy. (C-1)

2–1.54 Define how to ventilate with a patient with a stoma, including mouth-to-stoma and bag-valve-mask-to-stoma ventilation. (C-1)

2–1.55 Describe the special considerations in airway management and ventilation for patients with facial injuries. (C-1)

2–1.56 Describe the special considerations in airway management and ventilation for the pediatric patient. (C-1)

2–1.57 Differentiate endotracheal intubation from other methods of advanced airway management. (C-3)

2–1.58 Describe the indications, contraindications, advantages, disadvantages, and complications of endotracheal intubation. (C-1)

2–1.59 Describe laryngoscopy for the removal of a foreign body airway obstruction. (C-1)

2–1.60 Describe the indications, contraindications, advantages, disadvantages, complications, equipment, and technique for direct laryngoscopy. (C-1)

2–1.61   Describe visual landmarks for direct laryngoscopy. (C-1)
2–1.62   Describe use of cricoid pressure during intubation. (C-1)
2–1.63   Describe the indications, contraindications, advantages, disadvantages, complications, equipment, and technique for digital endotracheal intubation. (C-1)
2–1.64   Describe the indications, contraindications, advantages, disadvantages, complications, equipment, and technique for using a dual lumen airway. (C-3)
2–1.65   Describe the indications, contraindications, advantages, disadvantages, complications, and equipment for rapid sequence intubation with neuromuscular blockade. (C-1)
2–1.66   Identify neuromuscular blocking drugs and other agents used in rapid sequence intubation. (C-1)
2–1.67   Describe the indications, contraindications, advantages, disadvantages, complications, and equipment for sedation during intubation. (C-1)
2–1.68   Identify sedative agents used in airway management. (C-1)
2–1.69   Describe the indications, contraindications, advantages, disadvantages, complications, equipment, and technique for nasotracheal intubation. (C-1)
2–1.70   Describe the indications, contraindications, advantages, disadvantages, and complications for performing an open cricothyrotomy. (C-3)
2–1.71   Describe the equipment and technique for performing an open cricothyrotomy. (C-1)
2–1.72   Describe the indications, contraindications, advantages, disadvantages, complications, equipment, and technique for translaryngeal catheter ventilation (needle cricothyrotomy). (C-3)
2–1.73   Describe methods of assessment for confirming correct placement of an endotracheal tube. (C-1)
2–1.74   Describe methods for securing an endotracheal tube. (C-1)
2–1.75   Describe the indications, contraindications, advantages, disadvantages, complications, equipment, and technique for extubation. (C-1)
2–1.76   Describe methods of endotracheal intubation in the pediatric patient. (C-1)

AFFECTIVE OBJECTIVES

At the completion of this unit, the paramedic student will be able to:
2–1.77   Defend the need to oxygenate and ventilate a patient. (A-1)
2–1.78   Defend the necessity of establishing and/or maintaining patency of a patient's airway. (A-1)
2–1.79   Comply with standard precautions to defend against infectious and communicable diseases. (A-1)

PSYCHOMOTOR OBJECTIVES

At the completion of this unit, the paramedic student will be able to:
2–1.80   Perform body substance isolation (BSI) procedures during basic airway management, advanced airway management, and ventilation. (P-2)
2–1.81   Perform pulse oximetry. (P-2)
2–1.82   Perform end-tidal CO_2 detection. (P-2)
2–1.83   Perform peak expiratory flow testing. (P-2)
2–1.84   Perform manual airway maneuvers, including: (P-2)
   a.   Opening the mouth
   b.   Head-tilt/chin-lift maneuver
   c.   Jaw-thrust without head-tilt maneuver
   d.   Modified jaw-thrust maneuver
2–1.85   Perform manual airway maneuvers for pediatric patients, including: (P-2)
   a.   Opening the mouth
   b.   Head-tilt/chin-lift maneuver
   c.   Jaw-thrust without head-tilt maneuver
   d.   Modified jaw-thrust maneuver
2–1.86   Perform the Sellick maneuver (cricoid pressure). (P-2)
2–1.87   Perform complete airway obstruction maneuvers, including: (P-2)
   a.   Heimlich maneuver
   b.   Finger sweep
   c.   Chest thrusts
   d.   Removal with Magill forceps
2–1.88   Demonstrate suctioning the upper airway by selecting a suction device, catheter, and technique. (P-2)
2–1.89   Perform tracheobronchial suctioning in the intubated patient by selecting a suction device, catheter, and technique. (P-2)
2–1.90   Demonstrate insertion of a nasogastric tube. (P-2)
2–1.91   Demonstrate insertion of an orogastric tube. (P-2)
2–1.92   Perform gastric decompression by selecting a suction device, catheter, and technique. (P-2)
2–1.93   Demonstrate insertion of an oropharyngeal airway. (P-2)
2–1.94   Demonstrate insertion of a nasopharyngeal airway. (P-2)
2–1.95   Demonstrate ventilating a patient by the following techniques: (P-2)
   a.   Mouth-to-mask ventilation
   b.   One person bag-valve-mask
   c.   Two person bag-valve-mask
   d.   Three person bag-valve-mask
   e.   Flow-restricted, oxygen-powered ventilation device
   f.   Automatic transport ventilator
   g.   Mouth-to-stoma
   h.   Bag-valve-mask-to-stoma ventilation
2–1.96   Ventilate a pediatric patient using the one and two person techniques. (P-2)
2–1.97   Perform ventilation with a bag-valve-mask with an in-line small-volume nebulizer. (P-2)
2–1.98   Perform oxygen delivery from a cylinder and regulator with an oxygen delivery device. (P-2)
2–1.99   Perform oxygen delivery with an oxygen humidifier. (P-2)
2–1.100   Deliver supplemental oxygen to a breathing patient using the following devices: nasal cannula, simple face mask, partial rebreather mask, non-rebreather mask, and venturi mask. (P-2)
2–1.101   Perform stoma suctioning. (P-2)
2–1.102   Perform retrieval of foreign bodies from the upper airway. (P-2)
2–1.103   Perform assessment to confirm correct placement of the endotracheal tube. (P-2)
2–1.104   Intubate the trachea by the following methods: (P-2)
   a.   Orotracheal intubation
   b.   Nasotracheal intubation
   c.   Multi-lumen airways
   d.   Digital intubation
   e.   Transillumination
   f.   Open cricothyrotomy
2–1.105   Adequately secure an endotracheal tube. (P-1)

2–1.106 Perform endotracheal intubation in the pediatric patient. (P-2)

2–1.107 Perform transtracheal catheter ventilation (needle crico-thyrotomy). (P-2)

2–1.108 Perform extubation. (P-2)

2–1.109 Perform replacement of a tracheostomy tube through a stoma. (P-2)

UNIT TERMINAL OBJECTIVE

3–1 At the completion of this unit, the paramedic student will be able to use the appropriate techniques to obtain a medical history from a patient.

COGNITIVE OBJECTIVES

At the completion of this unit, the paramedic student will be able to:

3–1.1 Describe the techniques of history taking. (C-1)

3–1.2 Discuss the importance of using open-ended questions. (C-1)

3–1.3 Describe the use of facilitation, reflection, clarification, empathetic responses, confrontation, and interpretation. (C-1)

3–1.4 Differentiate between facilitation, reflection, clarification, sympathetic responses, confrontation, and interpretation. (C-3)

3–1.5 Describe the structure and purpose of a health history. (C-1)

3–1.6 Describe how to obtain a comprehensive health history. (C-1)

3–1.7 List the components of a comprehensive history of an adult patient. (C-1)

AFFECTIVE OBJECTIVES

At the completion of this unit, the paramedic student will be able to:

3–1.8 Demonstrate the importance of empathy when obtaining a health history. (A-1)

3–1.9 Demonstrate the importance of confidentiality when obtaining a health history. (A-1)

PSYCHOMOTOR OBJECTIVES

None identified for this unit.

UNIT TERMINAL OBJECTIVE

3–2 At the completion of this unit, the paramedic student will be able to explain the pathophysiological significance of physical exam findings.

COGNITIVE OBJECTIVES

At the completion of this unit, the paramedic student will be able to:

3–2.1 Define the terms inspection, palpation, percussion, and auscultation. (C-1)

3–2.2 Describe the techniques of inspection, palpation, percussion, and auscultation. (C-1)

3–2.3 Describe the evaluation of mental status. (C-1)

3–2.4 Evaluate the importance of a general survey. (C-3)

3–2.5 Describe the examination of skin, hair, and nails. (C-1)

3–2.6 Differentiate normal and abnormal findings of the assessment of the skin. (C-3)

3–2.7 Distinguish the importance of abnormal findings of the assessment of the skin. (C-3)

3–2.8 Describe the examination of the head and neck. (C-1)

3–2.9 Differentiate normal and abnormal findings of the scalp examination. (C-3)

3–2.10 Describe the normal and abnormal assessment findings of the skull. (C-1)

3–2.11 Describe the assessment of visual acuity. (C-1)

3–2.12 Explain the rationale for the use of an ophthalmoscope. (C-1)

3–2.13 Describe the examination of the eyes. (C-1)

3–2.14 Distinguish between normal and abnormal assessment findings of the eyes. (C-3)

3–2.15 Explain the rationale for the use of an otoscope. (C-1)

3–2.16 Describe the examination of the ears. (C-1)

3–2.17 Differentiate normal and abnormal assessment findings of the ears. (C-3)

3–2.18 Describe the examination of the nose. (C-1)

3–2.19 Differentiate normal and abnormal assessment findings of the nose. (C-3)

3–2.20 Describe the examination of the mouth and pharynx. (C-1)

3–2.21 Differentiate normal and abnormal assessment findings of the mouth and pharynx. (C-3)

3–2.22 Describe the examination of the neck. (C-1)

3–2.23 Differentiate normal and abnormal assessment findings of the neck. (C-3)

3–2.24 Describe the survey of the thorax and respiration. (C-1)

3–2.25 Describe the examination of the posterior chest. (C-1)

3–2.26 Describe percussion of the chest. (C-1)

3–2.27 Differentiate the percussion notes and their characteristics. (C-3)

3–2.28 Differentiate the characteristics of breath sounds. (C-3)

3–2.29 Describe the examination of the anterior chest. (C-1)

3–2.30 Differentiate normal and abnormal assessment findings of the chest examination. (C-3)

3–2.31 Describe special examination techniques related to the assessment of the chest. (C-1)

3–2.32 Describe the examination of the arterial pulse including rate, rhythm, and amplitude. (C-1)

3–2.33 Distinguish normal and abnormal findings of arterial pulse. (C-3)

3–2.34 Describe the assessment of jugular venous pressure and pulsations. (C-1)

3–2.35 Distinguish normal and abnormal examination findings of jugular venous pressure and pulsations. (C-3)

3–2.36 Describe the examination of the heart and blood vessels. (C-1)

3–2.37 Differentiate normal and abnormal assessment findings of the heart and blood vessels. (C-3)

3–2.38 Describe the auscultation of the heart. (C-1)

3–2.39 Differentiate the characteristics of normal and abnormal findings associated with the auscultation of the heart. (C-3)

3–2.40 Describe special examination techniques of the cardiovascular examination. (C-1)

3–2.41 Describe the examination of the abdomen. (C-1)

3–2.42 Differentiate normal and abnormal assessment findings of the abdomen. (C-3)

3–2.43 Describe auscultation of the abdomen. (C-1)

3–2.44 Distinguish normal and abnormal findings of the auscultation of the abdomen. (C-3)

3–2.45 Describe the examination of the female genitalia. (C-1)

3–2.46 Differentiate normal and abnormal assessment findings of the female genitalia. (C-3)

3–2.47 Describe the examination of the male genitalia. (C-1)

3–2.48 Differentiate normal and abnormal findings of the male genitalia. (C-3)

3–2.49 Describe the examination of the anus and rectum. (C-3)

3–2.50 Distinguish between normal and abnormal findings of the anus and rectum. (C-3)

3–2.51 Describe the examination of the peripheral vascular system. (C-1)

3–2.52 Differentiate normal and abnormal findings of the peripheral vascular system. (C-3)

3–2.53 Describe the examination of the musculoskeletal system. (C-1)

3–2.54 Differentiate normal and abnormal findings of the musculoskeletal system. (C-3)

3–2.55 Describe the examination of the nervous system. (C-1)

3–2.56 Differentiate normal and abnormal findings of the nervous system. (C-3)

3–2.57 Describe the assessment of the cranial nerves. (C-1)

3–2.58 Differentiate normal and abnormal findings of the cranial nerves. (C-3)

3–2.59 Describe the general guidelines of recording examination information. (C-1)

3–2.60 Discuss the considerations of examination of an infant or child. (C-1)

AFFECTIVE OBJECTIVES

At the completion of this unit, the paramedic student will be able to:

3–2.61 Demonstrate a caring attitude when performing physical examination skills. (A-3)

3–2.62 Discuss the importance of a professional appearance and demeanor when performing physical examination skills. (A-1)

3–2.63 Appreciate the limitations of conducting a physical exam in the out-of-hospital environment. (A-2)

PSYCHOMOTOR OBJECTIVES

At the completion of this unit, the paramedic student will be able to:

3–2.64 Demonstrate the examination of skin, hair, and nails. (P-2)

3–2.65 Demonstrate the examination of the head and neck. (P-2)

3–2.66 Demonstrate the examination of the eyes. (P-2)

3–2.67 Demonstrate the examination of the ears. (P-2)

3–2.68 Demonstrate the assessment of visual acuity. (P-2)

3–2.69 Demonstrate the examination of the nose. (P-2)

3–2.70 Demonstrate the examination of the mouth and pharynx. (P-2)

3–2.71 Demonstrate the examination of the neck. (P-2)

3–2.72 Demonstrate the examination of the thorax and ventilation. (P-2)

3–2.73 Demonstrate the examination of the posterior chest. (P-2)

3–2.74 Demonstrate auscultation of the chest. (P-2)

3–2.75 Demonstrate percussion of the chest. (P-2)

3–2.76 Demonstrate the examination of the anterior chest. (P-2)

3–2.77 Demonstrate special examination techniques related to the assessment of the chest. (P-2)

3–2.78 Demonstrate the examination of the arterial pulse including location, rate, rhythm, and amplitude. (P-2)

3–2.79 Demonstrate the assessment of jugular venous pressure and pulsations. (P-2)

3–2.80 Demonstrate the examination of the heart and blood vessels. (P-2)

3–2.81 Demonstrate special examination techniques of the cardiovascular examination. (P-2)

3–2.82 Demonstrate the examination of the abdomen. (P-2)

3–2.83 Demonstrate auscultation of the abdomen. (P-2)

3–2.84 Demonstrate the external visual examination of the female genitalia. (P-2)

3–2.85 Demonstrate the examination of the male genitalia. (P-2)

3–2.86 Demonstrate the examination of the peripheral vascular system. (P-2)

3–2.87 Demonstrate the examination of the musculoskeletal system. (P-2)

3–2.88 Demonstrate the examination of the nervous system. (P-2)

UNIT TERMINAL OBJECTIVE

3–3 At the completion of this unit, the paramedic student will be able to integrate the principles of history taking and techniques of physical exam to perform a patient assessment.

COGNITIVE OBJECTIVES

At the completion of this unit, the paramedic student will be able to:

3–3.1 Recognize hazards/potential hazards. (C-1)

3–3.2 Describe common hazards found at the scene of a trauma and a medical patient. (C-1)

3–3.3 Determine hazards found at the scene of a medical or trauma patient. (C-2)

3–3.4 Differentiate safe from unsafe scenes. (C-3)

3–3.5 Describe methods of making an unsafe scene safe. (C-1)

3–3.6 Discuss common mechanisms of injury/nature of illness. (C-1)

3–3.7 Predict patterns of injury based on mechanism of injury. (C-2)

3–3.8 Discuss the reason for identifying the total number of patients at the scene. (C-1)

3–3.9 Organize the management of a scene following size-up. (C-3)

3–3.10 Explain the reasons for identifying the need for additional help or assistance. (C-1)

3–3.11 Summarize the reasons for forming a general impression of the patient. (C-1)

3–3.12 Discuss methods of assessing mental status. (C-1)

3–3.13 Categorize levels of consciousness in the adult, infant, and child. (C-3)

3–3.14 Differentiate between assessing the altered mental status in the adult, child, and infant patient. (C-3)

3–3.15 Discuss methods of assessing the airway in the adult, child, and infant patient. (C-1)

3–3.16 State reasons for management of the cervical spine once the patient has been determined to be a trauma patient. (C-1)

3–3.17 Analyze a scene to determine if spinal precautions are required. (C-3)

3–3.18 Describe methods used for assessing if a patient is breathing. (C-1)

3–3.19 Differentiate between a patient with adequate and inadequate minute ventilation. (C-3)

3–3.20 Distinguish between methods of assessing breathing in the adult, child, and infant patient. (C-3)

3–3.21 Compare the methods of providing airway care to the adult, child, and infant patient. (C-3)

3–3.22 Describe the methods used to locate and assess a pulse. (C-1)

3–3.23 Differentiate between locating and assessing a pulse in an adult, child, and infant patient. (C-3)

3–3.24 Discuss the need for assessing the patient for external bleeding. (C-1)

3–3.25 Describe normal and abnormal findings when assessing skin color. (C-1)

3–3.26 Describe normal and abnormal findings when assessing skin temperature. (C-1)

3–3.27 Describe normal and abnormal findings when assessing skin condition. (C-1)

3–3.28 Explain the reason for prioritizing a patient for care and transport. (C-1)

3–3.29 Identify patients who require expeditious transport. (C-3)

3–3.30 Describe the evaluation of patient's perfusion status based on findings in the initial assessment. (C-1)

3–3.31 Describe orthostatic vital signs and evaluate their usefulness in assessing a patient in shock. (C-1)

3–3.32 Apply the techniques of physical examination to the medical patient. (C-1)

3–3.33 Differentiate between the assessment that is performed for a patient who is unresponsive or has an altered mental status and other medical patients requiring assessment. (C-3)

3–3.34 Discuss the reasons for reconsidering the mechanism of injury. (C-1)

3–3.35 State the reasons for performing a rapid trauma assessment. (C-1)

3–3.36 Recite examples and explain why patients should receive a rapid trauma assessment. (C-1)

3–3.37 Apply the techniques of physical examination to the trauma patient. (C-1)

3–3.38 Describe the areas included in the rapid trauma assessment and discuss what should be evaluated. (C-1)

3–3.39 Differentiate cases when the rapid assessment may be altered in order to provide patient care. (C-3)

3–3.40 Discuss the reason for performing a focused history and physical exam. (C-1)

3–3.41 Describe when and why a detailed physical examination is necessary. (C-1)

3–3.42 Discuss the components of the detailed physical exam in relation to the techniques of examination. (C-1)

3–3.43 State the areas of the body that are evaluated during the detailed physical exam. (C-1)

3–3.44 Explain what additional care should be provided while performing the detailed physical exam. (C-1)

3–3.45 Distinguish between the detailed physical exam that is performed on a trauma patient and that of the medical patient. (C-3)

3–3.46 Differentiate patients requiring a detailed physical exam from those who do not. (C-3)

3–3.47 Discuss the reasons for repeating the initial assessment as part of the ongoing assessment. (C-1)

3–3.48 Describe the components of the ongoing assessment. (C-1)

3–3.49 Describe trending of assessment components. (C-1)

3–3.50 Discuss medical identification devices/systems. (C-1)

AFFECTIVE OBJECTIVES

At the completion of this unit, the paramedic student will be able to:

3–3.51 Explain the rationale for crew members to evaluate scene safety prior to entering. (A-2)

3–3.52 Serve as a model for others explaining how patient situations affect your evaluation of mechanism of injury or illness. (A-3)

3–3.53 Explain the importance of forming a general impression of the patient. (A-1)

3–3.54 Explain the value of performing an initial assessment. (A-2)

3–3.55 Demonstrate a caring attitude when performing an initial assessment. (A-3)

3–3.56 Attend to the feelings that patients with medical conditions might be experiencing. (A-1)

3–3.57 Value the need for maintaining a professional caring attitude when performing a focused history and physical examination. (A-3)

3–3.58 Explain the rationale for the feelings that these patients might be experiencing. (A-3)

3–3.59 Demonstrate a caring attitude when performing a detailed physical examination. (A-3)

3–3.60 Explain the value of performing an on-going assessment. (A-2)

3–3.61 Recognize and respect the feelings that patients might experience during assessment. (A-1)

3–3.62 Explain the value of trending assessment components to other health professionals who assume care of the patient. (A-2)

PSYCHOMOTOR OBJECTIVES

At the completion of this unit, the paramedic student will be able to:

3–3.63 Observe various scenarios and identify potential hazards. (P-1)

3–3.64 Demonstrate the scene-size-up. (P-2)

3–3.65 Demonstrate the techniques for assessing mental status. (P-2)

3–3.66 Demonstrate the techniques for assessing the airway. (P-2)

3–3.67 Demonstrate the techniques for assessing if the patient is breathing. (P-2)

3–3.68 Demonstrate the techniques for assessing if the patient has a pulse. (P-2)

3–3.69 Demonstrate the techniques for assessing the patient for external bleeding. (P-2)

3–3.70 Demonstrate the techniques for assessing the patient's skin color, temperature, and condition. (P-2)

3–3.71 Demonstrate the ability to prioritize patients. (P-2)

3–3.72 Using the techniques of examination, demonstrate the assessment of a medical patient. (P-2)

3–3.73 Demonstrate the patient care skills that should be used to assist with a patient who is responsive with no known history. (P-2)

3–3.74 Demonstrate the patient care skills that should be used to assist with a patient who is unresponsive or has an altered mental status. (P-2)

3–3.75 Perform a rapid medical assessment. (P-2)

3–3.76 Perform a focused history and physical exam of the medical patient. (P-2)

3–3.77 Using the techniques of physical examination, demonstrate the assessment of a trauma patient. (P-2)

3–3.78 Demonstrate the rapid trauma assessment used to assess a patient based on mechanism of injury. (P-2)

3–3.79 Perform a focused history and physical exam on a non-critically injured patient. (P-2)

3–3.80 Perform a focused history and physical exam on a patient with life-threatening injuries. (P-2)

3–3.81 Perform a detailed physical examination. (P-2)

3–3.82 Demonstrate the skills involved in performing the ongoing assessment. (P-2)

UNIT TERMINAL OBJECTIVE

3–4 At the completion of this unit, the paramedic student will be able to apply a process of clinical decision making to use the assessment findings to help form a field impression.

COGNITIVE OBJECTIVES

At the completion of this unit, the paramedic student will be able to:

3–4.1 Compare the factors influencing medical care in the out-of-hospital environment to other medical settings. (C-2)

3–4.2 Differentiate between critical life-threatening, potentially life-threatening, and non-life-threatening patient presentations. (C-3)

3–4.3 Evaluate the benefits and shortfalls of protocols, standing orders, and patient care algorithms. (C-3)

3–4.4 Define the components, stages, and sequences of the critical thinking process for paramedics. (C-1)

3–4.5 Apply the fundamental elements of critical thinking for paramedics. (C-2)

3–4.6 Describe the effects of the "fight or flight" response and the positive and negative effects on a paramedic's decision making. (C-1)

3–4.7 Summarize the "six Rs" of putting it all together: Read the patient, Read the scene, React, Reevaluate, Revise the management plan, Review performance. (C-1)

AFFECTIVE OBJECTIVES

At the completion of this unit, the paramedic student will be able to:

3–4.8 Defend the position that clinical decision making is the cornerstone of effective paramedic practice. (A-3)

3–4.9 Practice facilitating behaviors when thinking under pressure. (A-1)

PSYCHOMOTOR OBJECTIVES

None identified for this unit.

UNIT TERMINAL OBJECTIVE

3–5 At the completion of this unit, the paramedic student will be able to follow an accepted format for dissemination of patient information in verbal form, either in person or over the radio.

COGNITIVE OBJECTIVES

At the completion of this unit, the paramedic student will be able to:

3–5.1 Identify the importance of communications when providing EMS. (C-1)

3–5.2 Identify the role of verbal, written, and electronic communications in the provision of EMS. (C-1)

3–5.3 Describe the phases of communications necessary to complete a typical EMS event. (C-1)

3–5.4 Identify the importance of proper terminology when communicating during an EMS event. (C-1)

3–5.5 Identify the importance of proper verbal communications during an EMS event. (C-1)

3–5.6 List factors that impede effective verbal communications. (C-1)

3–5.7 List factors that enhance verbal communications. (C-1)

3–5.8 Identify the importance of proper written communications during an EMS event. (C-1)

3–5.9 List factors that impede effective written communications. (C-1)

3–5.10 List factors that enhance written communications. (C-1)

3–5.11 Recognize the legal status of written communications related to an EMS event. (C-1)

3–5.12 State the importance of data collection during an EMS event. (C-1)

3–5.13 Identify technology used to collect and exchange patient and/or scene information electronically. (C-1)

3–5.14 Recognize the legal status of patient medical information exchanged electronically. (C-1)

3–5.15 Identify the components of the local EMS communications system and describe their function and use. (C-1)

3–5.16 Identify and differentiate among the following communications systems: (C-3)
   a. Simplex
   b. Multiplex
   c. Duplex
   d. Trunked
   e. Digital communications
   f. Cellular telephone
   g. Facsimile
   h. Computer

3–5.17 Identify the components of the local dispatch communications system and describe their function and use. (C-1)

3–5.18 Describe the functions and responsibilities of the Federal Communications Commission. (C-1)

3–5.19 Describe how an EMS dispatcher functions as an integral part of the EMS team. (C-1)

3–5.20 List appropriate information to be gathered by the Emergency Medical Dispatcher. (C-1)

3–5.21 Identify the role of Emergency Medical Dispatch in a typical EMS event. (C-1)

3–5.22 Identify the importance of pre-arrival instructions in a typical EMS event. (C-1)

3–5.23 Describe the purpose of verbal communication of patient information to the hospital. (C-1)

3–5.24 Describe information that should be included in patient assessment information verbally reported to medical direction. (C-1)

3–5.25 Diagram a basic model of communications. (C-3)

3–5.26 Organize a list of patient assessment information in the correct order for electronic transmission to medical direction according to the format used locally. (C-3)

AFFECTIVE OBJECTIVES

At the completion of this unit, the paramedic student will be able to:

3–5.27 Show appreciation for proper terminology when describing a patient or patient condition. (A-2)

PSYCHOMOTOR OBJECTIVES

At the completion of this unit, the paramedic student will be able to:

3–5.28 Demonstrate the ability to use the local dispatch communications system. (P-1)

3–5.29 Demonstrate the ability to use a radio. (P-1)

3–5.30 Demonstrate the ability to use the biotelemetry equipment used locally. (P-1)

UNIT TERMINAL OBJECTIVE

3–6 At the completion of this unit, the paramedic student will be able to effectively document the essential elements of patient assessment, care, and transport.

COGNITIVE OBJECTIVES

At the completion of this unit, the paramedic student will be able to:

3–6.1 Identify the general principles regarding the importance of EMS documentation and ways in which documents are used. (C-1)

3–6.2 Identify and use medical terminology correctly. (C-1)

3–6.3 Recite appropriate and accurate medical abbreviations and acronyms. (C-1)

3–6.4 Record all pertinent administrative information. (C-1)

3–6.5 Explain the role of documentation in agency reimbursement. (C-1)

3–6.6 Analyze the documentation for accuracy and completeness, including spelling. (C-3)

3–6.7 Identify and eliminate extraneous or nonprofessional information. (C-1)

3–6.8 Describe the differences between subjective and objective elements of documentation. (C-1)

3–6.9 Evaluate a finished document for errors and omissions. (C-3)

3–6.10 Evaluate a finished document for proper use and spelling of abbreviations and acronyms. (C-3)

3–6.11 Evaluate the confidential nature of an EMS report. (C-3)

3–6.12 Describe the potential consequences of illegible, incomplete, or inaccurate documentation. (C-1)

3–6.13 Describe the special considerations concerning patient refusal of transport. (C-3)

3–6.14 Record pertinent information using a consistent narrative format. (C-3)

3–6.15 Explain how to properly record direct patient or bystander comments. (C-1)

3–6.16 Describe the special considerations concerning mass casualty incident documentation. (C-1)

3–6.17 Apply the principles of documentation to computer charting, as access to this technology becomes available. (C-2)

3–6.18 Identify and record the pertinent, reportable clinical data of each patient interaction. (C-1)

3–6.19 Note and record "pertinent negative" clinical findings. (C-1)

3–6.20 Correct errors and omissions, using proper procedures as defined under local protocol. (C-1)

3–6.21 Revise documents, when necessary, using locally-approved procedures. (C-1)

3–6.22 Assume responsibility for self-assessment of all documentation. (C-3)

3–6.23 Demonstrate proper completion of an EMS event record used locally. (C-3)

AFFECTIVE OBJECTIVES

At the completion of this unit, the paramedic student will be able to:

3–6.24 Advocate among peers the relevance and importance of properly completed documentation. (A-3)

3–6.25 Resolve the common negative attitudes toward the task of documentation. (A-3)

PSYCHOMOTOR OBJECTIVES

None identified for this unit.

UNIT TERMINAL OBJECTIVE

4–1 At the completion of this unit, the paramedic student will be able to integrate the principles of kinematics to enhance the patient assessment and predict the likelihood of injuries based on the patient's mechanism of injury.

COGNITIVE OBJECTIVES

At the completion of this unit, the paramedic student will be able to:

4–1.1 List and describe the components of a comprehensive trauma system. (C-1)

4–1.2 Describe the role of and differences between levels of trauma centers. (C-3)

4–1.3 Describe the criteria for transport to a trauma center. (C-1)

4–1.4 Describe the criteria and procedure for air medical transport. (C-1)

4–1.5 Define energy and force as they relate to trauma. (C-1)

4–1.6 Define laws of motion and energy and understand the role that increased speed has in injuries. (C-1)

4–1.7 Describe each type of impact and its effect on unrestrained victims (e.g., "down and under," "up and over," compression, deceleration). (C-1)

4–1.8 Describe the pathophysiology of the head, spine, thorax, and abdomen that result from the above forces. (C-1)

4–1.9 List specific injuries and their causes as related to interior and exterior vehicle damage. (C-1)

4–1.10 Describe the kinematics of penetrating injuries. (C-1)

4–1.11 List the motion and energy considerations of mechanisms other than motor vehicle crashes. (C-1)

4–1.12 Define the role of kinematics as an additional tool for patient assessment. (C-1)

AFFECTIVE OBJECTIVES

None identified for this unit.

PSYCHOMOTOR OBJECTIVES

None identified for this unit.

UNIT TERMINAL OBJECTIVE

4–2 At the completion of this unit, the paramedic student will be able to integrate pathophysiological principles and assessment findings to formulate a field impression and implement the treatment plan for the patient with shock or hemorrhage.

COGNITIVE OBJECTIVES

At the completion of this unit, the paramedic student will be able to:

4–2.1 Describe the epidemiology, including the morbidity/mortality and prevention strategies, for shock and hemorrhage. (C-1)

4–2.2 Discuss the anatomy and physiology of the cardiovascular system. (C-1)

4 2.3 Predict shock and hemorrhage based on mechanism of injury. (C-1)

4–2.4 Discuss the various types and degrees of shock and hemorrhage. (C-1)

4–2.5 Discuss the pathophysiology of hemorrhage and shock. (C-1)

4–2.6 Discuss the assessment findings associated with hemorrhage and shock. (C-1)

4–2.7 Identify the need for intervention and transport of the patient with hemorrhage or shock. (C-1)

4–2.8 Discuss the treatment plan and management of hemorrhage and shock. (C-1)

4–2.9 Discuss the management of external hemorrhage. (C-1)

4–2.10 Differentiate between controlled and uncontrolled hemorrhage. (C-3)

4–2.11 Differentiate between the administration rate and amount of IV fluid in a patient with controlled versus uncontrolled hemorrhage. (C-3)

4–2.12 Relate internal hemorrhage to the pathophysiology of compensated and decompensated hemorrhagic shock. (C-3)

4–2.13 Relate internal hemorrhage to the assessment findings of compensated and decompensated hemorrhagic shock. (C-3)

4–2.14 Discuss the management of internal hemorrhage. (C-1)

4–2.15 Define shock based on aerobic and anaerobic metabolism. (C-1)

4–2.16 Describe the incidence, morbidity, and mortality of shock. (C-1)

4–2.17 Describe the body's physiologic response to changes in perfusion. (C-1)

4–2.18 Describe the effects of decreased perfusion at the capillary level. (C-1)

4–2.19 Discuss the cellular ischemic phase related to hemorrhagic shock. (C-1)

4–2.20 Discuss the capillary stagnation phase related to hemorrhagic shock. (C-1)

4–2.21 Discuss the capillary washout phase related to hemorrhagic shock. (C-1)

4–2.22 Discuss the assessment findings of hemorrhagic shock. (C-1)

4–2.23 Relate pulse pressure changes to perfusion status. (C-3)

4–2.24 Relate orthostatic vital sign changes to perfusion status. (C-3)

4–2.25 Define compensated and decompensated hemorrhagic shock. (C-1)

4–2.26 Discuss the pathophysiological changes associated with compensated shock. (C-1)

4–2.27 Discuss the assessment findings associated with compensated shock. (C-1)

4–2.28 Identify the need for intervention and transport of the patient with compensated shock. (C-1)

4–2.29 Discuss the treatment plan and management of compensated shock. (C-1)

4–2.30 Discuss the pathophysiological changes associated with decompensated shock. (C-1)

4–2.31 Discuss the assessment findings associated with decompensated shock. (C-1)

4–2.32 Identify the need for intervention and transport of the patient with decompensated shock. (C-1)

4–2.33 Discuss the treatment plan and management of the patient with decompensated shock. (C-1)

4–2.34 Differentiate between compensated and decompensated shock. (C-3)

4–2.35 Relate external hemorrhage to the pathophysiology of compensated and decompensated hemorrhagic shock. (C-3)

4–2.36 Relate external hemorrhage to the assessment findings of compensated and decompensated hemorrhagic shock. (C-3)

4–2.37 Differentiate between the normotensive, hypotensive, or profoundly hypotensive patient. (C-3)

4–2.38 Differentiate between the administration of fluid in the normotensive, hypotensive, or profoundly hypotensive patient. (C-3)

4–2.39 Discuss the physiologic changes associated with the pneumatic anti-shock garment (PASG). (C-1)

4–2.40 Discuss the indications and contraindications for the application and inflation of the PASG. (C-1)

4–2.41 Apply epidemiology to develop prevention strategies for hemorrhage and shock. (C-1)

4–2.42 Integrate the pathophysiological principles to the assessment of a patient with hemorrhage or shock. (C-3)

4–2.43 Synthesize assessment findings and patient history information to form a field impression for the patient with hemorrhage or shock. (C-3)

4–2.44 Develop, execute, and evaluate a treatment plan based on the field impression for the hemorrhage or shock patient. (C-3)

AFFECTIVE OBJECTIVES

None identified for this unit.

PSYCHOMOTOR OBJECTIVES

At the completion of this unit, the paramedic student will be able to:

4–2.45 Demonstrate the assessment of a patient with signs and symptoms of hemorrhagic shock. (P-2)

4–2.46 Demonstrate the management of a patient with signs and symptoms of hemorrhagic shock. (P-2)

4–2.47 Demonstrate the assessment of a patient with signs and symptoms of compensated hemorrhagic shock. (P-2)

4–2.48 Demonstrate the management of a patient with signs and symptoms of compensated hemorrhagic shock. (P-2)

4–2.49 Demonstrate the assessment of a patient with signs and symptoms of decompensated hemorrhagic shock. (P-2)

4–2.50 Demonstrate the management of a patient with signs and symptoms of decompensated hemorrhagic shock. (P-2)

4–2.51 Demonstrate the assessment of a patient with signs and symptoms of external hemorrhage. (P-2)

4–2.52 Demonstrate the management of a patient with signs and symptoms of external hemorrhage. (P-2)

4–2.53 Demonstrate the assessment of a patient with signs and symptoms of internal hemorrhage. (P-2)

4–2.54 Demonstrate the management of a patient with signs and symptoms of internal hemorrhage. (P-2)

UNIT TERMINAL OBJECTIVE

4–3 At the completion of this unit, the paramedic student will be able to integrate pathophysiological principles and the assessment findings to formulate a field impression and implement the treatment plan for the patient with soft tissue trauma.

COGNITIVE OBJECTIVES

At the completion of this unit, the paramedic student will be able to:

4–3.1 Describe the incidence, morbidity, and mortality of soft tissue injures. (C-1)

4–3.2 Describe the layers of the skin, specifically: (C-1)
   a. Epidermis and dermis (cutaneous)
   b. Superficial fascia (subcutaneous)
   c. Deep fascia

4–3.3 Identify the major functions of the integumentary system. (C-1)

4–3.4 Identify the skin tension lines of the body. (C-1)

4–3.5 Predict soft tissue injuries based on mechanism of injury. (C-1)

4–3.6 Discuss the pathophysiology of wound healing, including: (C-1)
   a. Hemostasis
   b. Inflammation phase
   c. Epithelialization
   d. Neovascularization
   e. Collagen synthesis

4–3.7 Discuss the pathophysiology of soft tissue injuries. (C-2)

4–3.8 Differentiate between the following types of closed soft tissue injuries: (C-3)
   a. Contusion

   b. Hematoma
   c. Crush injuries

4–3.9 Discuss the assessment findings associated with closed soft tissue injuries. (C-1)

4–3.10 Discuss the management of a patient with closed soft tissue injuries. (C-2)

4–3.11 Discuss the pathophysiology of open soft tissue injuries. (C-2)

4–3.12 Differentiate between the following types of open soft tissue injuries: (C-3)
   a. Abrasions
   b. Lacerations
   c. Major arterial lacerations
   d. Avulsions
   e. Impaled objects
   f. Amputations
   g. Incisions
   h. Crush injuries
   i. Blast injuries
   j. Penetrations/punctures

4–3.13 Discuss the incidence, morbidity, and mortality of blast injuries. (C-1)

4–3.14 Predict blast injuries based on mechanism of injury, including: (C-2)
   a. Primary
   b. Secondary
   c. Tertiary

4–3.15 Discuss types of trauma including: (C-1)
   a. Blunt
   b. Penetrating
   c. Barotrauma
   d. Burns

4–3.16 Discuss the pathophysiology associated with blast injuries. (C-1)

4–3.17 Discuss the effects of an explosion within an enclosed space on a patient. (C-1)

4–3.18 Discuss the assessment findings associated with blast injuries. (C-1)

4–3.19 Identify the need for rapid intervention and transport of the patient with a blast injury. (C-1)

4–3.20 Discuss the management of a patient with a blast injury. (C-1)

4–3.21 Discuss the incidence, morbidity, and mortality of crush injuries. (C-1)

4–3.22 Define the following conditions: (C-1)
   a. Crush injury
   b. Crush syndrome
   c. Compartment syndrome

4–3.23 Discuss the mechanisms of injury in a crush injury. (C-1)

4–3.24 Discuss the effects of reperfusion and rhabdomyolysis on the body. (C-1)

4–3.25 Discuss the assessment findings associated with crush injuries. (C-1)

4–3.26 Identify the need for rapid intervention and transport of the patient with a crush injury. (C-1)

4–3.27 Discuss the management of a patient with a crush injury. (C-1)

4–3.28 Discuss the pathophysiology of hemorrhage associated with soft tissue injuries, including: (C-2)
   a. Capillary

b. Venous

c. Arterial

4–3.29 Discuss the assessment findings associated with open soft tissue injuries. (C-1)

4–3.30 Discuss the assessment of hemorrhage associated with open soft tissue injuries. (C-1)

4–3.31 Differentiate between the various management techniques for hemorrhage control of open soft tissue injuries, including: (C-3)

a. Direct pressure

b. Elevation

c. Pressure dressing

d. Pressure point

e. Tourniquet application

4–3.32 Differentiate between the types of injuries requiring the use of an occlusive versus non-occlusive dressing. (C-3)

4–3.33 Identify the need for rapid assessment, intervention, and appropriate transport for the patient with a soft tissue injury. (C-2)

4–3.34 Discuss the management of the soft tissue injury patient. (C-2)

4–3.35 Define and discuss the following: (C-1)

a. Dressings

1. Sterile

2. Non-sterile

3. Occlusive

4. Non-occlusive

5. Adherent

6. Non-adherent

7. Absorbent

8. Non-absorbent

9. Wet

10. Dry

b. Bandages

1. Absorbent

2. Non-absorbent

3. Adherent

4. Non-adherent

c. Tourniquet

4–3.36 Predict the possible complications of an improperly applied dressing, bandage, or tourniquet. (C-2)

4–3.37 Discuss the assessment of wound healing. (C-1)

4–3.38 Discuss the management of wound healing. (C-1)

4–3.39 Discuss the pathophysiology of wound infection. (C-1)

4–3.40 Discuss the assessment of wound infection. (C-1)

4–3.41 Discuss the management of wound infection. (C-1)

4–3.42 Integrate pathophysiological principles into the assessment of a patient with a soft tissue injury. (C-3)

4–3.43 Formulate treatment priorities for patients with soft tissue injuries in conjunction with: (C-3)

a. Airway/face/neck trauma

b. Thoracic trauma (open/closed)

c. Abdominal trauma

4–3.44 Synthesize assessment findings and patient history information to form a field impression for the patient with soft tissue trauma. (C-3)

4–3.45 Develop, execute, and evaluate a treatment plan based on the field impression for the patient with soft tissue trauma. (C-3)

AFFECTIVE OBJECTIVES

At the completion of this unit, the paramedic student will be able to:

4–3.46 Defend the rationale explaining why immediate life-threats must take priority over wound closure. (A-3)

4–3.47 Defend the management regimens for various soft tissue injuries. (A-3)

4–3.48 Defend why immediate life-threatening conditions take priority over soft tissue management. (A-3)

4–3.49 Value the importance of a thorough assessment for patients with soft tissue injuries. (A-3)

4–3.50 Attend to the feelings that the patient with a soft tissue injury may experience. (A-2)

4–3.51 Appreciate the importance of good follow-up care for patients receiving sutures. (A-2)

4–3.52 Understand the value of the written report for soft tissue injuries, in the continuum of patient care. (A-2)

PSYCHOMOTOR OBJECTIVES

At the completion of this unit, the paramedic student will be able to:

4–3.53 Demonstrate the assessment and management of a patient with signs and symptoms of soft tissue injury, including: (P-2)

a. Contusion

b. Hematoma

c. Crushing

d. Abrasion

e. Laceration

f. Avulsion

g. Amputation

h. Impaled object

i. Penetration/puncture

j. Blast

UNIT TERMINAL OBJECTIVE

4–4 At the completion of this unit, the paramedic student will be able to integrate pathophysiological principles and the assessment findings to formulate a field impression and implement the management plan for the patient with a burn injury.

COGNITIVE OBJECTIVES

At the completion of this unit, the paramedic student will be able to:

4–4.1 Describe the anatomy and physiology pertinent to burn injuries. (C-1)

4–4.2 Describe the epidemiology, including incidence, mortality/morbidity, risk factors, and prevention strategies for the patient with a burn injury. (C-1)

4–4.3 Describe the pathophysiologic complications and systemic complications of a burn injury. (C-1)

4–4.4 Identify and describe types of burn injuries, including a thermal burn, an inhalation burn, a chemical burn, an electrical burn, and a radiation exposure. (C-1)

4–4.5 Identify and describe the depth classifications of burn injuries, including a superficial burn, a partial-thickness burn, a full-thickness burn, and other depth classifications described by local protocol. (C-1)

4–4.6   Identify and describe methods for determining body surface area percentage of a burn injury including the "rules of nines," the "rules of palms," and other methods described by local protocol. (C-1)

4–4.7   Identify and describe the severity of a burn including a minor burn, a moderate burn, a severe burn, and other severity classifications described by local protocol. (C-1)

4–4.8   Differentiate criteria for determining the severity of a burn injury between a pediatric patient and an adult patient. (C-3)

4–4.9   Describe special considerations for a pediatric patient with a burn injury. (C-1)

4–4.10   Discuss considerations which impact management and prognosis of the burn injured patient. (C-1)

4–4.11   Discuss mechanisms of burn injuries. (C-1)

4–4.12   Discuss conditions associated with burn injuries, including trauma, blast injuries, airway compromise, respiratory compromise, and child abuse. (C-1)

4–4.13   Describe the management of a burn injury, including airway and ventilation, circulation, pharmacological, non-pharmacological, transport considerations, psychological support/communication strategies, and other management described by local protocol. (C-1)

4–4.14   Describe the epidemiology of a thermal burn injury. (C-1)

4–4.15   Describe the specific anatomy and physiology pertinent to a thermal burn injury. (C-1)

4–4.16   Describe the pathophysiology of a thermal burn injury. (C-1)

4–4.17   Identify and describe the depth classifications of a thermal burn injury. (C-1)

4–4.18   Identify and describe the severity of a thermal burn injury. (C-1)

4–4.19   Describe considerations which impact management and prognosis of the patient with a thermal burn injury. (C-1)

4–4.20   Discuss mechanisms of burn injury and conditions associated with a thermal burn injury. (C-1)

4–4.21   Describe the management of a thermal burn injury, including airway and ventilation, circulation, pharmacological, non-pharmacological, transport considerations, and psychological support/communication strategies. (C-1)

4–4.22   Describe the epidemiology of an inhalation burn injury. (C-1)

4–4.23   Describe the specific anatomy and physiology pertinent to an inhalation burn injury. (C-1)

4–4.24   Describe the pathophysiology of an inhalation burn injury. (C-1)

4–4.25   Differentiate between supraglottic and infraglottic inhalation injuries. (C-3)

4–4.26   Identify and describe the depth classifications of an inhalation burn injury. (C-1)

4–4.27   Identify and describe the severity of an inhalation burn injury. (C-1)

4–4.28   Describe considerations which impact management and prognosis of the patient with an inhalation burn injury. (C-1)

4–4.29   Discuss mechanisms of burn injury and conditions associated with an inhalation burn injury. (C-1)

4–4.30   Describe the management of an inhalation burn injury, including airway and ventilation, circulation, pharmacological, non-pharmacological, transport considerations, and psychological support/communication strategies. (C-1)

4–4.31   Describe the epidemiology of a chemical burn injury and a chemical burn injury to the eye. (C-1)

4–4.32   Describe the specific anatomy and physiology pertinent to a chemical burn injury and a chemical burn injury to the eye. (C-1)

4–4.33   Describe the pathophysiology of a chemical burn injury, including types of chemicals and their burning processes and a chemical burn injury to the eye. (C-1)

4–4.34   Identify and describe the depth classifications of a chemical burn injury. (C-1)

4–4.35   Identify and describe the severity of a chemical burn injury. (C-1)

4–4.36   Describe considerations which impact management and prognosis of the patient with a chemical burn injury and a chemical burn injury to the eye. (C-1)

4–4.37   Discuss mechanisms of burn injury and conditions associated with a chemical burn injury. (C-1)

4–4.38   Describe the management of a chemical burn injury and a chemical burn injury to the eye, including airway and ventilation, circulation, pharmacological, non-pharmacological, transport considerations, and psychological support/communication strategies. (C-1)

4–4.39   Describe the epidemiology of an electrical burn injury. (C-1)

4–4.40   Describe the specific anatomy and physiology pertinent to an electrical burn injury. (C-1)

4–4.41   Describe the pathophysiology of an electrical burn injury. (C-1)

4–4.42   Identify and describe the depth classifications of an electrical burn injury. (C-1)

4–4.43   Identify and describe the severity of an electrical burn injury. (C-1)

4–4.44   Describe considerations which impact management and prognosis of the patient with an electrical burn injury. (C-1)

4–4.45   Discuss mechanisms of burn injury and conditions associated with an electrical burn injury. (C-1)

4–4.46   Describe the management of an electrical burn injury, including airway and ventilation, circulation, pharmacological, non-pharmacological, transport considerations, and psychological support/communication strategies. (C-1)

4–4.47   Describe the epidemiology of a radiation exposure. (C-1)

4–4.48   Describe the specific anatomy and physiology pertinent to a radiation exposure. (C-1)

4–4.49   Describe the pathophysiology of a radiation exposure, including the types and characteristics of ionizing radiation. (C-1)

4–4.50   Identify and describe the depth classifications of a radiation exposure. (C-1)

4–4.51   Identify and describe the severity of a radiation exposure. (C-1)

4–4.52   Describe considerations which impact management and prognosis of the patient with a radiation exposure. (C-1)

4–4.53   Discuss mechanisms of burn injury associated with a radiation exposure. (C-1)

4–4.54   Discuss conditions associated with a radiation exposure. (C-1)

4–4.55   Describe the management of a radiation exposure, including airway and ventilation, circulation, pharmacological, non-pharmacological, transport considerations, and psychological support/communication strategies. (C-1)

4–4.56 Integrate pathophysiological principles into the assessment of a patient with a thermal burn injury. (C-3)

4–4.57 Integrate pathophysiological principles into the assessment of a patient with an inhalation burn injury. (C-3)

4–4.58 Integrate pathophysiological principles into the assessment of a patient with a chemical burn injury. (C-3)

4–4.59 Integrate pathophysiological principles into the assessment of a patient with an electrical burn injury. (C-3)

4–4.60 Integrate pathophysiological principles into the assessment of a patient with a radiation exposure. (C-3)

4–4.61 Synthesize patient history information and assessment findings to form a field impression for the patient with a thermal burn injury. (C-3)

4–4.62 Synthesize patient history information and assessment findings to form a field impression for the patient with an inhalation burn injury. (C-3)

4–4.63 Synthesize patient history information and assessment findings to form a field impression for the patient with a chemical burn injury. (C-3)

4–4.64 Synthesize patient history information and assessment findings to form a field impression for the patient with an electrical burn injury. (C-3)

4–4.65 Synthesize patient history information and assessment findings to form a field impression for the patient with a radiation exposure. (C-3)

4–4.66 Develop, execute, and evaluate a management plan based on the field impression for the patient with a thermal burn injury. (C-3)

4–4.67 Develop, execute, and evaluate a management plan based on the field impression for the patient with an inhalation burn injury. (C-3)

4–4.68 Develop, execute, and evaluate a management plan based on the field impression for the patient with a chemical burn injury. (C-3)

4–4.69 Develop, execute, and evaluate a management plan based on the field impression for the patient with an electrical burn injury. (C-3)

4–4.70 Develop, execute, and evaluate a management plan based on the field impression for the patient with a radiation exposure. (C-3)

AFFECTIVE OBJECTIVES

At the completion of this unit, the paramedic student will be able to:

4–4.71 Value the changes of a patient's self-image associated with a burn injury. (A-2)

4–4.72 Value the impact of managing a burn injured patient. (A-2)

4–4.73 Advocate empathy for a burn injured patient. (A-2)

4–4.74 Assess safety at a burn injury incident. (A-3)

4–4.75 Characterize mortality and morbidity based on the pathophysiology and assessment findings of a patient with a burn injury. (A-3)

4–4.76 Value and defend the sense of urgency in burn injuries. (A-3)

4–4.77 Serve as a model for universal precautions and body substance isolation (BSI). (A-3)

PSYCHOMOTOR OBJECTIVES

At the completion of this unit, the paramedic student will be able to:

4–4.78 Take body substance isolation procedures during assessment and management of patients with a burn injury. (P-2)

4–4.79 Perform assessment of a patient with a burn injury. (P-2)

4–4.80 Perform management of a thermal burn injury, including airway and ventilation, circulation, pharmacological, non-pharmacological, transport considerations, psychological support/communication strategies, and other management described by local protocol. (P-2)

4–4.81 Perform management of an inhalation burn injury, including airway and ventilation, circulation, pharmacological, non-pharmacological, transport considerations, psychological support/communication strategies, and other management described by local protocol. (P-2)

4–4.82 Perform management of a chemical burn injury, including airway and ventilation, circulation, pharmacological, non-pharmacological, transport considerations, psychological support/communication strategies, and other management described by local protocol. (P-2)

4–4.83 Perform management of an electrical burn injury, including airway and ventilation, circulation, pharmacological, non-pharmacological, transport considerations, psychological support/communication strategies, and other management described by local protocol. (P-2)

4–4.84 Perform management of a radiation exposure, including airway and ventilation, circulation, pharmacological, non-pharmacological, transport considerations, psychological support/communication strategies, and other management described by local protocol. (P-2)

UNIT TERMINAL OBJECTIVE

4–5 At the completion of this unit, the paramedic student will be able to integrate pathophysiological principles and the assessment findings to formulate a field impression and implement a treatment plan for the trauma patient with a suspected head injury.

COGNITIVE OBJECTIVES

At the completion of this unit, the paramedic student will be able to:

4–5.1 Describe the incidence, morbidity, and mortality of facial injures. (C-1)

4–5.2 Explain facial anatomy and relate physiology to facial injuries. (C-1)

4–5.3 Predict facial injuries based on mechanism of injury. (C-1)

4–5.4 Predict other injuries commonly associated with facial injuries based on mechanism of injury. (C-2)

4–5.5 Differentiate between the following types of facial injuries, highlighting the defining characteristics of each: (C-3)
   a. Eye
   b. Ear
   c. Nose
   d. Throat
   e. Mouth

4–5.6 Integrate pathophysiological principles into the assessment of a patient with a facial injury. (C-3)

4–5.7 Differentiate between facial injuries based on the assessment and history. (C-3)

4–5.8 Formulate a field impression for a patient with a facial injury based on the assessment findings. (C-3)

4–5.9 Develop a patient management plan for a patient with a facial injury based on the field impression. (C-3)

4–5.10   Explain the pathophysiology of eye injuries. (C-1)

4–5.11   Relate assessment findings associated with eye injuries to pathophysiology. (C-3)

4–5.12   Integrate pathophysiological principles into the assessment of a patient with an eye injury. (C-3)

4–5.13   Formulate a field impression for a patient with an eye injury based on the assessment findings. (C-3)

4–5.14   Develop a patient management plan for a patient with an eye injury based on the field impression. (C-3)

4–5.15   Explain the pathophysiology of ear injuries. (C-1)

4–5.16   Relate assessment findings associated with ear injuries to pathophysiology. (C-3)

4–5.17   Integrate pathophysiological principles into the assessment of a patient with an ear injury. (C-3)

4–5.18   Formulate a field impression for a patient with an ear injury based on the assessment findings. (C-3)

4–5.19   Develop a patient management plan for a patient with an ear injury based on the field impression. (C-3)

4–5.20   Explain the pathophysiology of nose injuries. (C-1)

4–5.21   Relate assessment findings associated with nose injuries to pathophysiology. (C-3)

4–5.22   Integrate pathophysiological principles into the assessment of a patient with a nose injury. (C-3)

4–5.23   Formulate a field impression for a patient with a nose injury based on the assessment findings. (C-3)

4–5.24   Develop a patient management plan for a patient with a nose injury based on the field impression. (C-3)

4–5.25   Explain the pathophysiology of throat injuries. (C-1)

4–5.26   Relate assessment findings associated with throat injuries to pathophysiology. (C-3)

4–5.27   Integrate pathophysiological principles into the assessment of a patient with a throat injury. (C-3)

4–5.28   Formulate a field impression for a patient with a throat injury based on the assessment findings. (C-3)

4–5.29   Develop a patient management plan for a patient with a throat injury based on the field impression. (C-3)

4–5.30   Explain the pathophysiology of mouth injuries. (C-1)

4–5.31   Relate assessment findings associated with mouth injuries to pathophysiology. (C-3)

4–5.32   Integrate pathophysiological principles into the assessment of a patient with a mouth injury. (C-3)

4–5.33   Formulate a field impression for a patient with a mouth injury based on the assessment findings. (C-3)

4–5.34   Develop a patient management plan for a patient with a mouth injury based on the field impression. (C-3)

4–5.35   Describe the incidence, morbidity, and mortality of head injures. (C-1)

4–5.36   Explain anatomy and relate physiology of the CNS to head injuries. (C-1)

4–5.37   Predict head injuries based on mechanism of injury. (C-2)

4–5.38   Distinguish between head injury and brain injury. (C-3)

4–5.39   Explain the pathophysiology of head/brain injuries. (C-1)

4–5.40   Explain the concept of increasing intracranial pressure (ICP). (C-1)

4–5.41   Explain the effect of increased and decreased carbon dioxide on ICP. (C-1)

4–5.42   Define and explain the process involved with each of the levels of increasing ICP. (C-1)

4–5.43   Relate assessment findings associated with head/brain injuries to the pathophysiologic process. (C-3)

4–5.44   Classify head injuries (mild, moderate, severe) according to assessment findings. (C-2)

4–5.45   Identify the need for rapid intervention and transport of the patient with a head/brain injury. (C-1)

4–5.46   Describe and explain the general management of the head/brain injury patient, including pharmacological and non-pharmacological treatment. (C-1)

4–5.47   Analyze the relationship between carbon dioxide concentration in the blood and management of the airway in the head/brain injured patient. (C-3)

4–5.48   Explain the pathophysiology of diffuse axonal injury. (C-1)

4–5.49   Relate assessment findings associated with concussion, moderate and severe diffuse axonal injury to pathophysiology. (C-3)

4–5.50   Develop a management plan for a patient with a moderate and severe diffuse axonal injury. (C-3)

4–5.51   Explain the pathophysiology of skull fracture. (C-1)

4–5.52   Relate assessment findings associated with skull fracture to pathophysiology. (C-3)

4–5.53   Develop a management plan for a patient with a skull fracture. (C-3)

4–5.54   Explain the pathophysiology of cerebral contusion. (C-1)

4–5.55   Relate assessment findings associated with cerebral contusion to pathophysiology. (C-3)

4–5.56   Develop a management plan for a patient with a cerebral contusion. (C-3)

4–5.57   Explain the pathophysiology of intracranial hemorrhage, including: (C-1)
   a. Epidural
   b. Subdural
   c. Intracerebral
   d. Subarachnoid

4–5.58   Relate assessment findings associated with intracranial hemorrhage to pathophysiology, including: (C-3)
   a. Epidural
   b. Subdural
   c. Intracerebral
   d. Subarachnoid

4–5.59   Develop a management plan for a patient with an intracranial hemorrhage, including: (C-1)
   a. Epidural
   b. Subdural
   c. Intracerebral
   d. Subarachnoid

4–5.60   Describe the various types of helmets and their purposes. (C-1)

4–5.61   Relate priorities of care to factors determining the need for helmet removal in various field situations including sports related incidents. (C-3)

4–5.62   Develop a management plan for the removal of a helmet for a head injured patient. (C-3)

4–5.63   Integrate the pathophysiological principles into the assessment of a patient with head/brain injury. (C-3)

4–5.64   Differentiate between the types of head/brain injuries based on the assessment and history. (C-3)

4–5.65   Formulate a field impression for a patient with a head/brain injury based on the assessment findings. (C-3)

4–5.66   Develop a patient management plan for a patient with a head/brain injury based on the field impression. (C-3)

AFFECTIVE OBJECTIVES

None identified for this unit.

PSYCHOMOTOR OBJECTIVES

None identified for this unit.

UNIT TERMINAL OBJECTIVE

4–6   At the completion of this unit, the paramedic student will be able to integrate pathophysiological principles and the assessment findings to formulate a field impression and implement a treatment plan for the patient with a suspected spinal injury.

COGNITIVE OBJECTIVES

At the completion of this unit, the paramedic student will be able to:

4–6.1   Describe the incidence, morbidity, and mortality of spinal injuries in the trauma patient. (C-1)

4–6.2   Describe the anatomy and physiology of structures related to spinal injuries: (C-1)
a. Cervical
b. Thoracic
c. Lumbar
d. Sacrum
e. Coccyx
f. Head
g. Brain
h. Spinal cord
i. Nerve tract(s)
j. Dermatomes

4–6.3   Predict spinal injuries based on mechanism of injury. (C-2)

4–6.4   Describe the pathophysiology of spinal injuries. (C-1)

4–6.5   Explain traumatic and non-traumatic spinal injuries. (C-1)

4–6.6   Describe the assessment findings associated with spinal injuries. (C-1)

4–6.7   Describe the management of spinal injuries. (C-1)

4–6.8   Identify the need for rapid intervention and transport of the patient with spinal injuries. (C-1)

4–6.9   Integrate the pathophysiological principles into the assessment of a patient with a spinal injury. (C-3)

4–6.10   Differentiate between spinal injuries based on the assessment and history. (C-3)

4–6.11   Formulate a field impression based on the assessment findings. (C-3)

4–6.12   Develop a patient management plan based on the field impression. (C-3)

4–6.13   Describe the pathophysiology of traumatic spinal injury related to: (C-1)
a. Spinal shock
b. Spinal neurogenic shock
c. Quadriplegia/paraplegia
d. Incomplete cord injury/cord syndromes:
1. Central cord syndrome
2. Anterior cord syndrome
3. Brown-Séquard syndrome

4–6.14   Describe the assessment findings associated with traumatic spinal injuries. (C-1)

4–6.15   Describe the management of traumatic spinal injuries. (C-1)

4–6.16   Integrate pathophysiological principles into the assessment of a patient with a traumatic spinal injury. (C-3)

4–6.17   Differentiate between traumatic and non-traumatic spinal injuries based on the assessment and history. (C-3)

4–6.18   Formulate a field impression for traumatic spinal injury based on the assessment findings. (C-3)

4–6.19   Develop a patient management plan for traumatic spinal injury based on the field impression. (C-3)

4–6.20   Describe the pathophysiology of non-traumatic spinal injury, including: (C-1)
a. Low back pain
b. Herniated intervertebral disk
c. Spinal cord tumors

4–6.21   Describe the assessment findings associated with non-traumatic spinal injuries. (C-1)

4–6.22   Describe the management of non-traumatic spinal injuries. (C-1)

4–6.23   Integrate pathophysiological principles into the assessment of a patient with non-traumatic spinal injury. (C-3)

4–6.24   Differentiate between traumatic and non-traumatic spinal injuries based on the assessment and history. (C-3)

4–6.25   Formulate a field impression for non-traumatic spinal injury based on the assessment findings. (C-3)

4–6.26   Develop a patient management plan for non-traumatic spinal injury based on the field impression. (C-3)

AFFECTIVE OBJECTIVES

At the completion of this unit, the paramedic student will be able to:

4–6.27   Advocate the use of a thorough assessment when determining the proper management modality for spine injuries. (A-3)

4–6.28   Value the implications of failing to properly immobilize a spine injured patient. (A-2)

PSYCHOMOTOR OBJECTIVES

At the completion of this unit, the paramedic student will be able to:

4–6.29   Demonstrate a clinical assessment to determine the proper management modality for a patient with a suspected traumatic spinal injury. (P-1)

4–6.30   Demonstrate a clinical assessment to determine the proper management modality for a patient with a suspected non-traumatic spinal injury. (P-1)

4–6.31   Demonstrate immobilization of the urgent and non-urgent patient with assessment findings of spinal injury from the following presentations: (P-1)
a. Supine
b. Prone
c. Semi-prone
d. Sitting
e. Standing

4–6.32   Demonstrate documentation of suspected spinal cord injury to include: (P-1)
a. General area of spinal cord involved
b. Sensation
c. Dermatomes
d. Motor function
e. Area(s) of weakness

4–6.33 Demonstrate preferred methods for stabilization of a helmet from a potentially spine injured patient. (P-1)

4–6.34 Demonstrate helmet removal techniques. (P-1)

4–6.35 Demonstrate alternative methods for stabilization of a helmet from a potentially spine injured patient. (P-1)

4–6.36 Demonstrate documentation of assessment before spinal immobilization. (P-1)

4–6.37 Demonstrate documentation of assessment during spinal immobilization. (P-1)

4–6.38 Demonstrate documentation of assessment after spinal immobilization. (P-1)

UNIT TERMINAL OBJECTIVE

4–7 At the completion of this unit, the paramedic student will be able to integrate pathophysiological principles and the assessment findings to formulate a field impression and implement a treatment plan for a patient with a thoracic injury.

COGNITIVE OBJECTIVES

At the completion of this unit, the paramedic student will be able to:

4–7.1 Describe the incidence, morbidity, and mortality of thoracic injuries in the trauma patient. (C-1)

4–7.2 Discuss the anatomy and physiology of the organs and structures related to thoracic injuries. (C-1)

4–7.3 Predict thoracic injuries based on mechanism of injury. (C-2)

4–7.4 Discuss the types of thoracic injuries. (C-1)

4–7.5 Discuss the pathophysiology of thoracic injuries. (C-1)

4–7.6 Discuss the assessment findings associated with thoracic injuries. (C-1)

4–7.7 Discuss the management of thoracic injuries. (C-1)

4–7.8 Identify the need for rapid intervention and transport of the patient with thoracic injuries. (C-1)

4–7.9 Discuss the pathophysiology of specific chest wall injuries, including: (C-1)
   a. Rib fracture
   b. Flail segment
   c. Sternal fracture

4–7.10 Discuss the assessment findings associated with chest wall injuries. (C-1)

4–7.11 Identify the need for rapid intervention and transport of the patient with chest wall injuries. (C-1)

4–7.12 Discuss the management of chest wall injuries. (C-1)

4–7.13 Discuss the pathophysiology of injury to the lung, including: (C-1)
   a. Simple pneumothorax
   b. Open pneumothorax
   c. Tension pneumothorax
   d. Hemothorax
   e. Hemopneumothorax
   f. Pulmonary contusion

4–7.14 Discuss the assessment findings associated with lung injuries. (C-1)

4–7.15 Discuss the management of lung injuries. (C-1)

4–7.16 Identify the need for rapid intervention and transport of the patient with lung injuries. (C-1)

4–7.17 Discuss the pathophysiology of myocardial injuries, including: (C-1)
   a. Pericardial tamponade
   b. Myocardial contusion
   c. Myocardial rupture

4–7.18 Discuss the assessment findings associated with myocardial injuries. (C-1)

4–7.19 Discuss the management of myocardial injuries. (C-1)

4–7.20 Identify the need for rapid intervention and transport of the patient with myocardial injuries. (C-1)

4–7.21 Discuss the pathophysiology of vascular injuries, including injuries to: (C-1)
   a. Aorta
   b. Vena cava
   c. Pulmonary arteries/veins

4–7.22 Discuss the assessment findings associated with vascular injuries. (C-1)

4–7.23 Discuss the management of vascular injuries. (C-1)

4–7.24 Identify the need for rapid intervention and transport of the patient with vascular injuries. (C-1)

4–7.25 Discuss the pathophysiology of diaphragmatic injuries. (C-1)

4–7.26 Discuss the assessment findings associated with diaphragmatic injuries. (C-1)

4–7.27 Discuss the management of diaphragmatic injuries. (C-1)

4–7.28 Identify the need for rapid intervention and transport of the patient with diaphragmatic injuries. (C-1)

4–7.29 Discuss the pathophysiology of esophageal injuries. (C-1)

4–7.30 Discuss the assessment findings associated with esophageal injuries. (C-1)

4–7.31 Discuss the management of esophageal injuries. (C-1)

4–7.32 Identify the need for rapid intervention and transport of the patient with esophageal injuries. (C-1)

4–7.33 Discuss the pathophysiology of tracheo-bronchial injuries. (C-1)

4–7.34 Discuss the assessment findings associated with tracheo-bronchial injuries. (C-1)

4–7.35 Discuss the management of tracheo-bronchial injuries. (C-1)

4–7.36 Identify the need for rapid intervention and transport of the patient with tracheo-bronchial injuries. (C-1)

4–7.37 Discuss the pathophysiology of traumatic asphyxia. (C-1)

4–7.38 Discuss the assessment findings associated with traumatic asphyxia. (C-1)

4–7.39 Discuss the management of traumatic asphyxia. (C-1)

4–7.40 Identify the need for rapid intervention and transport of the patient with traumatic asphyxia. (C-1)

4–7.41 Integrate the pathophysiological principles into the assessment of a patient with thoracic injury. (C-1)

4–7.42 Differentiate between thoracic injuries based on the assessment and history. (C-3)

4–7.43 Formulate a field impression based on the assessment findings. (C-3)

4–7.44 Develop a patient management plan based on the field impression. (C-3)

AFFECTIVE OBJECTIVES

At the completion of this unit, the paramedic student will be able to:

4–7.45 Advocate the use of a thorough assessment to determine a differential diagnosis and treatment plan for thoracic trauma. (A-3)

4–7.46 Advocate the use of a thorough scene survey to determine the forces involved in thoracic trauma. (A-3)

4–7.47 Value the implications of failing to properly diagnose thoracic trauma. (A-2)

4–7.48 Value the implications of failing to initiate timely interventions to patients with thoracic trauma. (A-2)

PSYCHOMOTOR OBJECTIVES

At the completion of this unit, the paramedic student will be able to:

4–7.49 Demonstrate a clinical assessment for a patient with suspected thoracic trauma. (P-1)

4–7.50 Demonstrate the following techniques of management for thoracic injuries: (P-1)
 a. Needle decompression
 b. Fracture stabilization
 c. Elective intubation
 d. ECG monitoring
 e. Oxygenation and ventilation

UNIT TERMINAL OBJECTIVE

4–8 At the completion of this unit, the paramedic student will be able to integrate pathophysiologic principles and the assessment findings to formulate a field impression and implement the treatment plan for the patient with suspected abdominal trauma.

COGNITIVE OBJECTIVES

At the completion of this unit, the paramedic student will be able to:

4–8.1 Describe the epidemiology, including the morbidity/mortality and prevention strategies, for a patient with abdominal trauma. (C-1)

4–8.2 Describe the anatomy and physiology of organs and structures related to abdominal injuries. (C-1)

4–8.3 Predict abdominal injuries based on blunt and penetrating mechanisms of injury. (C-2)

4–8.4 Describe open and closed abdominal injuries. (C-1)

4–8.5 Explain the pathophysiology of abdominal injuries. (C-1)

4–8.6 Describe the assessment findings associated with abdominal injuries. (C-1)

4–8.7 Identify the need for rapid intervention and transport of the patient with abdominal injuries based on assessment findings. (C-1)

4–8.8 Describe the management of abdominal injuries. (C-1)

4–8.9 Integrate the pathophysiological principles to the assessment of a patient with abdominal injury. (C-3)

4–8.10 Differentiate between abdominal injuries based on the assessment and history. (C-3)

4–8.11 Formulate a field impression for patients with abdominal trauma based on the assessment findings. (C-3)

4–8.12 Develop a patient management plan for patients with abdominal trauma based on the field impression. (C-3)

4–8.13 Describe the epidemiology, including the morbidity/mortality and prevention strategies, for solid organ injuries. (C-1)

4–8.14 Explain the pathophysiology of solid organ injuries. (C-1)

4–8.15 Describe the assessment findings associated with solid organ injuries. (C-1)

4–8.16 Describe the treatment plan and management of solid organ injuries. (C-1)

4–8.17 Describe the epidemiology, including the morbidity/mortality and prevention strategies, for hollow organ injuries. (C-1)

4–8.18 Explain the pathophysiology of hollow organ injuries. (C-1)

4–8.19 Describe the assessment findings associated with hollow organ injuries. (C-1)

4–8.20 Describe the treatment plan and management of hollow organ injuries. (C-1)

4–8.21 Describe the epidemiology, including the morbidity/mortality and prevention strategies, for abdominal vascular injuries. (C-1)

4–8.22 Explain the pathophysiology of abdominal vascular injuries. (C-1)

4–8.23 Describe the assessment findings associated with abdominal vascular injuries. (C-1)

4–8.24 Describe the treatment plan and management of abdominal vascular injuries. (C-1)

4–8.25 Describe the epidemiology, including the morbidity/mortality and prevention strategies, for pelvic fractures. (C-1)

4–8.26 Explain the pathophysiology of pelvic fractures. (C-1)

4–8.27 Describe the assessment findings associated with pelvic fractures. (C-1)

4–8.28 Describe the treatment plan and management of pelvic fractures. (C-1)

4–8.29 Describe the epidemiology, including the morbidity/mortality and prevention strategies, for other related abdominal injuries. (C-1)

4–8.30 Explain the pathophysiology of other related abdominal injuries. (C-1)

4–8.31 Describe the assessment findings associated with other related abdominal injuries. (C-1)

4–8.32 Describe the treatment plan and management of other related abdominal injuries. (C-1)

4–8.33 Apply the epidemiologic principles to develop prevention strategies for abdominal injuries. (C-2)

4–8.34 Integrate the pathophysiological principles into the assessment of a patient with abdominal injuries. (C-3)

4–8.35 Differentiate between abdominal injuries based on the assessment and history. (C-3)

4–8.36 Formulate a field impression based upon the assessment findings for a patient with abdominal injuries. (C-3)

4–8.37 Develop a patient management plan for a patient with abdominal injuries, based upon field impression. (C-3)

AFFECTIVE OBJECTIVES

At the completion of this unit, the paramedic student will be able to:

4–8.38 Advocate the use of a thorough assessment to determine a differential diagnosis and treatment plan for abdominal trauma. (A-3)

4–8.39 Advocate the use of a thorough scene survey to determine the forces involved in abdominal trauma. (A-3)

4–8.40 Value the implications of failing to properly diagnose abdominal trauma and initiate timely interventions to patients with abdominal trauma. (A-2)

PSYCHOMOTOR OBJECTIVES

At the completion of this unit, the paramedic student will be able to:

4–8.41 Demonstrate a clinical assessment to determine the proper treatment plan for a patient with suspected abdominal trauma. (P-1)

4–8.42 Demonstrate the proper use of PASG in a patient with suspected abdominal trauma. (P-1)

4–8.43 Demonstrate the proper use of PASG in a patient with suspected pelvic fracture. (P-1)

UNIT TERMINAL OBJECTIVE

4–9 At the completion of this unit, the paramedic student will be able to integrate pathophysiological principles and the assessment findings to formulate a field impression and implement the treatment plan for the patient with a musculoskeletal injury.

COGNITIVE OBJECTIVES

At the completion of this unit, the paramedic student will be able to:

4–9.1 Describe the incidence, morbidity, and mortality of musculoskeletal injuries. (C-1)

4–9.2 Discuss the anatomy and physiology of the musculoskeletal system. (C-1)

4–9.3 Predict injuries based on the mechanism of injury, including: (C-3)
   a. Direct
   b. Indirect
   c. Pathologic

4–9.4 Discuss the types of musculoskeletal injuries: (C-1)
   a. Fracture (open and closed)
   b. Dislocation/fracture
   c. Sprain
   d. Strain

4–9.5 Discuss the pathophysiology of musculoskeletal injuries. (C-1)

4–9.6 Discuss the assessment findings associated with musculoskeletal injuries. (C-1)

4–9.7 List the six "P"s of musculoskeletal injury assessment. (C-1)

4–9.8 List the primary signs and symptoms of extremity trauma. (C-1)

4–9.9 List other signs and symptoms that can indicate less obvious extremity injury. (C-1)

4–9.10 Discuss the need for assessment of pulses, motor, and sensation before and after splinting. (C-1)

4–9.11 Identify the need for rapid intervention and transport when dealing with musculoskeletal injuries. (C-1)

4–9.12 Discuss the management of musculoskeletal injuries. (C-1)

4–9.13 Discuss the general guidelines for splinting. (C-1)

4–9.14 Explain the benefits of cold application for musculoskeletal injury. (C-1)

4–9.15 Explain the benefits of heat application for musculoskeletal injury. (C-1)

4–9.16 Describe age associated changes in the bones. (C-1)

4–9.17 Discuss the pathophysiology of open and closed fractures. (C-1)

4–9.18 Discuss the relationship between volume of hemorrhage and open or closed fractures. (C-3)

4–9.19 Discuss the assessment findings associated with fractures. (C-1)

4–9.20 Discuss the management of fractures. (C-1)

4–9.21 Discuss the usefulness of the pneumatic anti-shock garment (PASG) in the management of fractures. (C-1)

4–9.22 Describe the special considerations involved in femur fracture management. (C-1)

4–9.23 Discuss the pathophysiology of dislocations. (C-1)

4–9.24 Discuss the assessment findings of dislocations. (C-1)

4–9.25 Discuss the out-of-hospital management of dislocation/fractures, including splinting and realignment. (C-1)

4–9.26 Explain the importance of manipulating a knee dislocation/fracture with an absent distal pulse. (C-1)

4–9.27 Describe the procedure for reduction of a shoulder, finger, or ankle dislocation/fracture. (C-1)

4–9.28 Discuss the pathophysiology of sprains. (C-1)

4–9.29 Discuss the assessment findings of sprains. (C-1)

4–9.30 Discuss the management of sprains. (C-1)

4–9.31 Discuss the pathophysiology of strains. (C-1)

4–9.32 Discuss the assessment findings of strains. (C-1)

4–9.33 Discuss the management of strains. (C-1)

4–9.34 Discuss the pathophysiology of a tendon injury. (C-1)

4–9.35 Discuss the assessment findings of a tendon injury. (C-1)

4–9.36 Discuss the management of a tendon injury. (C-1)

4–9.37 Integrate the pathophysiological principles into the assessment of a patient with a musculoskeletal injury. (C-3)

4–9.38 Differentiate between musculoskeletal injuries based on the assessment findings and history. (C-3)

4–9.39 Formulate a field impression of a musculoskeletal injury based on the assessment findings. (C-3)

4–9.40 Develop a patient management plan for the musculoskeletal injury based on the field impression. (C-3)

AFFECTIVE OBJECTIVES

At the completion of this unit, the paramedic student will be able to:

4–9.41 Advocate the use of a thorough assessment to determine a working diagnosis and treatment plan for musculoskeletal injuries. (A-3)

4–9.42 Advocate for the use of pain management in the treatment of musculoskeletal injuries. (A-3)

PSYCHOMOTOR OBJECTIVES

At the completion of this unit, the paramedic student will be able to:

4–9.43 Demonstrate a clinical assessment to determine the proper treatment plan for a patient with a suspected musculoskeletal injury. (P-1)

4–9.44 Demonstrate the proper use of fixation, soft, and traction splints for a patient with a suspected fracture. (P-1)

UNIT TERMINAL OBJECTIVE

5–1 At the completion of this unit, the paramedic student will be able to integrate pathophysiological principles and assessment findings to formulate a field impression and implement the treatment plan for the patient with respiratory problems.

COGNITIVE OBJECTIVES

At the completion of this unit, the paramedic student will be able to:

5–1.1   Discuss the epidemiology of pulmonary diseases and conditions. (C-1)

5–1.2   Identify and describe the function of the structures located in the upper and lower airway. (C-1)

5–1.3   Discuss the physiology of ventilation and respiration. (C-1)

5–1.4   Identify common pathological events that affect the pulmonary system. (C-1)

5–1.5   Discuss abnormal assessment findings associated with pulmonary diseases and conditions. (C-1)

5–1.6   Compare various airway and ventilation techniques used in the management of pulmonary diseases. (C-3)

5–1.7   Review the pharmacological preparations that paramedics use for management of respiratory diseases and conditions. (C-1)

5–1.8   Review the pharmacological preparations used in managing patients with respiratory diseases that may be prescribed by physicians. (C-1)

5–1.9   Review the use of equipment used during the physical examination of patients with complaints associated with respiratory diseases and conditions. (C-1)

5–1.10 Identify the epidemiology, anatomy, physiology, pathophysiology, assessment findings, and management for the following respiratory diseases and conditions: (C-1)
  a. Adult respiratory distress syndrome
  b. Bronchial asthma
  c. Chronic bronchitis
  d. Emphysema
  e. Pneumonia
  f. Pulmonary edema
  g. Pulmonary thromboembolism
  h. Neoplasms of the lung
  i. Upper respiratory infections
  j. Spontaneous pneumothorax
  k. Hyperventilation syndrome

AFFECTIVE OBJECTIVES

At the completion of this unit, the paramedic student will be able to:

5–1.11 Recognize and value the assessment and treatment of patients with respiratory diseases. (A-2)

5–1.12 Indicate appreciation for the critical nature of accurate field impressions of patients with respiratory diseases and conditions. (A-2)

PSYCHOMOTOR OBJECTIVES

At the completion of this unit, the paramedic student will be able to:

5–1.13 Demonstrate proper use of airway and ventilation devices. (P-1)

5–1.14 Conduct a history and patient assessment for patients with pulmonary diseases and conditions. (P-1)

5–1.15 Demonstrate the application of a CPAP/BiPAP unit. (P-1)

UNIT TERMINAL OBJECTIVE

5–2   At the completion of this unit, the paramedic student will be able to integrate pathophysiological principles and assessment findings to formulate a field impression and implement the treatment plan for the patient with cardiovascular disease.

COGNITIVE OBJECTIVES

At the completion of this unit, the paramedic student will be able to:

5–2.1   Describe the incidence, morbidity, and mortality of cardiovascular disease. (C-1)

5–2.2   Discuss prevention strategies that may reduce the morbidity and mortality of cardiovascular disease. (C-1)

5–2.3   Identify the risk factors most predisposing to coronary artery disease. (C-1)

5–2.4   Describe the anatomy of the heart, including the position in the thoracic cavity, layers of the heart, chambers of the heart, and location and function of cardiac valves. (C-1)

5–2.5   Identify the major structures of the vascular system. (C-1)

5 2.6   Identify the factors affecting venous return. (C-1)

5–2.7   Identify and define the components of cardiac output. (C-1)

5–2.8   Identify phases of the cardiac cycle. (C-1)

5–2.9   Identify the arterial blood supply to any given area of the myocardium. (C-1)

5–2.10 Compare and contrast the coronary arterial distribution to the major portions of the cardiac conduction system. (C-3)

5–2.11 Identify the structure and course of all divisions and subdivisions of the cardiac conduction system. (C-1)

5–2.12 Identify and describe how the heart's pacemaking control, rate, and rhythm are determined. (C-2)

5–2.13 Explain the physiological basis of conduction delay in the AV node. (C-3)

5–2.14 Define the functional properties of cardiac muscle. (C-1)

5–2.15 Define the events comprising electrical potential. (C-1)

5–2.16 List the most important ions involved in myocardial action potential and their primary function in this process. (C-2)

5–2.17 Describe the events involved in the steps from excitation to contraction of cardiac muscle fibers. (C-1)

5–2.18 Describe the clinical significance of Starling's law. (C-3)

5–2.19 Identify the structures of the autonomic nervous system (ANS). (C-1)

5–2.20 Identify the effect of the ANS on heart rate, rhythm, and contractility. (C-1)

5–2.21 Define and give examples of positive and negative inotropism, chronotropism, and dromotropism. (C-2)

5–2.22 Discuss the pathophysiology of cardiac disease and injury. (C-1)

5–2.23 Identify and describe the details of inspection, auscultation, and palpation specific to the cardiovascular system. (C-1)

5–2.24 Define pulse deficit, pulsus paradoxus, and pulsus alternans. (C-1)

5–2.25 Identify the normal characteristics of the point of maximal impulse (PMI). (C-1)

5–2.26 Identify and define the heart sounds. (C-1)

5–2.27 Relate heart sounds to hemodynamic events in the cardiac cycle. (C-2)

5–2.28 Describe the differences between normal and abnormal heart sounds. (C-2)

5–2.29 Identify and describe the components of the focused history as it relates to the patient with cardiovascular compromise. (C-1)

5–2.30 Explain the purpose of ECG monitoring. (C-1)

5–2.31 Describe how ECG wave forms are produced. (C-2)

5–2.32 Correlate the electrophysiological and hemodynamic events occurring throughout the entire cardiac cycle with the various ECG wave forms, segments, and intervals. (C-2)

5–2.33 Identify how heart rates, durations, and amplitudes may be determined from ECG recordings. (C-3)

5–2.34 Relate the cardiac surfaces or areas represented by the ECG leads. (C-2)

5–2.35 Given an ECG, identify the arrhythmia. (C-3)

5–2.36 Identify the limitations to the ECG. (C-1)

5–2.37 Differentiate among the primary mechanisms responsible for producing cardiac arrhythmias. (C-1)

5–2.38 Describe a systematic approach to the analysis and interpretation of cardiac arrhythmias. (C-2)

5–2.39 Describe the arrhythmias originating in the sinus node, the AV junction, the atria, and the ventricles. (C-3)

5–2.40 Describe the arrhythmias originating or sustained in the AV junction. (C-3)

5–2.41 Describe the abnormalities originating within the bundle branch system. (C-3)

5–2.42 Describe the process of differentiating wide QRS complex tachycardias. (C-3)

5–2.43 Recognize the pitfalls in the differentiation of wide QRS complex tachycardias. (C-1)

5–2.44 Describe the conditions of pulseless electrical activity. (C-3)

5–2.45 Describe the phenomena of reentry, aberration, and accessory pathways. (C-1)

5–2.46 Identify the ECG changes characteristically produced by electrolyte imbalances and specify the clinical implications. (C-2)

5–2.47 Identify patient situations where ECG rhythm analysis is indicated. (C-1)

5–2.48 Recognize the changes on the ECG that may reflect evidence of myocardial ischemia and injury. (C-1)

5–2.49 Recognize the limitations of the ECG in reflecting evidence of myocardial ischemia and injury. (C-1)

5–2.50 Correlate abnormal ECG findings with clinical interpretation. (C-2)

5–2.51 Identify the major therapeutic objectives in the treatment of the patient with any arrhythmia. (C-1)

5–2.52 Identify the major mechanical, pharmacological, and electrical therapeutic interventions. (C-3)

5–2.53 Based on field impressions, identify the need for rapid intervention for the patient in cardiovascular compromise. (C-3)

5–2.54 Describe the incidence, morbidity, and mortality associated with myocardial conduction defects. (C-1)

5–2.55 Identify the clinical indications for transcutaneous and permanent artificial cardiac pacing. (C-1)

5–2.56 Describe the components and the functions of a transcutaneous pacing system. (C-1)

5–2.57 Explain what each setting and indicator on a transcutaneous pacing system represents and how the settings may be adjusted. (C-2)

5–2.58 Describe the techniques of applying a transcutaneous pacing system. (C-1)

5–2.59 Describe the characteristics of an implanted pacemaking system. (C-1)

5–2.60 Describe artifacts that may cause confusion when evaluating the ECG of a patient with a pacemaker. (C-2)

5–2.61 List the possible complications of pacing. (C-3)

5–2.62 List the causes and implications of pacemaker failure. (C-2)

5–2.63 Identify additional hazards that interfere with artificial pacemaker function. (C-1)

5–2.64 Recognize the complications of artificial pacemakers as evidenced on the ECG. (C-2)

5–2.65 Describe the epidemiology, morbidity and mortality, and pathophysiology of angina pectoris. (C-1)

5–2.66 List and describe the assessment parameters to be evaluated in a patient with angina pectoris. (C-1)

5–2.67 Identify what is meant by the OPQRST of chest pain assessment. (C-3)

5–2.68 List other clinical conditions that may mimic signs and symptoms of coronary artery disease and angina pectoris. (C-1)

5–2.69 Identify the ECG findings in patients with angina pectoris. (C-3)

5–2.70 Identify the paramedic responsibilities associated with management of the patient with angina pectoris. (C-2)

5–2.71 Based on the pathophysiology and clinical evaluation of the patient with chest pain, list the anticipated clinical problems according to their life-threatening potential. (C-3)

5–2.72 Describe the epidemiology, morbidity, and mortality of myocardial infarction. (C-1)

5–2.73 List the mechanisms by which an MI may be produced by traumatic and non-traumatic events. (C-2)

5–2.74 Identify the primary hemodynamic changes produced in myocardial infarction. (C-1)

5–2.75 List and describe the assessment parameters to be evaluated in a patient with a suspected myocardial infarction. (C-1)

5–2.76 Identify the anticipated clinical presentation of a patient with a suspected acute myocardial infarction. (C-3)

5–2.77 Differentiate the characteristics of the pain/discomfort occurring in angina pectoris and acute myocardial infarction. (C-2)

5–2.78 Identify the ECG changes characteristically seen during evolution of an acute myocardial infarction. (C-2)

5–2.79 Identify the most common complications of an acute myocardial infarction. (C-3)

5–2.80 List the characteristics of a patient eligible for thrombolytic therapy. (C-2)

5–2.81 Describe the "window of opportunity" as it pertains to reperfusion of a myocardial injury or infarction. (C-3)

5–2.82 Based on the pathophysiology and clinical evaluation of the patient with a suspected acute myocardial infarction, list the anticipated clinical problems according to their life-threatening potential. (C-3)

5–2.83 Specify the measures that may be taken to prevent or minimize complications in the patient suspected of myocardial infarction. (C-3)

5–2.84 Describe the most commonly used cardiac drugs in terms of therapeutic effect and dosages, routes of administration, side effects, and toxic effects. (C-3)

5–2.85 Describe the epidemiology, morbidity, and mortality of heart failure. (C-1)

5–2.86 Define the principal causes and terminology associated with heart failure. (C-1)

5–2.87 Identify the factors that may precipitate or aggravate heart failure. (C-3)

5–2.88 Describe the physiological effects of heart failure. (C-2)

5–2.89 Define the term "acute pulmonary edema" and describe its relationship to left ventricular failure. (C-3)

5–2.90 Define preload, afterload, and left ventricular end-diastolic pressure and relate each to the pathophysiology of heart failure. (C-3)

5–2.91 Differentiate between early and late signs and symptoms of left ventricular failure and those of right ventricular failure. (C-3)

5–2.92 Explain the clinical significance of paroxysmal nocturnal dyspnea. (C-1)

5–2.93 Explain the clinical significance of edema of the extremities and sacrum. (C-1)

5–2.94 List the interventions prescribed for the patient in acute congestive heart failure. (C-2)

5–2.95 Describe the most commonly used pharmacological agents in the management of congestive heart failure in terms of therapeutic effect, dosages, routes of administration, side effects, and toxic effects. (C-1)

5–2.96 Define the term "cardiac tamponade." (C-1)

5 2.97 List the mechanisms by which cardiac tamponade may be produced by traumatic and non-traumatic events. (C-2)

5–2.98 Identify the limiting factor of pericardial anatomy that determines intrapericardiac pressure. (C-1)

5–2.99 Identify the clinical criteria specific to cardiac tamponade. (C-2)

5–2.100 Describe how to determine if pulsus paradoxus, pulsus alternans, or electrical alternans is present. (C-2)

5–2.101 Identify the paramedic responsibilities associated with management of a patient with cardiac tamponade. (C-2)

5–2.102 Describe the incidence, morbidity, and mortality of hypertensive emergencies. (C-1)

5–2.103 Define the term "hypertensive emergency." (C-1)

5–2.104 Identify the characteristics of the patient population at risk for developing a hypertensive emergency. (C-1)

5–2.105 Explain the essential pathophysiological defect of hypertension in terms of Starling's law of the heart. (C-3)

5–2.106 Identify the progressive vascular changes associated with sustained hypertension. (C-1)

5–2.107 Describe the clinical features of the patient in a hypertensive emergency. (C-3)

5–2.108 Rank the clinical problems of patients in hypertensive emergencies according to their sense of urgency. (C-3)

5–2.109 From the priority of clinical problems identified, state the management responsibilities for the patient with a hypertensive emergency. (C-2)

5–2.110 Identify the drugs of choice for hypertensive emergencies, rationale for use, clinical precautions, and disadvantages of selected antihypertensive agents. (C-3)

5–2.111 Correlate abnormal findings with clinical interpretation of the patient with a hypertensive emergency. (C-3)

5–2.112 Define the term "cardiogenic shock." (C-1)

5–2.113 Describe the major systemic effects of reduced tissue perfusion caused by cardiogenic shock. (C-3)

5–2.114 Explain the primary mechanisms by which the heart may compensate for a diminished cardiac output and describe their efficiency in cardiogenic shock. (C-3)

5–2.115 Differentiate progressive stages of cardiogenic shock. (C-3)

5–2.116 Identify the clinical criteria for cardiogenic shock. (C-1)

5–2.117 Describe the characteristics of patients most likely to develop cardiogenic shock. (C-3)

5–2.118 Describe the most commonly used pharmacological agents in the management of cardiogenic shock in terms of therapeutic effects, dosages, routes of administration, side effects, and toxic effects. (C-2)

5–2.119 Correlate abnormal findings with clinical assessment of the patient in cardiogenic shock. (C-3)

5–2.120 Identify the paramedic responsibilities associated with management of a patient in cardiogenic shock. (C-2)

5–2.121 Define the term "cardiac arrest." (C-1)

5–2.122 Identify the characteristics of the patient population at risk for developing cardiac arrest from cardiac causes. (C-1)

5–2.123 Identify noncardiac causes of cardiac arrest. (C-1)

5–2.124 Describe the arrhythmias seen in cardiac arrest. (C-3)

5–2.125 Identify the critical actions necessary in caring for the patient with cardiac arrest. (C-3)

5–2.126 Explain how to confirm asystole using the 3-lead ECG. (C-1)

5–2.127 Define the terms "defibrillation" and "synchronized cardioversion." (C-1)

5–2.128 Specify the methods of supporting the patient with a suspected ineffective implanted defibrillation device. (C-2)

5–2.129 Describe the most commonly used pharmacological agents in the management of cardiac arrest in terms of therapeutic effects. (C-3)

5–2.130 Identify resuscitation. (C-1)

5–2.131 Identify circumstances and situations where resuscitation efforts would not be initiated. (C-1)

5–2.132 Identify and list the inclusion and exclusion criteria for termination of resuscitation efforts. (C-1)

5–2.133 Identify communication and documentation protocols with medical direction and law enforcement used for termination of resuscitation efforts. (C-1)

5–2.134 Describe the incidence, morbidity, and mortality of vascular disorders. (C-1)

5–2.135 Describe the pathophysiology of vascular disorders. (C-1)

5–2.136 List the traumatic and non-traumatic causes of vascular disorders. (C-1)

5–2.137 Define the terms "aneurysm," "claudication," and "phlebitis." (C-1)

5–2.138 Identify the peripheral arteries most commonly affected by occlusive disease. (C-1)

5–2.139 Identify the major factors involved in the pathophysiology of aortic aneurysm. (C-1)

5–2.140 Recognize the usual order of signs and symptoms that develop following peripheral artery occlusion. (C-3)

5–2.141 Identify the clinical significance of claudication and presence of arterial bruits in a patient with peripheral vascular disorders. (C-3)

5–2.142 Describe the clinical significance of unequal arterial blood pressure readings in the arms. (C-3)

5–2.143 Recognize and describe the signs and symptoms of dissecting thoracic or abdominal aneurysm. (C-3)

5–2.144 Describe the significant elements of the patient history in a patient with vascular disease. (C-2)

5–2.145 Identify the hemodynamic effects of vascular disorders. (C-1)

5–2.146 Identify the complications of vascular disorders. (C-1)

5–2.147 Identify the paramedic's responsibilities associated with management of patients with vascular disorders. (C-2)

5–2.148 Develop, execute, and evaluate a treatment plan based on the field impression for the patient with vascular disorders. (C-3)

5–2.149 Differentiate between signs and symptoms of cardiac tamponade, hypertensive emergencies, cardiogenic shock, and cardiac arrest. (C-3)

5–2.150 Based on the pathophysiology and clinical evaluation of the patient with chest pain, characterize the clinical problems according to their life-threatening potential. (C-3)

5–2.151 Apply knowledge of the epidemiology of cardiovascular disease to develop prevention strategies. (C-3)

5–2.152 Integrate pathophysiological principles into the assessment of a patient with cardiovascular disease. (C-3)

5–2.153 Apply knowledge of the epidemiology of cardiovascular disease to develop prevention strategies. (C-3)

5–2.154 Integrate pathophysiological principles into the assessment of a patient with cardiovascular disease. (C-3)

5–2.155 Synthesize patient history, assessment findings, and ECG analysis to form a field impression for the patient with cardiovascular disease. (C-3)

5–2.156 Integrate pathophysiological principles into the assessment of a patient in need of a pacemaker. (C-1)

5–2.157 Synthesize patient history, assessment findings, and ECG analysis to form a field impression for the patient in need of a pacemaker. (C-3)

5–2.158 Develop, execute, and evaluate a treatment plan based on field impression for the patient in need of a pacemaker. (C-3)

5–2.159 Based on the pathophysiology and clinical evaluation of the patient with chest pain, characterize the clinical problems according to their life-threatening potential. (C-3)

5–2.160 Integrate pathophysiological principles into the assessment of a patient with chest pain. (C-3)

5–2.161 Synthesize patient history, assessment findings, and ECG analysis to form a field impression for the patient with angina pectoris. (C-3)

5–2.162 Develop, execute, and evaluate a treatment plan based on the field impression for the patient with chest pain. (C-3)

5–2.163 Integrate pathophysiological principles into the assessment of a patient with a suspected myocardial infarction. (C-3)

5–2.164 Synthesize patient history, assessment findings, and ECG analysis to form a field impression for the patient with a suspected myocardial infarction. (C-3)

5–2.165 Develop, execute, and evaluate a treatment plan based on the field impression for the suspected myocardial infarction patient. (C-3)

5–2.166 Integrate pathophysiological principles into the assessment of the patient with heart failure. (C-3)

5–2.167 Synthesize assessment findings and patient history information to form a field impression of the patient with heart failure. (C-3)

5–2.168 Develop, execute, and evaluate a treatment plan based on the field impression for the heart failure patient. (C-3)

5–2.169 Integrate pathophysiological principles into the assessment of a patient with cardiac tamponade. (C-3)

5–2.170 Synthesize assessment findings and patient history information to form a field impression of the patient with cardiac tamponade. (C-3)

5–2.171 Develop, execute, and evaluate a treatment plan based on the field impression for the patient with cardiac tamponade. (C-3)

5–2.172 Integrate pathophysiological principles into the assessment of the patient with a hypertensive emergency. (C-3)

5–2.173 Synthesize assessment findings and patient history information to form a field impression of the patient with a hypertensive emergency. (C-3)

5–2.174 Develop, execute, and evaluate a treatment plan based on the field impression for the patient with a hypertensive emergency. (C-3)

5–2.175 Integrate pathophysiological principles into the assessment of the patient with cardiogenic shock. (C-3)

5–2.176 Synthesize assessment findings and patient history information to form a field impression of the patient with cardiogenic shock. (C-3)

5–2.177 Develop, execute, and evaluate a treatment plan based on the field impression for the patient with cardiogenic shock. (C-3)

5–2.178 Integrate the pathophysiological principles into the assessment of the patient with cardiac arrest. (C-3)

5–2.179 Synthesize assessment findings to formulate a rapid intervention for a patient in cardiac arrest. (C-3)

5–2.180 Synthesize assessment findings to formulate the termination of resuscitative efforts for a patient in cardiac arrest. (C-3)

5–2.181 Integrate pathophysiological principles into the assessment of a patient with vascular disorders. (C-3)

5–2.182 Synthesize assessment findings and patient history to form a field impression for the patient with vascular disorders. (C-3)

5–2.183 Integrate pathophysiological principles into the assessment and field management of a patient with chest pain. (C-3)

AFFECTIVE OBJECTIVES

At the completion of this unit, the paramedic student will be able to:

5–2.184 Value the sense of urgency for initial assessment and intervention in the patient with cardiac compromise. (A-3)

5–2.185 Value and defend the sense of urgency necessary to protect the window of opportunity for reperfusion in the patient with suspected myocardial infarction. (A-3)

5–2.186 Defend patient situations where ECG rhythm analysis is indicated. (A-3)

5–2.187 Value and defend the application of a transcutaneous pacing system. (A-3)

5–2.188 Value and defend the urgency in identifying pacemaker malfunction. (A-3)

5–2.189 Based on the pathophysiology and clinical evaluation of the patient with acute myocardial infarction, characterize the clinical problems according to their life-threatening potential. (A-3)

5–2.190 Defend the measures that may be taken to prevent or minimize complications in the patient with a suspected myocardial infarction. (A-3)

5–2.191 Defend the urgency based on the severity of the patient's clinical problems in a hypertensive emergency. (A-3)

5–2.192 From the priority of clinical problems identified, state the management responsibilities for the patient with a hypertensive emergency. (A-3)

5–2.193 Value and defend the urgency in rapid determination of and rapid intervention of patients in cardiac arrest. (A-3)

5–2.194 Value and defend the possibility of termination of resuscitative efforts in the out-of-hospital setting. (A-3)

5–2.195 Based on the pathophysiology and clinical evaluation of the patient with vascular disorders, characterize the clinical problems according to their life-threatening potential. (A-3)

5–2.196 Value and defend the sense of urgency in identifying peripheral vascular occlusion. (A-3)

5–2.197 Value and defend the sense of urgency in recognizing signs of aortic aneurysm. (A-3)

PSYCHOMOTOR OBJECTIVES

At the completion of this unit, the paramedic student will be able to:

5–2.198 Demonstrate how to set and adjust the ECG monitor settings to varying patient situations. (P-3)

5–2.199 Demonstrate a working knowledge of various ECG lead systems. (P-3)

5–2.200 Demonstrate how to record an ECG. (P-2)

5–2.201 Perform, document, and communicate a cardiovascular assessment. (P-1)

5–2.202 Set up and apply a transcutaneous pacing system. (P-3)

5–2.203 Given the model of a patient with signs and symptoms of heart failure, position the patient to afford comfort and relief. (P-2)

5–2.204 Demonstrate how to determine if pulsus paradoxus, pulsus alternans, or electrical alternans is present. (P-2)

5–2.205 Demonstrate satisfactory performance of psychomotor skills of basic and advanced life support techniques according to the current American Heart Association Standards and Guidelines, including: (P-3)
   a. Cardiopulmonary resuscitation
   b. Defibrillation
   c. Synchronized cardioversion
   d. Transcutaneous pacing

5–2.206 Complete a communication patch with medical direction and law enforcement used for termination of resuscitation efforts. (P-1)

5–2.207 Demonstrate how to evaluate major peripheral arterial pulses. (P-1)

UNIT TERMINAL OBJECTIVE

5–3 At the completion of this unit, the paramedic student will be able to integrate pathophysiological principles and assessment findings to formulate a field impression and implement the treatment plan for the patient with a neurological problem.

COGNITIVE OBJECTIVES

At the completion of this unit, the paramedic student will be able to:

5–3.1 Describe the incidence, morbidity, and mortality of neurological emergencies. (C-1)

5–3.2 Identify the risk factors most predisposing to the nervous system. (C-1)

5–3.3 Discuss the anatomy and physiology of the organs and structures related to the nervous system. (C-1)

5–3.4 Discuss the pathophysiology of non-traumatic neurologic emergencies. (C-1)

5–3.5 Discuss the assessment findings associated with non-traumatic neurologic emergencies. (C-1)

5–3.6 Identify the need for rapid intervention and the transport of the patient with non-traumatic emergencies. (C-1)

5–3.7 Discuss the management of non-traumatic neurological emergencies. (C-1)

5–3.8 Discuss the pathophysiology of coma and altered mental status. (C-1)

5–3.9 Discuss the assessment findings associated with coma and altered mental status. (C-1)

5–3.10 Discuss the management/treatment plan of coma and altered mental status. (C-1)

5–3.11 Describe the epidemiology, including the morbidity/mortality and prevention strategies, for seizures. (C-1)

5–3.12 Discuss the pathophysiology of seizures. (C-1)

5–3.13 Discuss the assessment findings associated with seizures. (C-1)

5–3.14 Define seizure. (C-1)

5–3.15 Describe and differentiate the major types of seizures. (C-3)

5–3.16 List the most common causes of seizures. (C-1)

5–3.17 Describe the phases of a generalized seizure. (C-1)

5–3.18 Discuss the pathophysiology of syncope. (C-1)

5–3.19 Discuss the assessment findings associated with syncope. (C-1)

5–3.20 Discuss the management/treatment plan of syncope. (C-1)

5–3.21 Discuss the pathophysiology of headache. (C-1)

5–3.22 Discuss the assessment findings associated with headache. (C-1)

5–3.23 Discuss the management/treatment plan of headache. (C-1)

5–3.24 Describe the epidemiology, including the morbidity/mortality and prevention strategies, for neoplasms. (C-1)

5–3.25 Discuss the pathophysiology of neoplasms. (C-1)

5–3.26 Describe the types of neoplasms. (C-1)

5–3.27 Discuss the assessment findings associated with neoplasms. (C-1)

5–3.28 Discuss the management/treatment plan of neoplasms. (C-1)

5–3.29 Define neoplasms. (C-1)

5–3.30 Recognize the signs and symptoms related to neoplasms. (C-1)

5–3.31 Correlate abnormal assessment findings with clinical significance in the patient with neoplasms. (C-3)

5–3.32 Differentiate among the various treatment and pharmacological interventions used in the management of neoplasms. (C-3)

5–3.33 Integrate the pathophysiological principles and the assessment findings to formulate a field impression and implement a treatment plan for the patient with neoplasms. (C-3)

5–3.34   Describe the epidemiology, including the morbidity/mortality and prevention strategies, for abscess. (C-1)

5–3.35   Discuss the pathophysiology of abscess. (C-1)

5–3.36   Discuss the assessment findings associated with abscess. (C-1)

5–3.37   Discuss the management/treatment plan of abscess. (C-1)

5–3.38   Define abscess. (C-1)

5–3.39   Recognize the signs and symptoms related to abscess. (C-1)

5–3.40   Correlate abnormal assessment findings with clinical significance in the patient with abscess. (C-3)

5–3.41   Differentiate among the various treatment and pharmacological interventions used in the management of abscess. (C-3)

5–3.42   Integrate the pathophysiological principles and the assessment findings to formulate a field impression and implement a treatment plan for the patient with abscess. (C-3)

5–3.43   Describe the epidemiology, including the morbidity/mortality and prevention strategies, for stroke and intracranial hemorrhage. (C-1)

5–3.44   Discuss the pathophysiology of stroke and intracranial hemorrhage. (C-1)

5–3.45   Describe the types of stroke and intracranial hemorrhage. (C-1)

5–3.46   Discuss the assessment findings associated with stroke and intracranial hemorrhage. (C-1)

5–3.47   Discuss the management/treatment plan of stroke and intracranial hemorrhage. (C-1)

5–3.48   Define stroke and intracranial hemorrhage. (C-1)

5–3.49   Recognize the signs and symptoms related to stroke and intracranial hemorrhage. (C-1)

5–3.50   Correlate abnormal assessment findings with clinical significance in the patient with stroke and intracranial hemorrhage. (C-3)

5–3.51   Differentiate among the various treatment and pharmacological interventions used in the management of stroke and intracranial hemorrhage. (C-3)

5–3.52   Integrate the pathophysiological principles and the assessment findings to formulate a field impression and implement a treatment plan for the patient with stroke and intracranial hemorrhage. (C-3)

5–3.53   Describe the epidemiology, including the morbidity/mortality and prevention strategies, for transient ischemic attack. (C-3)

5–3.54   Discuss the pathophysiology of transient ischemic attack. (C-1)

5–3.55   Discuss the assessment findings associated with transient ischemic attack. (C-1)

5–3.56   Discuss the management/treatment plan of transient ischemic attack. (C-1)

5–3.57   Define transient ischemic attack. (C-1)

5–3.58   Recognize the signs and symptoms related to transient ischemic attack. (C-1)

5–3.59   Correlate abnormal assessment findings with clinical significance in the patient with transient ischemic attack. (C-3)

5–3.60   Differentiate among the various treatment and pharmacological interventions used in the management of transient ischemic attack. (C-3)

5–3.61   Integrate the pathophysiological principles and the assessment findings to formulate a field impression and implement a treatment plan for the patient with transient ischemic attack. (C-3)

5–3.62   Describe the epidemiology, including the morbidity/mortality and prevention strategies, for degenerative neurological diseases. (C-1)

5–3.63   Discuss the pathophysiology of degenerative neurological diseases. (C-1)

5–3.64   Discuss the assessment findings associated with degenerative neurological diseases. (C-1)

5–3.65   Discuss the management/treatment plan of degenerative neurological diseases. (C-1)

5–3.66   Define the following: (C-1)
a. Muscular dystrophy
b. Multiple sclerosis
c. Dystonia
d. Parkinson's disease
e. Trigeminal neuralgia
f. Bell's palsy
g. Amyotrophic lateral sclerosis
h. Peripheral neuropathy
i. Myoclonus
j. Spina bifida
k. Poliomyelitis

5–3.67   Recognize the signs and symptoms related to degenerative neurological diseases. (C-1)

5–3.68   Correlate abnormal assessment findings with clinical significance in the patient with degenerative neurological diseases. (C-3)

5–3.69   Differentiate among the various treatment and pharmacological interventions used in the management of degenerative neurological diseases. (C-3)

5–3.70   Integrate the pathophysiological principles and the assessment findings to formulate a field impression and implement a treatment plan for the patient with degenerative neurological diseases. (C-3)

5–3.71   Integrate the pathophysiological principles of the patient with a neurological emergency. (C-3)

5–3.72   Differentiate between neurological emergencies based on assessment findings. (C-3)

5–3.73   Correlate abnormal assessment findings with the clinical significance in the patient with neurological complaints. (C-3)

5–3.74   Develop a patient management plan based on field impression in the patient with neurological emergencies. (C-3)

AFFECTIVE OBJECTIVES

At the completion of this unit, the paramedic student will be able to:

5–3.75   Characterize the feelings of a patient who regains consciousness among strangers. (A-2)

5–3.76   Formulate means of conveying empathy to patients whose ability to communicate is limited by their condition. (A-3)

PSYCHOMOTOR OBJECTIVES

At the completion of this unit, the paramedic student will be able to:

5–3.77   Perform an appropriate assessment of a patient with coma or altered mental status. (P-3)

5–3.78 Perform a complete neurological examination as part of the comprehensive physical examination of a patient with coma or altered mental status. (P-3)

5–3.79 Appropriately manage a patient with coma or altered mental status, including the administration of oxygen, oral glucose, 50% dextrose, and narcotic reversal agents. (P-3)

5–3.80 Perform an appropriate assessment of a patient with syncope. (P-3)

5–3.81 Appropriately manage a patient with syncope. (P-3)

5–3.82 Perform an appropriate assessment of a patient with seizures. (P-3)

5–3.83 Appropriately manage a patient with seizures, including the administration of diazepam or lorazepam. (P-3)

5–3.84 Perform an appropriate assessment of a patient with stroke and intracranial hemorrhage or TIA. (P-3)

5–3.85 Appropriately manage a patient with stroke and intracranial hemorrhage or TIA. (P-3)

5–3.86 Demonstrate an appropriate assessment of a patient with a chief complaint of weakness. (P-3)

UNIT TERMINAL OBJECTIVE

5–4 At the completion of this unit, the paramedic student will be able to integrate pathophysiological principles and assessment findings to formulate a field impression and implement a treatment plan for the patient with an endocrine problem.

COGNITIVE OBJECTIVES

At the completion of this unit, the paramedic student will be able to:

5–4.1 Describe the incidence, morbidity, and mortality of endocrinologic emergencies. (C-1)

5–4.2 Identify the risk factors most predisposing to endocrinologic disease. (C-1)

5–4.3 Discuss the anatomy and physiology of organs and structures related to endocrinologic diseases. (C-1)

5–4.4 Review the pathophysiology of endocrinologic emergencies. (C-1)

5–4.5 Discuss the general assessment findings associated with endocrinologic emergencies. (C-1)

5–4.6 Identify the need for rapid intervention of the patient with endocrinologic emergencies. (C-1)

5–4.7 Discuss the management of endocrinologic emergencies. (C-1)

5–4.8 Describe osmotic diuresis and its relationship to diabetes. (C-1)

5–4.9 Describe the pathophysiology of adult onset diabetes mellitus. (C-1)

5–4.10 Describe the pathophysiology of juvenile onset diabetes mellitus. (C-1)

5–4.11 Describe the effects of decreased levels of insulin on the body. (C-1)

5–4.12 Correlate abnormal findings in assessment with clinical significance in the patient with a diabetic emergency. (C-3)

5–4.13 Discuss the management of diabetic emergencies. (C-1)

5–4.14 Integrate the pathophysiological principles and the assessment findings to formulate a field impression and implement a treatment plan for the patient with a diabetic emergency. (C-3)

5–4.15 Differentiate between the pathophysiology of normal glucose metabolism and diabetic glucose metabolism. (C-3)

5–4.16 Describe the mechanism of ketone body formation and its relationship to ketoacidosis. (C-1)

5–4.17 Discuss the physiology of the excretion of potassium and ketone bodies by the kidneys. (C-1)

5–4.18 Describe the relationship of insulin to serum glucose levels. (C-1)

5–4.19 Describe the effects of decreased levels of insulin on the body. (C-1)

5–4.20 Describe the effects of increased serum glucose levels on the body. (C-1)

5–4.21 Discuss the pathophysiology of hypoglycemia. (C-1)

5–4.22 Discuss the utilization of glycogen by the human body as it relates to the pathophysiology of hypoglycemia. (C-3)

5–4.23 Describe the actions of epinephrine as it relates to the pathophysiology of hypoglycemia. (C-3)

5–4.24 Recognize the signs and symptoms of the patient with hypoglycemia. (C-1)

5–4.25 Describe the compensatory mechanisms utilized by the body to promote homeostasis relative to hypoglycemia. (C-1)

5–4.26 Describe the management of a responsive hypoglycemic patient. (C-1)

5–4.27 Correlate abnormal findings in assessment with clinical significance in the patient with hypoglycemia. (C-1)

5–4.28 Discuss the management of the hypoglycemic patient. (C-1)

5–4.29 Integrate the pathophysiological principles and the assessment findings to formulate a field impression and implement a treatment plan for the patient with hypoglycemia. (C-3)

5–4.30 Discuss the pathophysiology of hyperglycemia. (C-1)

5–4.31 Recognize the signs and symptoms of the patient with hyperglycemia. (C-1)

5–4.32 Describe the management of hyperglycemia. (C-1)

5–4.33 Correlate abnormal findings in assessment with clinical significance in the patient with hyperglycemia. (C-3)

5–4.34 Discuss the management of the patient with hyperglycemia. (C-1)

5–4.35 Integrate the pathophysiological principles and the assessment findings to formulate a field impression and implement a treatment plan for the patient with hyperglycemia. (C-3)

5–4.36 Discuss the pathophysiology of nonketotic hyperosmolar coma. (C-1)

5–4.37 Recognize the signs and symptoms of the patient with nonketotic hyperosmolar coma. (C-1)

5–4.38 Describe the management of nonketotic hyperosmolar coma. (C-1)

5–4.39 Correlate abnormal findings in assessment with clinical significance in the patient with nonketotic hyperosmolar coma. (C-3)

5–4.40 Integrate the pathophysiological principles and the assessment findings to formulate a field impression and implement a treatment plan for the patient with nonketotic hyperosmolar coma. (C-3)

5–4.41 Discuss the management of the patient with hyperglycemia. (C-1)

5–4.42 Integrate the pathophysiological principles and the assessment findings to formulate a field impression and implement a treatment plan for the patient with hyperglycemia. (C-3)

5–4.43 Discuss the pathophysiology of diabetic ketoacidosis. (C-1)

5–4.44 Recognize the signs and symptoms of the patient with diabetic ketoacidosis. (C-1)

5–4.45 Describe the management of diabetic ketoacidosis. (C-1)

5–4.46 Correlate abnormal findings in assessment with clinical significance in the patient with diabetic ketoacidosis. (C-3)

5–4.47 Discuss the management of the patient with diabetic ketoacidosis. (C-1)

5–4.48 Integrate the pathophysiological principles and the assessment findings to formulate a field impression and implement a treatment plan for the patient with diabetic ketoacidosis. (C-3)

5–4.49 Discuss the pathophysiology of thyrotoxicosis. (C-1)

5–4.50 Recognize signs and symptoms of the patient with thyrotoxicosis. (C-1)

5–4.51 Describe the management of thyrotoxicosis. (C-1)

5–4.52 Correlate abnormal findings in assessment with clinical significance in the patient with thyrotoxicosis. (C-3)

5–4.53 Discuss the management of the patient with thyrotoxicosis. (C-1)

5–4.54 Integrate the pathophysiological principles and the assessment findings to formulate a field impression and implement a treatment plan for the patient with thyrotoxicosis. (C-3)

5–4.55 Discuss the pathophysiology of myxedema. (C-1)

5–4.56 Recognize signs and symptoms of the patient with myxedema. (C-1)

5–4.57 Describe the management of myxedema. (C-1)

5–4.58 Correlate abnormal findings in assessment with clinical significance in the patient with myxedema. (C-3)

5–4.59 Discuss the management of the patient with myxedema. (C-1)

5–4.60 Integrate the pathophysiological principles and the assessment findings to formulate a field impression and implement a treatment plan for the patient with myxedema. (C-3)

5–4.61 Discuss the pathophysiology of Cushing's syndrome. (C-1)

5–4.62 Recognize signs and symptoms of the patient with Cushing's syndrome. (C-1)

5–4.63 Describe the management of Cushing's syndrome. (C-1)

5–4.64 Correlate abnormal findings in assessment with clinical significance in the patient with Cushing's syndrome. (C-3)

5–4.65 Discuss the management of the patient with Cushing's syndrome. (C-1)

5–4.66 Integrate the pathophysiological principles and the assessment findings to formulate a field impression and implement a treatment plan for the patient with Cushing's syndrome. (C-3)

5–4.67 Discuss the pathophysiology of adrenal insufficiency. (C-1)

5–4.68 Recognize signs and symptoms of the patient with adrenal insufficiency. (C-1)

5–4.69 Describe the management of adrenal insufficiency. (C-1)

5–4.70 Correlate abnormal findings in assessment with clinical significance in the patient with adrenal insufficiency. (C-3)

5–4.71 Discuss the management of the patient with adrenal insufficiency. (C-1)

5–4.72 Integrate the pathophysiological principles and the assessment findings to formulate a field impression and im-

plement a treatment plan for the patient with adrenal insufficiency. (C-3)

5–4.73 Integrate the pathophysiological principles into the assessment of a patient with an endocrinological emergency. (C-3)

5–4.74 Differentiate between endocrine emergencies based on assessment and history. (C-3)

5–4.75 Correlate abnormal findings in the assessment with clinical significance in the patient with endocrinologic emergencies. (C-3)

5–4.76 Develop a patient management plan based on field impression in the patient with an endocrinologic emergency. (C-3)

AFFECTIVE OBJECTIVES

None identified for this unit.

PSYCHOMOTOR OBJECTIVES

None identified for this unit.

UNIT TERMINAL OBJECTIVE

5–5 At the completion of this unit, the paramedic student will be able to integrate pathophysiological principles and assessment findings to formulate a field impression and implement a treatment plan for the patient with an allergic or anaphylactic reaction.

COGNITIVE OBJECTIVES

At the completion of this unit, the paramedic student will be able to:

5–5.1 Define allergic reaction. (C-1)

5–5.2 Define anaphylaxis. (C-1)

5–5.3 Describe the incidence, morbidity, and mortality of anaphylaxis. (C-1)

5–5.4 Identify the risk factors most predisposing to anaphylaxis. (C-1)

5–5.5 Discuss the anatomy and physiology of the organs and structures related to anaphylaxis. (C-1)

5–5.6 Describe the prevention of anaphylaxis and appropriate patient education. (C-1)

5–5.7 Discuss the pathophysiology of allergy and anaphylaxis. (C-1)

5–5.8 Describe the common methods of entry of substances into the body. (C-1)

5–5.9 Define natural and acquired immunity. (C-1)

5–5.10 Define antigens and antibodies. (C-1)

5–5.11 List common antigens most frequently associated with anaphylaxis. (C-1)

5–5.12 Discuss the formation of antibodies in the body. (C-1)

5–5.13 Describe physical manifestations in anaphylaxis. (C-1)

5–5.14 Differentiate manifestations of an allergic reaction from anaphylaxis. (C-3)

5–5.15 Recognize the signs and symptoms related to anaphylaxis. (C-1)

5–5.16 Differentiate among the various treatment and pharmacological interventions used in the management of anaphylaxis. (C-3)

5–5.17 Integrate the pathophysiological principles of the patient with anaphylaxis. (C-3)

5–5.18 Correlate the abnormal findings in assessment with the clinical significance in the patient with anaphylaxis. (C-3)

5–5.19 Develop a treatment plan based on field impression in the patient with allergic reaction and anaphylaxis. (C-3)

AFFECTIVE OBJECTIVES

None identified for this unit.

PSYCHOMOTOR OBJECTIVES

None identified for this unit.

UNIT TERMINAL OBJECTIVE

5–6 At the completion of this unit, the paramedic student will be able to integrate pathophysiological principles and assessment findings to formulate a field impression and implement the treatment plan for the patient with a gastroenterologic problem.

COGNITIVE OBJECTIVES

At the conclusion of this unit, the paramedic student will be able to:

5–6.1 Describe the incidence, morbidity, and mortality of gastrointestinal emergencies. (C-1)

5–6.2 Identify the risk factors most predisposing to gastrointestinal emergencies. (C-1)

5–6.3 Discuss the anatomy and physiology of the organs and structures related to gastrointestinal diseases. (C-1)

5–6.4 Discuss the pathophysiology of inflammation and its relationship to acute abdominal pain. (C-1)

5–6.5 Define somatic pain as it relates to gastroenterology. (C-1)

5–6.6 Define visceral pain as it relates to gastroenterology. (C-1)

5–6.7 Define referred pain as it relates to gastroenterology. (C-1)

5–6.8 Differentiate between hemorrhagic and non-hemorrhagic abdominal pain. (C-3)

5–6.9 Discuss the signs and symptoms of local inflammation relative to acute abdominal pain. (C-1)

5–6.10 Discuss the signs and symptoms of peritoneal inflammation relative to acute abdominal pain. (C-1)

5–6.11 List the signs and symptoms of general inflammation relative to acute abdominal pain. (C-1)

5–6.12 Based on assessment findings, differentiate between local, peritoneal, and general inflammation as they relate to acute abdominal pain. (C-3)

5–6.13 Describe the questioning technique and specific questions the paramedic should ask when gathering a focused history in a patient with abdominal pain. (C-1)

5–6.14 Describe the technique for performing a comprehensive physical examination on a patient complaining of abdominal pain. (C-1)

5–6.15 Define upper gastrointestinal bleeding. (C-1)

5–6.16 Discuss the pathophysiology of upper gastrointestinal bleeding. (C-1)

5–6.17 Recognize the signs and symptoms related to upper gastrointestinal bleeding. (C-1)

5–6.18 Describe the management for upper gastrointestinal bleeding. (C-1)

5–6.19 Integrate pathophysiological principles and assessment findings to formulate a field impression and implement a treatment plan for the patient with upper GI bleeding. (C-3)

5–6.20 Define lower gastrointestinal bleeding. (C-1)

5–6.21 Discuss the pathophysiology of lower gastrointestinal bleeding. (C-1)

5–6.22 Recognize the signs and symptoms related to lower gastrointestinal bleeding. (C-1)

5–6.23 Describe the management for lower gastrointestinal bleeding. (C-1)

5–6.24 Integrate pathophysiological principles and assessment findings to formulate a field impression and implement a treatment plan for the patient with lower GI bleeding. (C-3)

5–6.25 Define acute gastroenteritis. (C-1)

5–6.26 Discuss the pathophysiology of acute gastroenteritis. (C-1)

5–6.27 Recognize the signs and symptoms related to acute gastroenteritis. (C-1)

5–6.28 Describe the management for acute gastroenteritis. (C-1)

5–6.29 Integrate pathophysiological principles and assessment findings to formulate a field impression and implement a treatment plan for the patient with acute gastroenteritis. (C-3)

5–6.30 Define colitis. (C-1)

5–6.31 Discuss the pathophysiology of colitis. (C-1)

5–6.32 Recognize the signs and symptoms related to colitis. (C-1)

5–6.33 Describe the management for colitis. (C-1)

5–6.34 Integrate pathophysiological principles and assessment findings to formulate a field impression and implement a treatment plan for the patient with colitis. (C-3)

5–6.35 Define gastroenteritis. (C-1)

5–6.36 Discuss the pathophysiology of gastroenteritis. (C-1)

5–6.37 Recognize the signs and symptoms related to gastroenteritis. (C-1)

5–6.38 Describe the management for gastroenteritis. (C-1)

5–6.39 Integrate pathophysiological principles and assessment findings to formulate a field impression and implement a treatment plan for the patient with gastroenteritis. (C-3)

5–6.40 Define diverticulitis. (C-1)

5–6.41 Discuss the pathophysiology of diverticulitis. (C-1)

5–6.42 Recognize the signs and symptoms related to diverticulitis. (C-1)

5–6.43 Describe the management for diverticulitis. (C-1)

5–6.44 Integrate pathophysiological principles and assessment findings to formulate a field impression and implement a treatment plan for the patient with diverticulitis. (C-3)

5–6.45 Define appendicitis. (C-1)

5–6.46 Discuss the pathophysiology of appendicitis. (C-1)

5–6.47 Recognize the signs and symptoms related to appendicitis. (C-1)

5–6.48 Describe the management for appendicitis. (C-1)

5–6.49 Integrate pathophysiological principles and assessment findings to formulate a field impression and implement a treatment plan for the patient with appendicitis. (C-3)

5–6.50 Define peptic ulcer disease. (C-1)

5–6.51 Discuss the pathophysiology of peptic ulcer disease. (C-1)

5–6.52 Recognize the signs and symptoms related to peptic ulcer disease. (C-1)

5–6.53 Describe the management for peptic ulcer disease. (C-1)

5–6.54 Integrate pathophysiological principles and assessment findings to formulate a field impression and implement a treatment plan for the patient with peptic ulcer disease. (C-3)

5–6.55 Define bowel obstruction. (C-1)

5–6.56 Discuss the pathophysiology of bowel obstruction. (C-1)

5–6.57 Recognize the signs and symptoms related to bowel obstruction. (C-1)

5–6.58 Describe the management for bowel obstruction. (C-1)

5–6.59 Integrate pathophysiological principles and assessment findings to formulate a field impression and implement a treatment plan for the patient with bowel obstruction. (C-3)

5–6.60 Define Crohn's disease. (C-1)

5–6.61 Discuss the pathophysiology of Crohn's disease. (C-1)

5–6.62 Recognize the signs and symptoms related to Crohn's disease. (C-1)

5–6.63 Describe the management for Crohn's disease. (C-1)

5–6.64 Integrate pathophysiological principles and assessment findings to formulate a field impression and implement a treatment plan for the patient with Crohn's disease. (C-3)

5–6.65 Define pancreatitis. (C-1)

5–6.66 Discuss the pathophysiology of pancreatitis. (C-1)

5–6.67 Recognize the signs and symptoms related to pancreatitis. (C-1)

5–6.68 Describe the management for pancreatitis. (C-1)

5–6.69 Integrate pathophysiological principles and assessment findings to formulate a field impression and implement a treatment plan for the patient with pancreatitis. (C-3)

5–6.70 Define esophageal varices. (C-1)

5–6.71 Discuss the pathophysiology of esophageal varices. (C-1)

5–6.72 Recognize the signs and symptoms related to esophageal varices. (C-1)

5–6.73 Describe the management for esophageal varices. (C-1)

5–6.74 Integrate pathophysiological principles and assessment findings to formulate a field impression and implement a treatment plan for the patient with esophageal varices. (C-3)

5–6.75 Define hemorrhoids. (C-1)

5–6.76 Discuss the pathophysiology of hemorrhoids. (C-1)

5–6.77 Recognize the signs and symptoms related to hemorrhoids. (C-1)

5–6.78 Describe the management for hemorrhoids. (C-1)

5–6.79 Integrate pathophysiological principles and assessment findings to formulate a field impression and implement a treatment plan for the patient with hemorrhoids. (C-3)

5–6.80 Define cholecystitis. (C-1)

5–6.81 Discuss the pathophysiology of cholecystitis. (C-1)

5–6.82 Recognize the signs and symptoms related to cholecystitis. (C-1)

5–6.83 Describe the management for cholecystitis. (C-1)

5–6.84 Integrate pathophysiological principles and assessment findings to formulate a field impression and implement a treatment plan for the patient with cholecystitis. (C-3)

5–6.85 Define acute hepatitis. (C-1)

5–6.86 Discuss the pathophysiology of acute hepatitis. (C-1)

5–6.87 Recognize the signs and symptoms related to acute hepatitis. (C-1)

5–6.88 Describe the management for acute hepatitis. (C-1)

5–6.89 Integrate pathophysiological principles and assessment findings to formulate a field impression and implement a treatment plan for the patient with acute hepatitis. (C-3)

5–6.90 Integrate pathophysiological principles of the patient with a gastrointestinal emergency. (C-3)

5–6.91 Differentiate between gastrointestinal emergencies based on assessment findings. (C-3)

5–6.92 Correlate abnormal findings in the assessment with the clinical significance in the patient with abdominal pain. (C-3)

5–6.93 Develop a patient management plan based on field impression in the patient with abdominal pain. (C-3)

AFFECTIVE OBJECTIVES

None identified for this unit.

PSYCHOMOTOR OBJECTIVES

None identified for this unit.

UNIT TERMINAL OBJECTIVE

5–7 At the completion of this unit, the paramedic student will be able to integrate pathophysiological principles and the assessment findings to formulate a field impression and implement a treatment plan for the patient with a renal or urologic problem.

COGNITIVE OBJECTIVES

At the completion of this unit, the paramedic student will be able to:

5–7.1 Describe the incidence, morbidity, mortality, and risk factors predisposing to urological emergencies. (C-1)

5–7.2 Discuss the anatomy and physiology of the organs and structures related to urogenital diseases. (C-1)

5–7.3 Define referred pain and visceral pain as it relates to urology. (C-1)

5–7.4 Describe the questioning technique and specific questions the paramedic should utilize when gathering a focused history in a patient with abdominal pain. (C-1)

5–7.5 Describe the technique for performing a comprehensive physical examination of a patient complaining of abdominal pain. (C-1)

5–7.6 Define acute renal failure. (C-1)

5–7.7 Discuss the pathophysiology of acute renal failure. (C-1)

5–7.8 Recognize the signs and symptoms related to acute renal failure. (C-1)

5–7.9 Describe the management for acute renal failure. (C-1)

5–7.10 Integrate pathophysiological principles and assessment findings to formulate a field impression and implement a treatment plan for the patient with acute renal failure. (C-3)

5–7.11 Define chronic renal failure. (C-1)

5–7.12 Discuss the pathophysiology of chronic renal failure. (C-1)

5–7.13 Recognize the signs and symptoms related to chronic renal failure. (C-1)

5–7.14 Describe the management for chronic renal failure. (C-1)

5–7.15 Integrate pathophysiological principles and assessment findings to formulate a field impression and implement a treatment plan for the patient with chronic renal failure. (C-3)

5–7.16 Define renal dialysis. (C-1)

5–7.17 Discuss the common complication of renal dialysis. (C-1)

5–7.18 Define renal calculi. (C-1)

5–7.19 Discuss the pathophysiology of renal calculi. (C-1)

5–7.20 Recognize the signs and symptoms related to renal calculi. (C-1)

5–7.21 Describe the management for renal calculi. (C-1)

5–7.22 Integrate pathophysiological principles and assessment findings to formulate a field impression and implement a treatment plan for the patient with renal calculi. (C-3)

5–7.23 Define urinary tract infection. (C-1)

5–7.24 Discuss the pathophysiology of urinary tract infection. (C-1)

5–7.25 Recognize the signs and symptoms related to urinary tract infection. (C-1)

5–7.26 Describe the management for a urinary tract infection. (C-1)

5–7.27 Integrate pathophysiological principles and assessment findings to formulate a field impression and implement a treatment plan for the patient with a urinary tract infection. (C-3)

5–7.28 Apply the epidemiology to develop prevention strategies for urological emergencies. (C-2)

5–7.29 Integrate pathophysiological principles into the assessment of a patient with abdominal pain. (C-3)

5–7.30 Synthesize assessment findings and patient history information to accurately differentiate between pain of a urogenital emergency and that of other origins. (C-3)

5–7.31 Develop, execute, and evaluate a treatment plan based on the field impression made in the assessment. (C-3)

AFFECTIVE OBJECTIVES

None identified for this unit.

PSYCHOMOTOR OBJECTIVES

None identified for this unit.

UNIT TERMINAL OBJECTIVE

5–8 At the completion of this unit, the paramedic student will be able to integrate pathophysiological principles and assessment findings to formulate a field impression and implement a treatment plan for the patient with a toxic exposure.

COGNITIVE OBJECTIVES

At the completion of this unit, the paramedic student will be able to:

5–8.1 Describe the incidence, morbidity, and mortality of toxic emergencies. (C-1)

5–8.2 Identify the risk factors most predisposing to toxic emergencies. (C-1)

5–8.3 Discuss the anatomy and physiology of the organs and structures related to toxic emergencies. (C-1)

5–8.4 Describe the routes of entry of toxic substances into the body. (C-1)

5–8.5 Discuss the role of the Poison Control Center in the United States. (C-1)

5–8.6 List the toxic substances that are specific to your region. (C-1)

5–8.7 Discuss the pathophysiology of the entry of toxic substances into the body. (C-1)

5–8.8 Discuss the assessment findings associated with various toxidromes. (C-1)

5–8.9 Identify the need for rapid intervention and transport of the patient with a toxic substance emergency. (C-1)

5–8.10 Discuss the management of toxic substances. (C-1)

5–8.11 Define poisoning by ingestion. (C-1)

5–8.12 List the most common poisonings by ingestion. (C-1)

5–8.13 Describe the pathophysiology of poisoning by ingestion. (C-1)

5–8.14 Recognize the signs and symptoms related to the most common poisonings by ingestion. (C-1)

5–8.15 Correlate the abnormal findings in assessment with the clinical significance in the patient with the most common poisonings by ingestion. (C-1)

5–8.16 Differentiate among the various treatments and pharmacological interventions in the management of the most common poisonings by ingestion. (C-3)

5–8.17 Discuss the factors affecting the decision to induce vomiting in a patient with ingested poison. (C-1)

5–8.18 Integrate pathophysiological principles and the assessment findings to formulate a field impression and implement a treatment plan for the patient with the most common poisonings by ingestion. (C-3)

5–8.19 Define poisoning by inhalation. (C-1)

5–8.20 List the most common poisonings by inhalation. (C-1)

5–8.21 Describe the pathophysiology of poisoning by inhalation. (C-1)

5–8.22 Recognize the signs and symptoms related to the most common poisonings by inhalation. (C-1)

5–8.23 Correlate the abnormal findings in assessment with the clinical significance in patients with the most common poisonings by inhalation. (C-1)

5–8.24 Differentiate among the various treatments and pharmacological interventions in the management of the most common poisonings by inhalation. (C-3)

5–8.25 Integrate pathophysiological principles and the assessment findings to formulate a field impression and implement a treatment plan for the patient with the most common poisonings by inhalation. (C-3)

5–8.26 Define poisoning by injection. (C-1)

5–8.27 List the most common poisonings by injection. (C-1)

5–8.28 Describe the pathophysiology of poisoning by injection. (C-1)

5–8.29 Recognize the signs and symptoms related to the most common poisonings by injection. (C-1)

5–8.30 Correlate the abnormal findings in assessment with the clinical significance in the patient with the most common poisonings by injection. (C-3)

5–8.31 Differentiate among the various treatments and pharmacological interventions in the management of the most common poisonings by injection. (C-3)

5–8.32 Integrate pathophysiological principles and the assessment findings to formulate a field impression and implement a treatment plan for the patient with the most common poisonings by injection. (C-3)

5–8.33 Define poisoning by surface absorption. (C-1)

5–8.34 List the most common poisonings by surface absorption. (C-1)

5–8.35 Describe the pathophysiology of poisoning by surface absorption. (C-1)

5–8.36 Recognize the signs and symptoms related to the most common poisonings by surface absorption. (C-1)

5–8.37 Correlate the abnormal findings in assessment with the clinical significance in patients with the most common poisonings by surface absorption. (C-3)

5–8.38 Differentiate among the various treatments and pharmacological interventions in the management of the most common poisonings by surface absorption. (C-3)

5–8.39 Integrate pathophysiological principles and the assessment findings to formulate a field impression and implement a treatment plan for patients with the most common poisonings by surface absorption. (C-3)

5–8.40 Define poisoning by overdose. (C-1)

5–8.41 List the most common poisonings by overdose. (C-1)

5–8.42 Describe the pathophysiology of poisoning by overdose. (C-1)

5–8.43 Recognize the signs and symptoms related to the most common poisonings by overdose. (C-1)

5–8.44 Correlate the abnormal findings in assessment with the clinical significance in patients with the most common poisonings by overdose. (C-3)

5–8.45 Differentiate among the various treatments and pharmacological interventions in the management of the most common poisonings by overdose. (C-3)

5–8.46 Integrate pathophysiological principles and the assessment findings to formulate a field impression and implement a treatment plan for patients with the most common poisonings by overdose. (C-3)

5–8.47 Define drug abuse. (C-1)

5–8.48 Discuss the incidence of drug abuse in the United States. (C-1)

5–8.49 Define the following terms: (C-1)
a. Substance or drug abuse
b. Substance or drug dependence
c. Tolerance
d. Withdrawal
e. Addiction

5–8.50 List the most commonly abused drugs (both by chemical name and street names). (C-1)

5–8.51 Describe the pathophysiology of commonly used drugs. (C-1)

5–8.52 Recognize the signs and symptoms related to the most commonly abused drugs. (C-1)

5–8.53 Correlate the abnormal findings in assessment with the clinical significance in patients using the most commonly abused drugs. (C-3)

5–8.54 Differentiate among the various treatments and pharmacological interventions in the management of the most commonly abused drugs. (C-3)

5–8.55 Integrate pathophysiological principles and the assessment findings to formulate a field impression and implement a treatment plan for patients using the most commonly abused drugs. (C-3)

5–8.56 List the clinical uses, street names, pharmacology, assessment finding, and management for patients who have taken the following drugs or been exposed to the following substances: (C-1)
a. Cocaine
b. Marijuana and cannabis compounds
c. Amphetamines and amphetamine-like drugs
d. Barbiturates
e. Sedative-hypnotics
f. Cyanide
g. Narcotics/opiates
h. Cardiac medications
i. Caustics
j. Common household substances
k. Drugs abused for sexual purposes/sexual gratification
l. Carbon monoxide
m. Alcohols
n. Hydrocarbons
o. Psychiatric medications
p. Newer antidepressants and serotonin syndromes
q. Lithium
r. MAO inhibitors
s. Nonprescription pain medications
   1. Nonsteroidal anti-inflammatory agents
   2. Salicylates
   3. Acetaminophen
t. Theophylline
u. Metals
v. Plants and mushrooms

5–8.57 Discuss common causative agents, pharmacology, assessment findings, and management for a patient with food poisoning. (C-1)

5–8.58 Discuss common offending organisms, pharmacology, assessment findings, and management for a patient with a bite or sting. (C-1)

5–8.59 Integrate pathophysiological principles of the patient with a toxic substance exposure. (C-1)

5–8.60 Differentiate between toxic substance emergencies based on assessment findings. (C-3)

5–8.61 Correlate abnormal findings in the assessment with the clinical significance in the patient exposed to a toxic substance. (C-3)

5–8.62 Develop a patient management plan based on field impression in the patient exposed to a toxic substance. (C-3)

AFFECTIVE OBJECTIVES

None identified for this unit.

PSYCHOMOTOR OBJECTIVES

None identified for this unit.

UNIT TERMINAL OBJECTIVE

5–9 At the completion of this unit, the paramedic student will be able to integrate the pathophysiological principles of the hematopoietic system to formulate a field impression and implement a treatment plan.

COGNITIVE OBJECTIVES

At the completion to this unit, the paramedic student will be able to:

5–9.1 Identify the anatomy of the hematopoietic system. (C-1)

5–9.2 Describe volume and volume-control related to the hematopoietic system. (C-1)

5–9.3 Identify and describe the blood-forming organs. (C-1)

5–9.4 Describe normal red blood cell (RBC) production, function, and destruction. (C-1)

5–9.5 Explain the significance of the hematocrit with respect to red cell size and number. (C-1)

5–9.6 Explain the correlation of the RBC count, hematocrit, and hemoglobin values. (C-1)

5–9.7 Define anemia. (C-1)

5–9.8 Describe normal white blood cell (WBC) production, function, and destruction. (C-1)

5–9.9 Identify the characteristics of the inflammatory process. (C-1)

5–9.10 Identify the difference between cellular and humoral immunity. (C-1)

5–9.11 Identify alterations in immunologic response. (C-1)

5–9.12 Describe the number, normal function, types, and life span of leukocytes. (C-1)

5–9.13 List the leukocyte disorders. (C-1)

5–9.14 Describe platelets with respect to normal function, life span, and numbers. (C-1)

5–9.15 Describe the components of the hemostatic mechanism. (C-1)

5–9.16 Describe the function of coagulation factors, platelets, and blood vessels necessary for normal coagulation. (C-1)

5–9.17 Describe the intrinsic and extrinsic clotting systems with respect to identification of factor deficiencies in each stage. (C-3)

5–9.18 Identify blood groups. (C-1)

5–9.19 Describe how acquired factor deficiencies may occur. (C-3)

5–9.20 Define fibrinolysis. (C-1)

5–9.21 Identify the components of physical assessment as they relate to the hematologic system. (C-1)

5–9.22 Describe the pathology and clinical manifestations and prognosis associated with: (C-3)
   a. Anemia
   b. Leukemia
   c. Lymphomas
   d. Polycythemia
   e. Disseminated intravascular coagulopathy
   f. Hemophilia
   g. Sickle cell disease
   h. Multiple myeloma

5–9.23 Integrate pathophysiological principles into the assessment of a patient with hematologic disease. (C-3)

AFFECTIVE OBJECTIVES

At the completion of this unit, the paramedic student will be able to:

5–9.24 Value the sense of urgency for initial assessment and interventions for patients with hematologic crises.

PSYCHOMOTOR OBJECTIVES

At the completion of this unit, the paramedic student will be able to:

5–9.25 Perform an assessment of the patient with hematologic disorder. (P-1)

UNIT TERMINAL OBJECTIVE

5–10 At the completion of this unit, the paramedic student will be able to integrate pathophysiological principles and assessment findings to formulate a field impression and implement the treatment plan for the patient with an environmentally induced or exacerbated medical or traumatic condition.

COGNITIVE OBJECTIVES

At the completion of this unit, the paramedic student will be able to:

5–10.1 Define "environmental emergency." (C-1)

5–10.2 Describe the incidence, morbidity, and mortality associated with environmental emergencies. (C-1)

5–10.3 Identify risk factors most predisposing to environmental emergencies. (C-1)

5–10.4 Identify environmental factors that may cause illness or exacerbate a preexisting illness. (C-1)

5–10.5 Identify environmental factors that may complicate treatment or transport decisions. (C-1)

5–10.6 List the principal types of environmental illnesses. (C-1)

5–10.7 Define "homeostasis" and relate the concept to environmental influences. (C-1)

5–10.8 Identify normal, critically high, and critically low body temperatures. (C-1)

5–10.9 Describe several methods of temperature monitoring. (C-1)

5–10.10 Identify the components of the body's thermoregulatory mechanism. (C-1)

5–10.11 Describe the general process of thermal regulation, including substances used and wastes generated. (C-1)

5–10.12 Describe the body's compensatory process for overheating. (C-1)

5–10.13 Describe the body's compensatory process for excess heat loss. (C-1)

5–10.14 List the common forms of heat and cold disorders. (C-1)

5–10.15 List the common predisposing factors associated with heat and cold disorders. (C-1)

5–10.16 List the common preventative measures associated with heat and cold disorders. (C-1)

5–10.17 Integrate the pathophysiological principles and complicating factors common to environmental emergencies and discuss differentiating features between emergent and urgent presentations. (C-3)

5–10.18 Define heat illness. (C-1)

5–10.19 Describe the pathophysiology of heat illness. (C-1)

5–10.20 Identify signs and symptoms of heat illness. (C-1)

5–10.21 List the predisposing factors for heat illness. (C-1)

5–10.22 List measures to prevent heat illness. (C-1)

5–10.23 Discuss the symptomatic variations presented in progressive heat disorders. (C-1)

5–10.24 Relate symptomatic findings to the commonly used terms: heat cramps, heat exhaustion, and heatstroke. (C-3)

5–10.25 Correlate the abnormal findings in assessment with their clinical significance in the patient with heat illness. (C-3)

5–10.26 Describe the contribution of dehydration to the development of heat disorders. (C-1)

5–10.27 Describe the differences between classical and exertional heatstroke. (C-1)

5–10.28 Define fever and discuss its pathophysiologic mechanism. (C-1)

5–10.29 Identify the fundamental thermoregulatory difference between fever and heatstroke. (C-1)

5–10.30 Discuss how one may differentiate between fever and heatstroke. (C-1)

5–10.31 Discuss the role of fluid therapy in the treatment of heat disorders. (C-1)

5–10.32 Differentiate among the various treatments and interventions in the management of heat disorders. (C-3)

5–10.33 Integrate the pathophysiological principles and the assessment findings to formulate a field impression and implement a treatment plan for the patient who has dehydration, heat exhaustion, or heatstroke. (C-3)

5–10.34 Define hypothermia. (C-1)

5–10.35 Describe the pathophysiology of hypothermia. (C-1)

5–10.36 List predisposing factors for hypothermia. (C-1)

5–10.37 List measures to prevent hypothermia. (C-1)

5–10.38 Identify differences between mild and severe hypothermia. (C-1)

5–10.39 Describe differences between chronic and acute hypothermia. (C-1)

5–10.40 List signs and symptoms of hypothermia. (C-1)

5–10.41 Correlate abnormal findings in assessment with their clinical significance in the patient with hypothermia. (C-3)

5–10.42 Discuss the impact of severe hypothermia on standard BCLS and ACLS algorithms and transport considerations. (C-1)

5–10.43 Integrate pathophysiological principles and the assessment findings to formulate a field impression and implement a treatment plan for the patient who has either mild or severe hypothermia. (C-3)

5–10.44 Define frostbite. (C-1)

5–10.45 Define superficial frostbite (frostnip). (C-1)

5–10.46 Differentiate between superficial frostbite and deep frostbite. (C-3)

5–10.47 List predisposing factors for frostbite. (C-1)

5–10.48 List measures to prevent frostbite. (C-1)

5–10.49 Correlate abnormal findings in assessment with their clinical significance in the patient with frostbite. (C-3)

5–10.50 Differentiate among the various treatments and interventions in the management of frostbite. (C-3)

5–10.51 Integrate pathophysiological principles and the assessment findings to formulate a field impression and implement a treatment plan for the patient with superficial or deep frostbite. (C-3)

5–10.52 Define near-drowning. (C-1)

5–10.53 Describe the pathophysiology of near-drowning. (C-1)

5–10.54 List signs and symptoms of near-drowning. (C-1)

5–10.55 Describe the lack of significance of fresh versus saltwater immersion, as it relates to near-drowning. (C-3)

5–10.56 Discuss the incidence of "wet" versus "dry" drownings and the differences in their management. (C-3)

5–10.57 Discuss the complications and protective role of hypothermia in the context of near-drowning. (C-1)

5–10.58 Correlate the abnormal findings in assessment with the clinical significance in the patient with near-drowning. (C-3)

5–10.59 Differentiate among the various treatments and interventions in the management of near-drowning. (C-3)

5–10.60 Integrate pathophysiological principles and assessment findings to formulate a field impression and implement a treatment plan for the near-drowning patient. (C-3)

5–10.61 Define self contained underwater breathing apparatus (SCUBA). (C-1)

5–10.62 Describe the laws of gasses and relate them to diving emergencies. (C-1)

5–10.63 Describe the pathophysiology of diving emergencies. (C-1)

5–10.64 Define decompression illness (DCI). (C-1)

5–10.65 Identify the various forms of DCI. (C-1)

5–10.66 Identify the various conditions that may result from pulmonary over-pressure accidents. (C-1)

5–10.67 Differentiate between the various diving emergencies. (C-3)

5–10.68 List signs and symptoms of diving emergencies. (C-1)

5–10.69 Correlate abnormal findings in assessment with their clinical significance in the patient with a diving related illness. (C-3)

5–10.70 Describe the function of the Divers Alert Network (DAN) and how its members may aid in the management of diving related illnesses. (C-1)

5–10.71 Differentiate among the various treatments and interventions for the management of diving accidents. (C-3)

5–10.72 Describe the specific function and benefit of hyperbaric oxygen therapy for the management of diving accidents. (C-1)

5–10.73 Integrate pathophysiological principles and assessment findings to formulate a field impression and implement a management plan for the patient who has had a diving accident. (C-3)

5–10.74 Define altitude illness. (C-1)

5–10.75 Describe the application of gas laws to altitude illness. (C-2)

5–10.76 Describe the etiology and epidemiology of altitude illness. (C-1)

5–10.77 List predisposing factors for altitude illness. (C-1)

5–10.78 List measures to prevent altitude illness. (C-1)

5–10.79 Define acute mountain sickness (AMS). (C-1)

5–10.80 Define high altitude pulmonary edema (HAPE). (C-1)

5–10.81 Define high altitude cerebral edema (HACE). (C-1)

5–10.82 Discuss the symptomatic variations presented in progressive altitude illnesses. (C-1)

5–10.83 List signs and symptoms of altitude illnesses. (C-1)

5–10.84 Correlate abnormal findings in assessment with their clinical significance in the patient with altitude illness. (C-3)

5–10.85 Discuss the pharmacology appropriate for the treatment of altitude illnesses. (C-1)

5–10.86 Differentiate among the various treatments and interventions for the management of altitude illness. (C-3)

5–10.87 Integrate pathophysiological principles and assessment findings to formulate a field impression and implement a treatment plan for the patient who has altitude illness. (C-1)

5–10.88 Integrate the pathophysiological principles of the patient affected by an environmental emergency. (C-3)

5–10.89 Differentiate between environmental emergencies based on assessment findings. (C-3)

5–10.90 Correlate abnormal findings in the assessment with their clinical significance in the patient affected by an environmental emergency. (C-3)

5–10.91 Develop a patient management plan based on the field impression of the patient affected by an environmental emergency. (C-3)

AFFECTIVE OBJECTIVES

None identified for this unit.

PSYCHOMOTOR OBJECTIVES

None identified for this unit.

UNIT TERMINAL OBJECTIVE

5–11 At the completion of this unit, the paramedic student will be able to integrate pathophysiological principles and assessment findings to formulate a field impression and implement a management plan for the patient with infectious and communicable diseases.

COGNITIVE OBJECTIVES

At the completion of this unit, the paramedic student will be able to:

5–11.1 Review the specific anatomy and physiology pertinent to infectious and communicable diseases. (C-1)

5–11.2 Define specific terminology identified with infectious/communicable diseases. (C-1)

5–11.3 Discuss public health principles relevant to infectious/communicable disease. (C-1)

5–11.4 Identify public health agencies involved in the prevention and management of disease outbreaks. (C-1)

5–11.5 List and describe the steps of an infectious process. (C-1)

5–11.6 Discuss the risks associated with infection. (C-1)

5–11.7 List and describe the stages of infectious diseases. (C-1)

5–11.8 List and describe infectious agents, including bacteria, viruses, fungi, protozoans, and helminths (worms). (C-1)

5–11.9 Describe host defense mechanisms against infection. (C-1)

5–11.10 Describe characteristics of the immune system, including the categories of white blood cells, the reticuloendothelial system (RES), and the complement system. (C-1)

5–11.11 Describe the processes of the immune system defenses, to include humoral and cell-mediated immunity. (C-1)

5–11.12 In specific diseases, identify and discuss the issues of personal isolation. (C-1)

5–11.13 Describe and discuss the rationale for the various types of PPE. (C-1)

5–11.14 Discuss what constitutes a significant exposure to an infectious agent. (C-1)

5–11.15 Describe the assessment of a patient suspected of, or identified as having, an infectious/communicable disease. (C-1)

5–11.16 Discuss the proper disposal of contaminated supplies (sharps, gauze sponges, tourniquets, etc.). (C-1)

5–11.17 Discuss disinfection of patient care equipment, and areas in which care of the patient occurred. (C-1)

5–11.18 Discuss the following relative to HIV—causative agent, body systems affected and potential secondary complications, modes of transmission, the seroconversion rate after direct significant exposure, susceptibility and resistance, signs and symptoms, specific patient management and personal protective measures, and immunization. (C-1)

5–11.19 Discuss Hepatitis A (infectious hepatitis), including the causative agent, body systems affected and potential secondary complications, routes of transmission, susceptibility and resistance, signs and symptoms, patient management and protective measures, and immunization. (C-1)

5–11.20 Discuss Hepatitis B (serum hepatitis), including the causative agent, the organ affected and potential secondary complications, routes of transmission, signs and symptoms, patient management and protective measures, and immunization. (C-1)

5–11.21 Discuss the susceptibility and resistance to Hepatits B. (C-1)

5–11.22 Discuss Hepatitis C, including the causative agent, the organ affected, routes of transmission, susceptibility and resistance, signs and symptoms, patient management and protective measures, and immunization and control measures. (C-1)

5–11.23 Discuss Hepatitis D (Hepatitis delta virus), including the causative agent, the organ affected, routes of transmission, susceptibility and resistance, signs and symptoms, patient management and protective measures, and immunization and control measures. (C-1)

5–11.24 Discuss Hepatitis E, including the causative agent, the organ affected, routes of transmission, susceptibility and resistance, signs and symptoms, patient management and protective measures, and immunization and control measures. (C-1)

5–11.25 Discuss tuberculosis, including the causative agent, body systems affected and secondary complications, routes of transmission, susceptibility and resistance, signs and symptoms, patient management and protective measures, and immunization and control measures. (C-1)

5–11.26 Discuss meningococcal meningitis (spinal meningitis), including causative organisms, tissues affected, modes of transmission, susceptibility and resistance, signs and symptoms, patient management and protective measures, and immunization and control measures. (C-1)

5–11.27 Discuss other infectious agents known to cause meningitis including streptococcus pneumonia, hemophilus influenza type b, and other varieties of viruses. (C-1)

5–11.28 Discuss pneumonia, including causative organisms, body systems affected, routes of transmission, susceptibility and resistance, signs and symptoms, patient management and protective measures, and immunization. (C-1)

5–11.29 Discuss tetanus, including the causative organism, the body system affected, modes of transmission, susceptibility and resistance, signs and symptoms, patient management and protective measures, and immunization. (C-1)

5–11.30 Discuss rabies and hantavirus as they apply to regional environmental exposures, including the causative organisms, the body systems affected, routes of transmission, susceptibility and resistance, signs and symptoms, patient management and protective measures, and immunization and control measures. (C-1)

5–11.31   Identify pediatric viral diseases. (C-3)

5–11.32   Discuss chickenpox, including the causative organism, the body system affected, mode of transmission, susceptibility and resistance, signs and symptoms, patient management and protective measures, and immunization and control measures. (C-1)

5–11.33   Discuss mumps, including the causative organism, the body organs and systems affected, mode of transmission, susceptibility and resistance, signs and symptoms, patient management and protective measures, and immunization. (C-1)

5–11.34   Discuss rubella (German measles), including the causative agent, the body tissues and systems affected, modes of transmission, susceptibility and resistance, signs and symptoms, patient management and protective measures, and immunization. (C-1)

5–11.35   Discuss measles (rubeola, hard measles), including the causative organism, the body tissues, organs, and systems affected, mode of transmission, susceptibility and resistance, signs and symptoms, patient management and protective measures, and immunization. (C-1)

5–11.36   Discuss the importance of immunization, and those diseases, especially in the pediatric population, which warrant widespread immunization (MMR). (C-1)

5–11.37   Discuss pertussis (whooping cough), including the causative organism, the body organs affected, mode of transmission, susceptibility and resistance, signs and symptoms, patient management and protective measures, and immunization. (C-1)

5–11.38   Discuss influenza, including causative organisms, the body system affected, mode of transmission, susceptibility and resistance, signs and symptoms, patient management and protective measures, and immunization. (C-1)

5–11.39   Discuss mononucleosis, including the causative organisms, the body regions, organs, and systems affected, modes of transmission, susceptibility and resistance, signs and symptoms, patient management and protective measures, and immunization. (C-1)

5–11.40   Discuss herpes simplex type 1, including the causative organism, the body regions and system affected, modes of transmission, susceptibility and resistance, signs and symptoms, patient management and protective measures, and immunization. (C-1)

5–11.41   Discuss the characteristics of, and organisms associated with, febrile and afebrile respiratory disease, to include bronchiolitis, bronchitis, laryngitis, croup, epiglottitis, and the common cold. (C-1)

5–11.42   Discuss syphilis, including the causative organism, the body regions, organs, and systems affected, modes of transmission, susceptibility and resistance, stages of signs and symptoms, patient management and protective measures, and immunization. (C-1)

5–11.43   Discuss gonorrhea, including the causative organism, the body organs and associated structures affected, mode of transmission, susceptibility and resistance, signs and symptoms, patient management and protective measures, and immunization. (C-1)

5–11.44   Discuss chlamydia, including the causative organism, the body regions, organs, and systems affected, modes of transmission, susceptibility and resistance, signs and symptoms, patient management and protective measures, and immunization. (C-1)

5–11.45   Discuss herpes simplex 2 (genital herpes), including the causative organism, the body regions, tissues, and structures affected, mode of transmission, susceptibility and resistance, signs and symptoms, patient management and protective measures, and immunization. (C-1)

5–11.46   Discuss scabies, including the etiologic agent, the body organs affected, modes of transmission, susceptibility and resistance, signs and symptoms, patient management and protective measures, and immunization. (C-1)

5–11.47   Discuss lice, including the infesting agents, the body regions affected, modes of transmission and host factors, susceptibility and resistance, signs and symptoms, patient management and protective measures, and prevention. (C-1)

5–11.48   Describe Lyme disease, including the causative organism, the body organs and systems affected, mode of transmission, susceptibility and resistance, phases of signs and symptoms, patient management and control measures, and immunization. (C-1)

5–11.49   Discuss gastroenteritis, including the causative organisms, the body system affected, modes of transmission, susceptibility and resistance, signs and symptoms, patient management and protective measures, and immunization. (C-1)

5–11.50   Discuss the local protocol for reporting and documenting an infectious/communicable disease exposure. (C-1)

5–11.51   Articulate the pathophysiological principles of an infectious process given a case study of a patient with an infectious/ communicable disease. (C-3)

5–11.52   Articulate the field assessment and management, to include safety considerations, of a patient presenting with signs and symptoms suggestive of an infectious/ communicable disease. (C-3)

AFFECTIVE OBJECTIVES

At the completion of this unit, the paramedic student will be able to:

5–11.53   Advocate compliance with standards and guidelines by role modeling adherence to universal/standard precautions and BSI. (A-1)

5–11.54   Value the importance of immunization, especially in children and populations at risk. (A-1)

5–11.55   Value the safe management of a patient with an infectious/communicable disease. (A-2)

5–11.56   Advocate respect for the feelings of patients, family, and others at the scene of an infectious/communicable disease. (A-2)

5–11.57   Advocate empathy for a patient with an infectious/communicable disease. (A-2)

5–11.58   Value the importance of infectious/communicable disease control. (A-2)

5–11.59   Consistently demonstrate the use of body substance isolation. (A-2)

PSYCHOMOTOR OBJECTIVES

At the completion of this unit, the paramedic student will be able to:

5–11.60 Demonstrate the ability to comply with body substance isolation guidelines. (P-2)

5–11.61 Perform an assessment of a patient with an infectious/ communicable disease. (P-2)

5–11.62 Effectively and safely manage a patient with an infectious/ communicable disease, including airway and ventilation care, support of circulation, pharmacological intervention, transport considerations, psychological support/ communication strategies, and other considerations as mandated by local protocol. (P-2)

UNIT TERMINAL OBJECTIVE

5–12 At the completion of this unit, the paramedic student will be able to describe and demonstrate safe, empathetic competence in caring for patients with behavioral emergencies.

COGNITIVE OBJECTIVES

At the completion of this unit, the paramedic student will be able to:

5–12.1 Define behavior and distinguish between normal and abnormal behavior. (C-1)

5–12.2 Define behavioral emergency. (C-1)

5–12.3 Discuss the prevalence of behavior and psychiatric disorders. (C-1)

5–12.4 Discuss the factors that may alter the behavior or emotional status of an ill or injured individual. (C-1)

5–12.5 Describe the medical legal considerations for management of emotionally disturbed patients. (C-1)

5–12.6 Discuss the pathophysiology of behavioral and psychiatric disorders. (C-1)

5–12.7 Describe the overt behaviors associated with behavioral and psychiatric disorders. (C-1)

5–12.8 Define the following terms: (C-1)
   a. Affect
   b. Anger
   c. Anxiety
   d. Confusion
   e. Depression
   f. Fear
   g. Mental status
   h. Open-ended question
   i. Posture

5–12.9 Describe the verbal techniques useful in managing the emotionally disturbed patient. (C-1)

5–12.10 List the reasons for taking appropriate measures to ensure the safety of the patient, paramedic, and others. (C-1)

5–12.11 Describe the circumstances when relatives, bystanders, and others should be removed from the scene. (C-1)

5–12.12 Describe the techniques that facilitate the systematic gathering of information from the disturbed patient. (C-1)

5–12.13 List situations in which the EMT-P is expected to transport a patient forcibly and against his will. (C-1)

5–12.14 Identify techniques for physical assessment in a patient with behavioral problems. (C-1)

5–12.15 Describe methods of restraint that may be necessary in managing the emotionally disturbed patient. (C-1)

5–12.16 List the risk factors for suicide. (C-1)

5–12.17 List the behaviors that may be seen as indicating that a patient may be at risk for suicide. (C-1)

5–12.18 Integrate the pathophysiological principles with the assessment of the patient with behavioral and psychiatric disorders. (C-3)

5–12.19 Differentiate between the various behavioral and psychiatric disorders based on the assessment and history. (C-3)

5–12.20 Formulate a field impression based on the assessment findings. (C-3)

5–12.21 Develop a patient management plan based on the field impressions. (C-3)

AFFECTIVE OBJECTIVES

At the completion of this unit, the paramedic student will be able to:

5–12.22 Advocate for empathetic and respectful treatment for individuals experiencing behavioral emergencies. (A-3)

PSYCHOMOTOR OBJECTIVES

At the completion of this unit, the paramedic student will be able to:

5–12.23 Demonstrate safe techniques for managing and restraining a violent patient. (P-1)

UNIT TERMINAL OBJECTIVE

5–13 At the completion of this unit, the paramedic student will be able to utilize gynecological principles and assessment findings to formulate a field impression and implement the management plan for the patient experiencing a gynecological emergency.

COGNITIVE OBJECTIVES

At the completion of this unit, the paramedic student will be able to:

5–13.1 Review the anatomic structures and physiology of the female reproductive system. (C-1)

5–13.2 Identify the normal events of the menstrual cycle. (C-1)

5–13.3 Describe how to assess a patient with a gynecological complaint. (C-1)

5–13.4 Explain how to recognize a gynecological emergency. (C-1)

5–13.5 Describe the general care for any patient experiencing a gynecological emergency. (C-1)

5–13.6 Describe the pathophysiology, assessment, and management of specific gynecological emergencies. (C-1)

AFFECTIVE OBJECTIVES

At the completion of this unit, the paramedic student will be able to:

5–13.7 Value the importance of maintaining a patient's modesty and privacy while still being able to obtain necessary information. (A-2)

5–13.8 Defend the need to provide care for a patient of sexual assault, while still preventing destruction of crime scene information. (A-3)

5–13.9   Serve as a role model for other EMS providers when discussing or caring for patients with gynecological emergencies. (A-3)

PSYCHOMOTOR OBJECTIVES

At the completion of this unit, the paramedic student will be able to:

5–13.10   Demonstrate how to assess a patient with a gynecological complaint. (P-2)
5–13.11   Demonstrate how to provide care for a patient with: (P-2)
          a. Excessive vaginal bleeding
          b. Abdominal pain
          c. Sexual assault

UNIT TERMINAL OBJECTIVE

5–14   At the completion of this unit, the paramedic student will be able to apply an understanding of the anatomy and physiology of the female reproductive system to the assessment and management of a patient experiencing normal or abnormal labor.

COGNITIVE OBJECTIVES

At the completion of this unit, the paramedic student will be able to:

5–14.1   Review the anatomic structures and physiology of the reproductive system. (C-1)
5–14.2   Identify the normal events of pregnancy. (C-1)
5–14.3   Describe how to assess an obstetrical patient. (C-1)
5–14.4   Identify the stages of labor and the paramedic's role in each stage. (C-1)
5–14.5   Differentiate between normal and abnormal delivery. (C-3)
5–14.6   Identify and describe complications associated with pregnancy and delivery. (C-1)
5–14.7   Identify predelivery emergencies. (C-1)
5–14.8   State indications of an imminent delivery. (C-1)
5–14.9   Explain the use of the contents of an obstetrics kit. (C-2)
5–14.10   Differentiate the management of a patient with predelivery emergencies from a normal delivery. (C-3)
5–14.11   State the steps in the predelivery preparation of the mother. (C-1)
5–14.12   Establish the relationship between body substance isolation and childbirth. (C-3)
5–14.13   State the steps to assist in the delivery of a newborn. (C-1)
5–14.14   Describe how to care for the newborn. (C-1)
5–14.15   Describe how and when to cut the umbilical cord. (C-1)
5–14.16   Discuss the steps in the delivery of the placenta. (C-1)
5–14.17   Describe the management of the mother postdelivery. (C-1)
5–14.18   Summarize neonatal resuscitation procedures. (C-1)
5–14.19   Describe the procedures for handling abnormal deliveries. (C-1)
5–14.20   Describe the procedures for handling complications of pregnancy. (C-1)
5–14.21   Describe the procedures for handling maternal complications of labor. (C-1)
5–14.22   Describe special considerations when meconium is present in amniotic fluid or during delivery. (C-1)
5–14.23   Describe special considerations of a premature baby. (C-1)

AFFECTIVE OBJECTIVES

At the completion of this unit, the paramedic student will be able to:

5–14.24   Advocate the need for treating two patients (mother and baby). (A-2)
5–14.25   Value the importance of maintaining a patient's modesty and privacy during assessment and management. (A-2)
5–14.26   Serve as a role model for other EMS providers when discussing or performing the steps of childbirth. (A-3)

PSYCHOMOTOR OBJECTIVES

At the completion of this unit, the paramedic student will be able to:

5–14.27   Demonstrate how to assess an obstetric patient. (P-2)
5–14.28   Demonstrate how to provide care for a patient with: (P-2)
          a. Excessive vaginal bleeding
          b. Abdominal pain
          c. Hypertensive crisis
5–14.29   Demonstrate how to prepare the obstetric patient for delivery. (P-2)
5–14.30   Demonstrate how to assist in the normal cephalic delivery of the fetus. (P-2)
5–14.31   Demonstrate how to deliver the placenta. (P-2)
5–14.32   Demonstrate how to provide postdelivery care of the mother. (P-2)
5–14.33   Demonstrate how to assist with abnormal deliveries. (P-2)
5–14.34   Demonstrate how to care for the mother with delivery complications. (P-2)

UNIT TERMINAL OBJECTIVE

6–1.1   At the completion of this unit, the paramedic student will be able to integrate pathophysiological principles and assessment findings to formulate a field impression and implement a treatment plan for a neonatal patient.

COGNITIVE OBJECTIVES

At the completion of this unit, the paramedic student will be able to:

6–1.2   Define the term newborn. (C-1)
6–1.3   Define the term neonate. (C-1)
6–1.4   Identify important antepartum factors that can affect childbirth. (C-1)
6–1.5   Identify important intrapartum factors that can term the newborn high risk. (C-1)
6–1.6   Identify the factors that lead to premature birth and low birth weight newborns. (C-1)
6–1.7   Distinguish between primary and secondary apnea. (C-3)
6–1.8   Discuss pulmonary perfusion and asphyxia. (C-1)
6–1.9   Identify the primary signs utilized for evaluating a newborn during resuscitation. (C-1)
6–1.10   Formulate an appropriate treatment plan for providing initial care to a newborn. (C-3)
6–1.11   Identify the appropriate use of the APGAR score in caring for a newborn. (C-1)
6–1.12   Calculate the APGAR score given various newborn situations. (C-3)
6–1.13   Determine when ventilatory assistance is appropriate for a newborn. (C-1)
6–1.14   Prepare appropriate ventilation equipment, adjuncts, and technique for a newborn. (C-1)

6–1.15 Determine when chest compressions are appropriate for a newborn. (C-1)

6–1.16 Discuss appropriate chest compression techniques for a newborn. (C-1)

6–1.17 Assess patient improvement due to chest compressions and ventilations. (C-1)

6–1.18 Determine when endotracheal intubation is appropriate for a newborn. (C-1)

6–1.19 Discuss appropriate endotracheal intubation techniques for a newborn. (C-1)

6–1.20 Assess patient improvement due to endotracheal intubation. (C-1)

6–1.21 Identify complications related to endotracheal intubation for a newborn. (C-1)

6–1.22 Determine when vascular access is indicated for a newborn. (C-1)

6–1.23 Discuss the routes of medication administration for a newborn. (C-1)

6–1.24 Determine when blow-by oxygen delivery is appropriate for a newborn. (C-1)

6–1.25 Discuss appropriate blow-by oxygen delivery devices and technique for a newborn. (C-1)

6–1.26 Assess patient improvement due to assisted ventilations. (C-1)

6–1.27 Determine when an orogastric tube should be inserted during positive-pressure ventilation. (C-1)

6–1.28 Discuss the signs of hypovolemia in a newborn. (C-1)

6–1.29 Discuss the initial steps in resuscitation of a newborn. (C-1)

6–1.30 Assess patient improvement due to blow-by oxygen delivery. (C-1)

6–1.31 Discuss the effects maternal narcotic usage has on the newborn. (C-1)

6–1.32 Determine the appropriate treatment for the newborn with narcotic depression. (C-1)

6–1.33 Discuss appropriate transport guidelines for a newborn. (C-1)

6–1.34 Determine appropriate receiving facilities for low and high risk newborns. (C-1)

6–1.35 Describe the epidemiology, including the incidence, morbidity/mortality, risk factors, and prevention strategies for meconium aspiration. (C-1)

6–1.36 Discuss the pathophysiology of meconium aspiration. (C-1)

6–1.37 Discuss the assessment findings associated with meconium aspiration. (C-1)

6–1.38 Discuss the management/treatment plan for meconium aspiration. (C-1)

6–1.39 Describe the epidemiology, including the incidence, morbidity/mortality, risk factors, and prevention strategies for apnea in the neonate. (C-1)

6–1.40 Discuss the pathophysiology of apnea in the neonate. (C-1)

6–1.41 Discuss the assessment findings associated with apnea in the neonate. (C-1)

6–1.42 Discuss the management/treatment plan for apnea in the neonate. (C-1)

6–1.43 Describe the epidemiology, pathophysiology, assessment findings, and management/treatment plan for diaphragmatic hernia. (C-1)

6–1.44 Describe the epidemiology, including the incidence, morbidity/mortality, and risk factors, for bradycardia in the neonate. (C-1)

6–1.45 Discuss the pathophysiology of bradycardia in the neonate. (C-1)

6–1.46 Discuss the assessment findings associated with bradycardia in the neonate. (C-1)

6–1.47 Discuss the management/treatment plan for bradycardia in the neonate. (C-1)

6–1.48 Describe the epidemiology, including the incidence, morbidity/mortality, and risk factors, for premature infants.

6–1.49 Discuss the pathophysiology of premature infants. (C-1)

6–1.50 Discuss the assessment findings associated with premature infants. (C-1)

6–1.51 Discuss the management/treatment plan for premature infants. (C-1)

6–1.52 Describe the epidemiology, including the incidence, morbidity/mortality, and risk factors, for respiratory distress/cyanosis in the neonate. (C-1)

6–1.53 Discuss the pathophysiology of respiratory distress/cyanosis in the neonate. (C-1)

6–1.54 Discuss the assessment findings associated with respiratory distress/cyanosis in the neonate. (C-1)

6–1.55 Discuss the management/treatment plan for respiratory distress/cyanosis in the neonate. (C-1)

6–1.56 Describe the epidemiology, including the incidence, morbidity/mortality, and risk factors, for seizures in the neonate. (C-1)

6–1.57 Discuss the pathophysiology of seizures in the neonate. (C-1)

6–1.58 Discuss the assessment findings associated with seizures in the neonate. (C-1)

6–1.59 Discuss the management/treatment plan for seizures in the neonate. (C-1)

6–1.60 Describe the epidemiology, including the incidence, morbidity/mortality, and risk factors, for fever in the neonate. (C-1)

6–1.61 Discuss the pathophysiology of fever in the neonate. (C-1)

6–1.62 Discuss the assessment findings associated with fever in the neonate. (C-1)

6–1.63 Discuss the management/treatment plan for fever in the neonate. (C-1)

6–1.64 Describe the epidemiology, including the incidence, morbidity/mortality, and risk factors, for hypothermia in the neonate. (C-1)

6–1.65 Discuss the pathophysiology of hypothermia in the neonate. (C-1)

6–1.66 Discuss the assessment findings associated with hypothermia in the neonate. (C-1)

6–1.67 Discuss the management/treatment plan for hypothermia in the neonate. (C-1)

6–1.68 Describe the epidemiology, including the incidence, morbidity/mortality, and risk factors, for hypoglycemia in the neonate. (C-1)

6–1.69 Discuss the pathophysiology of hypoglycemia in the neonate. (C-1)

6–1.70 Discuss the assessment findings associated with hypoglycemia in the neonate. (C-1)

6–1.71 Discuss the management/treatment plan for hypoglycemia in the neonate. (C-1)

6–1.72 Describe the epidemiology, including the incidence, morbidity/mortality, and risk factors, for vomiting in the neonate. (C-1)

6–1.73 Discuss the pathophysiology of vomiting in the neonate. (C-1)

6–1.74 Discuss the assessment findings associated with vomiting in the neonate. (C-1)

6–1.75 Discuss the management/treatment plan for vomiting in the neonate. (C-1)

6–1.76 Describe the epidemiology, including the incidence, morbidity/mortality, and risk factors, for diarrhea in the neonate. (C-1)

6–1.77 Discuss the pathophysiology of diarrhea in the neonate. (C-1)

6–1.78 Discuss the assessment findings associated with diarrhea in the neonate. (C-1)

6–1.79 Discuss the management/treatment plan for diarrhea in the neonate. (C-1)

6–1.80 Describe the epidemiology, including the incidence, morbidity/mortality, and risk factors, for common birth injuries in the neonate. (C-1)

6–1.81 Discuss the pathophysiology of common birth injuries in the neonate. (C-1)

6–1.82 Discuss the assessment findings associated with common birth injuries in the neonate. (C-1)

6–1.83 Discuss the management/treatment plan for common birth injuries in the neonate. (C-1)

6–1.84 Describe the epidemiology, including the incidence, morbidity/mortality, and risk factors, for cardiac arrest in the neonate. (C-1)

6–1.85 Discuss the pathophysiology of cardiac arrest in the neonate. (C-1)

6–1.86 Discuss the assessment findings associated with cardiac arrest in the neonate. (C-1)

6–1.87 Discuss the management/treatment plan for cardiac arrest in the neonate. (C-1)

6–1.88 Discuss the pathophysiology of post–arrest management of the neonate. (C-1)

6–1.89 Discuss the assessment findings associated with post–arrest situations in the neonate. (C-1)

6–1.90 Discuss the management/treatment plan to stabilize the post–arrest neonate. (C-1)

AFFECTIVE OBJECTIVES

At the completion of this unit, the paramedic student will be able to:

6–1.91 Demonstrate and advocate appropriate interaction with a newborn/neonate that conveys respect for their position in life. (A-3)

6–1.92 Recognize the emotional impact of newborn/neonate injuries/illnesses on parents/guardians. (A-1)

6–1.93 Recognize and appreciate the physical and emotional difficulties associated with separation of the parent/guardian and a newborn/neonate. (A-3)

6–1.94 Listen to the concerns expressed by parents/guardians. (A-1)

6–1.95 Attend to the need for reassurance, empathy, and compassion for the parent/guardian. (A-1)

PSYCHOMOTOR OBJECTIVES

At the completion of this unit, the paramedic student will be able to:

6–1.96 Demonstrate preparation of a newborn resuscitation area. (P-2)

6–1.97 Demonstrate appropriate assessment technique for examining a newborn. (P-2)

6–1.98 Demonstrate appropriate assisted ventilations for a newborn. (P-2)

6–1.99 Demonstrate appropriate endotracheal intubation technique for a newborn. (P-2)

6–1.100 Demonstrate appropriate meconium aspiration suctioning technique for a newborn. (P-2)

6–1.101 Demonstrate appropriate insertion of an orogastric tube. (P-2)

6–1.102 Demonstrate needle chest decompression for a newborn or neonate. (P-2)

6–1.103 Demonstrate appropriate chest compression and ventilation technique for a newborn. (P-2)

6–1.104 Demonstrate appropriate techniques to improve or eliminate endotracheal intubation complications. (P-2)

6–1.105 Demonstrate vascular access cannulation techniques for a newborn. (P-2)

6–1.106 Demonstrate the initial steps in resuscitation of a newborn. (P-2)

6–1.107 Demonstrate blow-by oxygen delivery for a newborn. (P-2)

UNIT TERMINAL OBJECTIVE

6–2.1 At the completion of this unit, the paramedic student will be able to integrate pathophysiological principles and assessment findings to formulate a field impression and implement a treatment plan for the pediatric patient.

COGNITIVE OBJECTIVES

At the completion of this unit, the paramedic student will be able to:

6–2.2 Discuss the paramedic's role in the reduction of infant and childhood morbidity and mortality from acute illness and injury. (C-1)

6–2.3 Identify methods/mechanisms that prevent injuries to infants and children. (C-1)

6–2.4 Describe Emergency Medical Services for Children (EMSC). (C-1)

6–2.5 Discuss how an integrated EMSC system can affect patient outcome. (C-2)

6–2.6 Identify key growth and developmental characteristics of infants and children and their implications. (C-2)

6–2.7 Identify key anatomical and physiological characteristics of infants and children and their implications. (C-2)

6–2.8 Describe techniques for successful assessment of infants and children. (C-1)

6–2.9 Describe techniques for successful treatment of infants and children. (C-1)

6–2.10 Identify the common responses of families to acute illness and injury of an infant or child. (C-1)

6–2.11 Describe techniques for successful interaction with families of acutely ill or injured infants and children. (C-1)

6–2.12 Outline differences in adult and childhood anatomy and physiology. (C-3)

6–2.13 Identify "normal" age group related vital signs. (C-1)

6–2.14 Discuss the appropriate equipment utilized to obtain pediatric vital signs. (C-1)

6–2.15 Determine appropriate airway adjuncts for infants and children. (C-1)

6–2.16 Discuss complications of improper utilization of airway adjuncts with infants and children. (C-1)

6–2.17 Discuss appropriate ventilation devices for infants and children. (C-1)

6–2.18 Discuss complications of improper utilization of ventilation devices with infants and children. (C-1)

6–2.19 Discuss appropriate endotracheal intubation equipment for infants and children. (C-1)

6–2.20 Identify complications of improper endotracheal intubation procedure in infants and children. (C-1)

6–2.21 List the indications and methods for gastric decompression for infants and children. (C-1)

6–2.22 Define respiratory distress. (C-1)

6–2.23 Define respiratory failure. (C-1)

6–2.24 Define respiratory arrest. (C-1)

6–2.25 Differentiate between upper airway obstruction and lower airway disease. (C-3)

6–2.26 Describe the general approach to the treatment of children with respiratory distress, failure, or arrest from upper airway obstruction or lower airway disease. (C-3)

6–2.27 Discuss the common causes of hypoperfusion in infants and children. (C-1)

6–2.28 Evaluate the severity of hypoperfusion in infants and children. (C-3)

6–2.29 Identify the major classifications of pediatric cardiac rhythms. (C-1)

6–2.30 Discuss the primary etiologies of cardiopulmonary arrest in infants and children. (C-1)

6–2.31 Discuss age appropriate vascular access sites for infants and children. (C-1)

6–2.32 Discuss the appropriate equipment for vascular access in infants and children. (C-1)

6–2.33 Identify complications of vascular access for infants and children. (C-1)

6–2.34 Describe the primary etiologies of altered level of consciousness in infants and children. (C-1)

6–2.35 Identify common lethal mechanisms of injury in infants and children. (C-1)

6–2.36 Discuss anatomical features of children that predispose or protect them from certain injuries. (C-1)

6–2.37 Describe aspects of infant and child airway management that are affected by potential cervical spine injury. (C-1)

6–2.38 Identify infant and child trauma patients who require spinal immobilization. (C-1)

6–2.39 Discuss fluid management and shock treatment for infant and child trauma patients. (C-1)

6–2.40 Determine when pain management and sedation are appropriate for infants and children. (C-1)

6–2.41 Define child abuse. (C-1)

6–2.42 Define child neglect. (C-1)

6–2.43 Define sudden infant death syndrome (SIDS). (C-1)

6–2.44 Discuss the parent/caregiver responses to the death of an infant or child. (C-1)

6–2.45 Define children with special health care needs. (C-1)

6–2.46 Define technology assisted children. (C-1)

6–2.47 Discuss basic cardiac life support (CPR) guidelines for infants and children. (C-1)

6–2.48 Identify appropriate parameters for performing infant and child CPR. (C-1)

6–2.49 Integrate advanced life support skills with basic cardiac life support for infants and children. (C-3)

6–2.50 Discuss the indications, dosage, route of administration, and special considerations for medication administration in infants and children. (C-1)

6–2.51 Discuss appropriate transport guidelines for infants and children. (C-1)

6–2.52 Discuss appropriate receiving facilities for low and high risk infants and children. (C-1)

6–2.53 Describe the epidemiology, including the incidence, morbidity/mortality, risk factors, and prevention strategies for respiratory distress/failure in infants and children. (C-1)

6–2.54 Discuss the pathophysiology of respiratory distress/failure in infants and children. (C-1)

6–2.55 Discuss the assessment findings associated with respiratory distress/failure in infants and children. (C-1)

6–2.56 Discuss the management/treatment plan for respiratory distress/failure in infants and children. (C-1)

6–2.57 Describe the epidemiology, including the incidence, morbidity/mortality, risk factors, and prevention strategies, for hypoperfusion in infants and children. (C-1)

6–2.58 Discuss the pathophysiology of hypoperfusion in infants and children. (C-1)

6–2.59 Discuss the assessment findings associated with hypoperfusion in infants and children. (C-1)

6–2.60 Discuss the management/treatment plan for hypoperfusion in infants and children. (C-1)

6–2.61 Describe the epidemiology, including the incidence, morbidity/mortality, risk factors, and prevention strategies, for cardiac dysrhythmias in infants and children. (C-1)

6–2.62 Discuss the pathophysiology of cardiac dysrhythmias in infants and children. (C-1)

6–2.63 Discuss the assessment findings associated with cardiac dysrhythmias in infants and children. (C-1)

6–2.64 Discuss the management/treatment plan for cardiac dysrhythmias in infants and children. (C-1)

6–2.65 Describe the epidemiology, including the incidence, morbidity/ mortality, risk factors, and prevention strategies, for neurological emergencies in infants and children. (C-1)

6–2.66 Discuss the pathophysiology of neurological emergencies in infants and children. (C-1)

6–2.67 Discuss the assessment findings associated with neurological emergencies in infants and children. (C-1)

6–2.68 Discuss the management/treatment plan for neurological emergencies in infants and children. (C-1)

6–2.69 Describe the epidemiology, including the incidence, morbidity/mortality, risk factors, and prevention strategies, for trauma in infants and children. (C-1)

6–2.70 Discuss the pathophysiology of trauma in infants and children. (C-1)

6–2.71 Discuss the assessment findings associated with trauma in infants and children. (C-1)

6–2.72 Discuss the management/treatment plan for trauma in infants and children. (C-1)

6–2.73 Describe the epidemiology, including the incidence, morbidity/mortality, risk factors, and prevention strategies, for abuse and neglect in infants and children. (C-1)

6–2.74 Discuss the pathophysiology of abuse and neglect in infants and children. (C-1)

6–2.75 Discuss the assessment findings associated with abuse and neglect in infants and children. (C-1)

6–2.76 Discuss the management/treatment plan for abuse and neglect in infants and children, including documentation and reporting. (C-1)

6–2.77 Describe the epidemiology, including the incidence, morbidity/mortality, risk factors, and prevention strategies, for SIDS infants. (C-1)

6–2.78 Describe the epidemiology, including the incidence, morbidity/mortality, risk factors, and prevention strategies, for children with special health care needs including technology assisted children. (C-1)

6–2.79 Discuss the pathophysiology of children with special health care needs including technology assisted children. (C-1)

6–2.80 Discuss the assessment findings associated with children with special health care needs including technology assisted children. (C-1)

6–2.81 Discuss the management/treatment plan for children with special health care needs including technology assisted children. (C-1)

6–2.82 Describe the epidemiology, including the incidence, morbidity/mortality, risk factors, and prevention strategies, for SIDS infants. (C-1)

6–2.83 Discuss the pathophysiology of SIDS in infants. (C-1)

6–2.84 Discuss the assessment findings associated with SIDS infants. (C-1)

6–2.85 Discuss the management/treatment plan for SIDS in infants. (C-1)

AFFECTIVE OBJECTIVES

At the completion of this unit, the paramedic student will be able to:

6–2.86 Demonstrate and advocate appropriate interactions with the infant/child that convey an understanding of their developmental stage. (A-3)

6–2.87 Recognize the emotional dependance of the infant/child on their parent/guardian. (A-1)

6–2.88 Recognize the emotional impact of the infant/child injuries and illnesses on the parent/guardian. (A-1)

6–2.89 Recognize and appreciate the physical and emotional difficulties associated with separation of the parent/guardian of a special needs child. (A-3)

6–2.90 Demonstrate the ability to provide reassurance, empathy, and compassion for the parent/guardian. (A-1)

PSYCHOMOTOR OBJECTIVES

At the completion of this unit, the paramedic student will be able to:

6–2.91 Demonstrate the appropriate approach for treating infants and children. (P-2)

6–2.92 Demonstrate appropriate intervention techniques with families of acutely ill or injured infants and children. (P-2)

6–2.93 Demonstrate an appropriate assessment for different developmental age groups. (P-2)

6–2.94 Demonstrate an appropriate technique for measuring pediatric vital signs. (P-2)

6–2.95 Demonstrate the use of a length-based resuscitation device for determining equipment sizes, drug doses, and other pertinent information for a pediatric patient. (P-2)

6–2.96 Demonstrate the appropriate approach for treating infants and children with respiratory distress, failure, and arrest. (P-2)

6–2.97 Demonstrate proper technique for administering blow-by oxygen to infants and children. (P-2)

6–2.98 Demonstrate the proper utilization of a pediatric non-rebreather oxygen mask. (P-2)

6–2.99 Demonstrate proper technique for suctioning of infants and children. (P-2)

6–2.100 Demonstrate appropriate use of airway adjuncts with infants and children. (P-2)

6–2.101 Demonstrate appropriate use of ventilation devices for infants and children. (P-2)

6–2.102 Demonstrate endotracheal intubation procedures in infants and children. (P-2)

6–2.103 Demonstrate appropriate treatment/management of intubation complications for infants and children. (P-2)

6–2.104 Demonstrate appropriate needle cricothyroidotomy in infants and children. (P-2)

6–2.105 Demonstrate proper placement of a gastric tube in infants and children. (P-2)

6–2.106 Demonstrate an appropriate technique for insertion of peripheral intravenous catheters for infants and children. (P-2)

6–2.107 Demonstrate an appropriate technique for administration of intramuscular, inhalation, subcutaneous, rectal, endotracheal, and oral medication for infants and children. (P-2)

6–2.108 Demonstrate an appropriate technique for insertion of an intraosseous line for infants and children. (P-2)

6–2.109 Demonstrate appropriate interventions for infants and children with a partially obstructed airway. (P-2)

6–2.110 Demonstrate age appropriate basic airway clearing maneuvers for infants and children with a completely obstructed airway. (P-2)

6–2.111 Demonstrate proper technique for direct laryngoscopy and foreign body retrieval in infants and children with a completely obstructed airway. (P-2)

6–2.112 Demonstrate appropriate airway and breathing control maneuvers for infant and child trauma patients. (P-2)

6–2.113 Demonstrate appropriate treatment of infants and children requiring advanced airway and breathing control. (P-2)

6–2.114 Demonstrate appropriate immobilization techniques for infant and child trauma patients. (P-2)

6–2.115 Demonstrate treatment of infants and children with head injuries. (P-2)

6–2.116 Demonstrate appropriate treatment of infants and children with chest injuries. (P-2)

6–2.117 Demonstrate appropriate treatment of infants and children with abdominal injuries. (P-2)

6–2.118 Demonstrate appropriate treatment of infants and children with extremity injuries. (P-2)

6–2.119 Demonstrate appropriate treatment of infants and children with burns. (P-2)

6–2.120 Demonstrate appropriate parent/caregiver interviewing techniques for infant and child death situations.(P-2)

6–2.121 Demonstrate proper infant CPR. (P-2)

6–2.122 Demonstrate proper child CPR. (P-2)

6–2.123 Demonstrate proper techniques for performing infant and child defibrillation and synchronized cardioversion. (P-2)

UNIT TERMINAL OBJECTIVE

6–3 At the completion of this unit, the paramedic student will be able to integrate the pathophysiological principles and the assessment findings to formulate and implement a treatment plan for the geriatric patient.

COGNITIVE OBJECTIVES

At the completion of this unit, the paramedic student will be able to:

6–3.1 Discuss population demographics demonstrating the rise in elderly population in the U.S. (C-1)

6–3.2 Discuss society's view of aging and the social, financial, and ethical issues facing the elderly. (C-1)

6–3.3 Assess the various living environments of elderly patients. (C-3)

6–3.4 Describe the local resources available to assist the elderly and create strategies to refer at-risk patients to appropriate community services. (C-3)

6–3.5 Discuss issues facing society concerning the elderly. (C-1)

6–3.6 Discuss common emotional and psychological reactions to aging to include causes and manifestations. (C-1)

6–3.7 Apply the pathophysiology of multi-system failure to the assessment and management of medical conditions in the elderly patient. (C-2)

6–3.8 Discuss the problems with mobility in the elderly and develop strategies to prevent falls. (C-1)

6–3.9 Discuss the implications of problems with sensation to communication and patient assessment. (C-2)

6–3.10 Discuss the problems with continence and elimination and develop communication strategies to provide psychological support. (C-3)

6–3.11 Discuss factors that may complicate the assessment of the elderly patient. (C-1)

6–3.12 Describe principles that should be employed when assessing and communicating with the elderly. (C-1)

6–3.13 Compare the assessment of a young patient with that of an elderly patient. (C-3)

6–3.14 Discuss common complaints of elderly patients. (C-1)

6–3.15 Compare the pharmacokinetics of an elderly patient to that of a young adult. (C-2)

6–3.16 Discuss the impact of polypharmacy and medication noncompliance on patient assessment and management. (C-1)

6–3.17 Discuss drug distribution, metabolism, and excretion in the elderly patient. (C-1)

6–3.18 Discuss medication issues of the elderly including polypharmacy, dosing errors, and increased drug sensitivity. (C-1)

6–3.19 Discuss the use and effects of commonly prescribed drugs for the elderly patient. (C-1)

6–3.20 Discuss the normal and abnormal changes with age of the pulmonary system. (C-1)

6–3.21 Describe the epidemiology of pulmonary diseases in the elderly, including incidence, morbidity/mortality, risk factors, and prevention strategies, for patients with pneumonia, chronic obstructive pulmonary diseases, and pulmonary embolism. (C-1)

6–3.22 Compare and contrast the pathophysiology of pulmonary diseases in the elderly with that of a younger adult, including pneumonia, chronic obstructive pulmonary diseases, and pulmonary embolism. (C-3)

6–3.23 Discuss the assessment of the elderly patient with pulmonary complaints, including pneumonia, chronic obstructive pulmonary diseases, and pulmonary embolism. (C-1)

6–3.24 Identify the need for intervention and transport of the elderly patient with pulmonary complaints. (C-1)

6–3.25 Develop a treatment and management plan of the elderly patient with pulmonary complaints, including pneumonia, chronic obstructive pulmonary diseases, and pulmonary embolism. (C-3)

6–3.26 Discuss the normal and abnormal cardiovascular system changes with age. (C-1)

6–3.27 Describe the epidemiology for cardiovascular diseases in the elderly, including incidence, morbidity/mortality, risk factors, and prevention strategies for patients with myocardial infarction, heart failure, dysrhythmias, aneurysm, and hypertension. (C-1)

6–3.28 Compare and contrast the pathophysiology of cardiovascular diseases in the elderly with that of a younger adult, including myocardial infarction, heart failure, dysrhythmias, aneurysm, and hypertension. (C-3)

6–3.29 Discuss the assessment of the elderly patient with complaints related to the cardiovascular system, including myocardial infarction, heart failure, dysrhythmias, aneurysm, and hypertension. (C-1)

6–3.30 Identify the need for intervention and transportation of the elderly patient with cardiovascular complaints. (C-1)

6–3.31 Develop a treatment and management plan of the elderly patient with cardiovascular complaints, including myocardial infarction, heart failure, dysrhythmias, aneurysm, and hypertension. (C-3)

6–3.32 Discuss the normal and abnormal changes with age of the nervous system. (C-1)

6–3.33 Describe the epidemiology for nervous system diseases in the elderly, including incidence, morbidity/mortality, risk factors, and prevention strategies for patients with cerebral vascular disease, delirium, dementia, Alzheimer's disease, and Parkinson's disease. (C-1)

6–3.34 Compare and contrast the pathophysiology of nervous system diseases in the elderly with that of a younger adult, including cerebral vascular disease, delirium, dementia, Alzheimer's disease, and Parkinson's disease. (C-3)

6–3.35 Discuss the assessment of the elderly patient with complaints related to the nervous system, including cerebral vascular disease, delirium, dementia, Alzheimer's disease, and Parkinson's disease. (C-1)

6–3.36 Identify the need for intervention and transportation of the patient with complaints related to the nervous system. (C-1)

6–3.37 Develop a treatment and management plan of the elderly patient with complaints related to the nervous system, including cerebral vascular disease, delirium, dementia, Alzheimer's disease, and Parkinson's disease. (C-3)

6–3.38 Discuss the normal and abnormal changes of the endocrine system with age. (C-1)

6–3.39 Describe the epidemiology for endocrine diseases in the elderly, including incidence, morbidity/mortality, risk factors, and prevention strategies for patients with diabetes and thyroid diseases. (C-1)

6–3.40 Compare and contrast the pathophysiology of diabetes and thyroid diseases in the elderly with that of a younger adult. (C-3)

6–3.41 Discuss the assessment of the elderly patient with complaints related to the endocrine system, including diabetes and thyroid diseases. (C-1)

6–3.42 Identify the need for intervention and transportation of the patient with endocrine problems. (C-1)

6–3.43 Develop a treatment and management plan of the elderly patient with endocrine problems, including diabetes and thyroid diseases. (C-3)

6–3.44 Discuss the normal and abnormal changes of the gastrointestinal system with age. (C-1)

6–3.45 Discuss the assessment of the elderly patient with complaints related to the gastrointestinal system. (C-1)

6–3.46 Identify the need for intervention and transportation of the patient with gastrointestinal complaints. (C-1)

6–3.47 Develop and execute a treatment and management plan of the elderly patient with gastrointestinal problems. (C-3)

6–3.48 Discuss the assessment and management of an elderly patient with GI hemorrhage and bowel obstruction. (C-1)

6–3.49 Compare and contrast the pathophysiology of GI hemorrhage and bowel obstruction in the elderly with that of a young adult. (C-3)

6–3.50 Discuss the normal and abnormal changes with age related to toxicology. (C-1)

6–3.51 Discuss the assessment of the elderly patient with complaints related to toxicology. (C-1)

6–3.52 Identify the need for intervention and transportation of the patient with toxicological problems. (C-1)

6–3.53 Develop and execute a treatment and management plan of the elderly patient with toxicological problems. (C-3)

6–3.54 Describe the epidemiology in the elderly, including the incidence, morbidity/mortality, risk factors, and prevention strategies, for patients with drug toxicity. (C-1)

6–3.55 Compare and contrast the pathophysiology of drug toxicity in the elderly with that of a younger adult. (C-3)

6–3.56 Discuss the assessment findings common in elderly patients with drug toxicity. (C-1)

6–3.57 Discuss the management/considerations when treating an elderly patient with drug toxicity. (C-1)

6–3.58 Describe the epidemiology for drug and alcohol abuse in the elderly, including incidence, morbidity/mortality, risk factors, and prevention strategies. (C-1)

6–3.59 Compare and contrast the pathophysiology of drug and alcohol abuse in the elderly with that of a younger adult. (C-3)

6–3.60 Discuss the assessment findings common in elderly patients with drug and alcohol abuse. (C-1)

6–3.61 Discuss the management/considerations when treating an elderly patient with drug and alcohol abuse. (C-1)

6–3.62 Discuss the normal and abnormal changes of thermoregulation with age. (C-1)

6–3.63 Discuss the assessment of the elderly patient with complaints related to thermoregulation. (C-1)

6–3.64 Identify the need for intervention and transportation of the patient with environmental considerations. (C-1)

6–3.65 Develop and execute a treatment and management plan of the elderly patient with environmental considerations. (C-3)

6–3.66 Compare and contrast the pathophysiology of hypothermia and hyperthermia in the elderly with that of a younger adult. (C-3)

6–3.67 Discuss the assessment findings and management plan for elderly patients with hypothermia and hyperthermia. (C-1)

6–3.68 Discuss the normal and abnormal psychiatric changes of age. (C-1)

6–3.69 Describe the epidemiology of depression and suicide in the elderly, including incidence, morbidity/mortality, risk factors, and prevention strategies. (C-1)

6–3.70 Compare and contrast the psychiatry of depression and suicide in the elderly with that of a younger adult. (C-3)

6–3.71 Discuss the assessment of the elderly patient with psychiatric complaints, including depression and suicide. (C-1)

6–3.72 Identify the need for intervention and transport of the elderly psychiatric patient. (C-1)

6–3.73 Develop a treatment and management plan of the elderly psychiatric patient, including depression and suicide. (C-3)

6–3.74 Discuss the normal and abnormal changes of the integumentary system with age. (C-1)

6–3.75 Describe the epidemiology for pressure ulcers in the elderly, including incidence, morbidity/mortality, risk factors, and prevention strategies. (C-1)

6–3.76 Compare and contrast the pathophysiology of pressure ulcers in the elderly with that of a younger adult. (C-3)

6–3.77 Discuss the assessment of the elderly patient with complaints related to the integumentary system, including pressure ulcers. (C-1)

6–3.78 Identify the need for intervention and transportation of the patient with complaints related to the integumentary system. (C-1)

6–3.79 Develop a treatment and management plan of the elderly patient with complaints related to the integumentary system, including pressure ulcers. (C-3)

6–3.80 Discuss the normal and abnormal changes of the musculoskeletal system with age. (C-1)

6–3.81 Describe the epidemiology for osteoarthritis and osteoporosis, including incidence, morbidity/mortality, risk factors, and prevention strategies. (C-1)

6–3.82 Compare and contrast the pathophysiology of osteoarthritis and osteoporosis with that of a younger adult. (C-3)

6–3.83 Discuss the assessment of the elderly patient with complaints related to the musculoskeletal system, including osteoarthritis and osteoporosis. (C-1)

6–3.84 Identify the need for intervention and transportation of the patient with musculoskeletal complaints. (C-1)

6–3.85 Develop a treatment and management plan of the elderly patient with musculoskeletal complaints, including osteoarthritis and osteoporosis. (C-3)

6–3.86 Describe the epidemiology for trauma in the elderly, including incidence, morbidity/mortality, risk factors, and prevention strategies, for patients with orthopedic injuries, burns, and head injuries. (C-1)

6–3.87 Compare and contrast the pathophysiology of trauma in the elderly with that of a younger adult, including orthopedic injuries, burns, and head injuries. (C-3)

6–3.88 Discuss the assessment findings common in elderly patients with traumatic injuries, including orthopedic injuries, burns, and head injuries. (C-1)

6–3.89 Discuss the management/considerations when treating an elderly patient with traumatic injuries, including orthopedic injuries, burns, and head injuries. (C-1)

6–3.90 Identify the need for intervention and transport of the elderly patient with trauma. (C-1)

AFFECTIVE OBJECTIVES

At the completion of this unit, the paramedic student will be able to:

6–3.91 Demonstrate and advocate appropriate interactions with the elderly that convey respect for their position in life. (A-3)

6–3.92 Recognize the emotional need for independence in the elderly while simultaneously attending to their apparent acute dependence. (A-1)

6–3.93 Recognize and appreciate the many impediments to physical and emotional well-being in the elderly. (A-2)

6–3.94 Recognize and appreciate the physical and emotional difficulties associated with being a caretaker of an impaired elderly person, particularly the patient with Alzheimer's disease. (A-3)

PSYCHOMOTOR OBJECTIVES

At the completion of this unit, the paramedic student will be able to:

6–3.95 Demonstrate the ability to assess a geriatric patient. (P-2)

6–3.96 Demonstrate the ability to adjust their assessment to a geriatric patient. (P-3)

UNIT TERMINAL OBJECTIVE

6–4 At the completion of this unit, the paramedic student will be able to integrate the assessment findings to formulate a field impression and implement a treatment plan for the patient who has sustained abuse or assault.

COGNITIVE OBJECTIVES

At the completion of this unit, the paramedic student will be able to:

6–4.1 Discuss the incidence of abuse and assault. (C-1)

6–4.2 Describe the categories of abuse. (C-1)

6–4.3 Discuss examples of spouse abuse. (C-1)

6–4.4 Discuss examples of elder abuse. (C-1)

6–4.5 Discuss examples of child abuse. (C-1)

6–4.6 Discuss examples of sexual assault. (C-1)

6–4.7 Describe the characteristics associated with the profile of the typical abuser of a spouse. (C-1)

6–4.8 Describe the characteristics associated with the profile of the typical abuser of the elder. (C-1)

6–4.9 Describe the characteristics associated with the profile of the typical abuser of children. (C-1)

6–4.10 Describe the characteristics associated with the profile of the typical assailant of sexual assault. (C-1)

6–4.11 Identify the profile of the "at-risk" spouse. (C-1)

6–4.12 Identify the profile of the "at-risk" elder. (C-1)

6–4.13 Identify the profile of the "at-risk" child. (C-1)

6–4.14 Discuss the assessment and management of the abused patient. (C-1)

6–4.15 Discuss the legal aspects associated with abuse situations. (C-1)

6–4.16 Identify community resources that are able to assist victims of abuse and assault. (C-1)

6–4.17 Discuss the documentation associated with abused and assaulted patients. (C-1)

AFFECTIVE OBJECTIVES

At the completion of this unit, the paramedic student will be able to:

6–4.18 Demonstrate sensitivity to the abused patient. (A-1)

6–4.19 Value the behavior of the abused patient. (A-2)

6–4.20 Attend to the emotional state of the abused patient. (A-1)

6–4.21 Recognize the value of nonverbal communication with the abused patient. (A-1)

6–4.22 Attend to the needs for reassurance, empathy, and compassion with the abused patient. (A-1)

6–4.23 Listen to the concerns expressed by the abused patient. (A-1)

6–4.24 Listen and value the concerns expressed by the sexually assaulted patient. (A-2)

PSYCHOMOTOR OBJECTIVES

At the completion of this unit, the paramedic student will be able to:

6–4.25 Demonstrate the ability to assess a spouse, elder, or child abused patient. (P-1)

6–4.26 Demonstrate the ability to assess a sexually assaulted patient. (P-1)

UNIT TERMINAL OBJECTIVE

6–5 At the completion of this unit the paramedic student will be able to integrate pathophysiological and psychosocial principles to adapt the assessment and treatment plan for diverse patients and those who face physical, mental, social, and financial challenges.

COGNITIVE OBJECTIVES

At the completion of this unit, the paramedic student will be able to:

6–5.1 Describe the various etiologies and types of hearing impairments. (C-1)

6–5.2 Recognize the patient with a hearing impairment. (C-1)

6–5.3 Anticipate accommodations that may be needed in order to properly manage the patient with a hearing impairment. (C-3)

6–5.4 Describe the various etiologies of visual impairments. (C-1)

6–5.5 Recognize the patient with a visual impairment. (C-1)

6–5.6 Anticipate accommodations that may be needed in order to properly manage the patient with a visual impairment. (C-3)

6–5.7 Describe the various etiologies and types of speech impairments. (C-1)

6–5.8 Recognize the patient with a speech impairment. (C-1)

6–5.9 Anticipate accommodations that may be needed in order to properly manage the patient with a speech impairment. (C-3)

6–5.10 Describe the various etiologies of obesity. (C-1)

6–5.11 Anticipate accommodations that may be needed in order to properly manage the patient with obesity. (C-3)

6–5.12 Describe paraplegia/quadriplegia. (C-1)

6–5.13 Anticipate accommodations that may be needed in order to properly manage the patient with paraplegia/ quadriplegia. (C-3)

6–5.14 Define mental illness. (C-1)

6–5.15 Describe the various etiologies of mental illness. (C-1)

6–5.16 Recognize the presenting signs of the various mental illnesses. (C-1)

6–5.17 Anticipate accommodations that may be needed in order to properly manage the patient with a mental illness. (C-3)

6–5.18 Define the term developmentally disabled. (C-1)

6–5.19 Recognize the patient with a developmental disability. (C-1)

6–5.20 Anticipate accommodations that may be needed in order to properly manage the patient with a developmental disability. (C-3)

6–5.21 Describe Down's syndrome. (C-1)

6–5.22 Recognize the patient with Down's syndrome. (C-1)

6–5.23 Anticipate accommodations that may be needed in order to properly manage the patient with Down's syndrome. (C-3)

6–5.24 Describe the various etiologies of emotional impairment. (C-1)

6–5.25 Recognize the patient with an emotional impairment. (C-1)

6–5.26 Anticipate accommodations that may be needed in order to properly manage the patient with an emotional impairment. (C-3)

6–5.27 Define emotional/mental impairment (EMI). (C-1)

6–5.28 Recognize the patient with an emotional or mental impairment. (C-1)

6–5.29 Anticipate accommodations that may be needed in order to properly manage patients with an emotional or mental impairment. (C-3)

6–5.30 Describe the following diseases/illnesses: (C-1)
   a. Arthritis
   b. Cancer
   c. Cerebral palsy
   d. Cystic fibrosis
   e. Multiple sclerosis
   f. Muscular dystrophy
   g. Myasthenia gravis
   h. Poliomyelitis
   i. Spina bifida
   j. Patients with a previous head injury

6–5.31 Identify the possible presenting sign(s) for the following diseases/illnesses: (C-1)
   a. Arthritis
   b. Cancer
   c. Cerebral palsy
   d. Cystic fibrosis
   e. Multiple sclerosis
   f. Muscular dystrophy
   g. Myasthenia gravis
   h. Poliomyelitis
   i. Spina bifida
   j. Patients with a previous head injury

6–5.32 Anticipate accommodations that may be needed in order to properly manage the following patients: (C-3)
   a. Arthritis
   b. Cancer
   c. Cerebral palsy
   d. Cystic fibrosis
   e. Multiple sclerosis
   f. Muscular dystrophy
   g. Myasthenia gravis
   h. Poliomyelitis
   i. Spina bifida
   j. Patients with a previous head injury

6–5.33 Define cultural diversity. (C-1)

6–5.34 Recognize a patient who is culturally diverse. (C-1)

6–5.35 Anticipate accommodations that may be needed in order to properly manage a patient who is culturally diverse. (C-3)

6–5.36 Identify a patient that is terminally ill. (C-1)

6–5.37 Anticipate accommodations that may be needed in order to properly manage a patient who is terminally ill. (C-3)

6–5.38 Identify a patient with a communicable disease. (C-1)

6–5.39 Recognize the presenting signs of a patient with a communicable disease. (C-1)

6–5.40 Anticipate accommodations that may be needed in order to properly manage a patient with a communicable disease. (C-3)

6–5.41 Recognize sign(s) of financial impairments. (C-1)

6–5.42 Anticipate accommodations that may be needed in order to properly manage the patient with a financial impairment. (C-3)

AFFECTIVE OBJECTIVES

None identified for this unit.

PSYCHOMOTOR OBJECTIVES

None identified for this unit.

UNIT TERMINAL OBJECTIVE

6–6 At the completion of this unit, the paramedic student will be able to integrate the pathophysiological principles and the assessment findings to formulate a field impression and implement a treatment plan for the acute deterioration of a chronic care patient.

COGNITIVE OBJECTIVES

At the completion of this unit, the paramedic student will be able to:

6–6.1 Compare and contrast the primary objectives of the ALS professional and the home care professional. (C-3)

6–6.2 Identify the importance of home health care medicine as related to the ALS level of care. (C-1)

6–6.3 Differentiate between the role of EMS provider and the role of the home care provider. (C-3)

6–6.4 Compare and contrast the primary objectives of acute care, home care and hospice care. (C-3)

6–6.5 Summarize the types of home health care available in your area and the services provided. (C-3)

6–6.6 Discuss the aspects of home care that result in enhanced quality of care for a given patient. (C-1)

6–6.7 Discuss the aspects of home care that have a potential to become a detriment to the quality of care for a given patient. (C-1)

6–6.8 List complications commonly seen in the home care patients which result in their hospitalization. (C-1)

6–6.9 Compare the cost, mortality, and quality of care for a given patient in the hospital versus the home care setting. (C-3)

6–6.10 Discuss the significance of palliative care programs as related to a patient in a home health care setting. (C-1)

6–6.11 Define hospice care, comfort care, and DNR/DNAR as they relate to local practice, law, and policy. (C-1)

6–6.12 List the stages of the grief process and relate them to an individual in hospice care. (C-1)

6–6.13 List pathologies and complications typical to home care patients. (C-1)

6–6.14 Given a home care scenario, predict complications requiring ALS intervention. (C-3)

6–6.15 Given a series of home care scenarios, determine which patients should receive follow-up home care and which should be transported to an emergency care facility. (C-3)

6–6.16 Describe airway maintenance devices typically found in the home care environment. (C-1)

6–6.17 Describe devices that provide or enhance alveolar ventilation in the home care setting. (C-1)

6–6.18 List modes of artificial ventilation and an out-of-hospital situation where each might be employed. (C-1)

6–6.19 List vascular access devices found in the home care setting. (C-1)

6–6.20 Recognize standard central venous access devices utilized in home health care. (C-1)

6–6.21 Describe the basic universal characteristics of central venous catheters. (C-1)

6–6.22 Describe the basic universal characteristics of implantable injection devices. (C-1)

6–6.23 List devices found in the home care setting that are used to empty, irrigate, or deliver nutrition or medication to the GI/GU tract. (C-1)

6–6.24 Describe complications of assessing each of the airway, vascular access, and GI/GU devices described above. (C-1)

6–6.25 Given a series of scenarios, demonstrate the appropriate ALS interventions. (C-3)

6–6.26 Given a series of scenarios, demonstrate interaction and support with the family members/support persons for a patient who has died. (C-3)

6–6.27 Describe common complications with central venous access and implantable drug administration ports in the out-of-hospital setting. (C-1)

6–6.28 Describe the indications and contraindications for urinary catheter insertion in an out-of-hospital setting. (C-1)

6–6.29 Identify the proper anatomy for placement of urinary catheters in males or females. (C-2)

6–6.30 Identify failure of GI/GU devices found in the home care setting. (C-2)

6–6.31 Identify failure of ventilatory devices found in the home care setting. (C-2)

6–6.32 Identify failure of vascular access devices found in the home care setting. (C-2)

6–6.33 Identify failure of drains. (C-2)

6–6.34 Differentiate between home care and acute care as preferable situations for a given patient scenario. (C-3)

6–6.35 Discuss the relationship between local home care treatment protocols/SOPs and local EMS protocols/SOPs. (C-3)

6–6.36 Discuss differences in individuals' ability to accept and cope with their own impending death. (C-3)

6–6.37 Discuss the rights of the terminally ill. (C-1)

AFFECTIVE OBJECTIVES

At the completion of this unit, the paramedic student will be able to:

6–6.38 Value the role of the home-care professional and understand their role in patient care along the life-span continuum. (A-2)

6–6.39 Value the patient's desire to remain in the home setting. (A-2)

6–6.40 Value the patient's desire to accept or deny hospice care. (A-2)

6–6.41 Value the uses of long term venous access in the home health setting, including but not limited to: (A-2)
  a. Chemotherapy
  b. Home pain management
  c. Nutrition therapy
  d. Congestive heart therapy
  e. Antibiotic therapy

PSYCHOMOTOR OBJECTIVES

At the completion of this unit, the paramedic student will be able to:

6–6.42 Observe for an infected or otherwise complicated venous access point. (P-1)

6–6.43 Demonstrate proper tracheotomy care. (P-1)

6–6.44 Demonstrate the insertion of a new inner cannula and/or the use of an endotracheal tube to temporarily maintain an airway in a tracheostomy patient. (P-1)

6–6.45 Demonstrate proper technique for drawing blood from a central venous line. (P-1)

6–6.46 Demonstrate the method of accessing vascular access devices found in the home health care setting. (P-1)

UNIT TERMINAL OBJECTIVE

7–1 At the completion of this unit, the paramedic student will be able to integrate the principles of assessment based management to perform an appropriate assessment and implement the management plan for patients with common complaints.

COGNITIVE OBJECTIVES

At the completion of this unit, the paramedic student will be able to:

7–1.1 Explain how effective assessment is critical to clinical decision making. (C-1)

7–1.2 Explain how the paramedic's attitude affects assessment and decision making. (C-1)

7–1.3 Explain how uncooperative patients affect assessment and decision making. (C-1)

7–1.4 Explain strategies to prevent labeling and tunnel vision. (C-1)

7–1.5 Develop strategies to decrease environmental distractions. (C-1)

7–1.6 Describe how manpower considerations and staffing configurations affect assessment and decision making. (C-1)

7–1.7 Synthesize concepts of scene management and choreography to simulated emergency calls. (C-3)

7–1.8 Explain the roles of the team leader and the patient care person. (C-1)

7–1.9 List and explain the rationale for carrying out the essential patient care items. (C-3)

7–1.10 When given a simulated call, list the appropriate equipment to be taken to the patient. (C-2)

7–1.11 Explain the general approach to the emergency patient. (C-1)

7–1.12 Explain the general approach, patient assessment, differentials, and management priorities for patients with the following problems: (C-3)
  a. Chest pain
  b. Medical and traumatic cardiac arrest
  c. Acute abdominal pain
  d. GI bleed
  e. Altered mental status
  f. Dyspnea
  g. Syncope
  h. Seizures
  i. Environmental or thermal problem
  j. Hazardous material or toxic exposure
  k. Trauma or multi-trauma patients
  l. Allergic reactions
  m. Behavioral problems
  n. Obstetric or gynecological problems
  o. Pediatric patients

7–1.13 Describe how to effectively communicate patient information face to face, over the telephone, by radio, and in writing. (C-1)

AFFECTIVE OBJECTIVES

At the completion of this unit, the paramedic student will be able to:

7–1.14 Appreciate the use of scenarios to develop high level clinical decision-making skills. (A-2)

7–1.15 Defend the importance of considering differentials in patient care. (A-3)

7–1.16 Advocate and practice the process of complete patient assessment on all patients. (A-3)

7–1.17 Value the importance of presenting the patient accurately and clearly. (A-2)

PSYCHOMOTOR OBJECTIVES

At the completion of this unit, the paramedic student will be able to:

7–1.18 While serving as team leader, choreograph the EMS response team, perform a patient assessment, provide local/regionally appropriate treatment, and present cases verbally and in writing, given a moulaged and programed simulated patient. (P-3)

7–1.19 While serving as team leader, assess a programmed patient or mannequin, consider differentials, make decisions relative to interventions and transportation, provide the interventions, patient packaging and transportation, work as a team, and practice various roles for the following common emergencies: (P-3)
  a. Chest pain
  b. Cardiac arrest
    1. Traumatic arrest
    2. Medical arrest
  c. Acute abdominal pain
  d. GI bleed
  e. Altered mental status
  f. Dyspnea
  g. Syncope
  h. Seizure
  i. Thermal/environmental problem
  j. Hazardous materials/toxicology
  k. Trauma
    1. Isolated extremity fracture (tibia/ fibula or radius/ ulna)
    2. Femur fracture
    3. Shoulder dislocation
    4. Clavicular fracture or A-C separation
    5. Minor wound (no sutures required, sutures required, high risk wounds, with tendon and/or nerve injury)
    6. Spine injury (no neurologic deficit, with neurologic deficit)
    7. Multiple trauma–blunt
    8. Penetrating trauma
    9. Impaled object
    10. Elderly fall
    11. Athletic injury
    12. Head injury (concussion, subdural/ epidural)
  l. Allergic reactions/bites/envenomation
    1. Local allergic reaction
    2. Systemic allergic reaction
    3. Envenomation
  m. Behavioral
    1. Mood disorders
    2. Schizophrenic and delusional disorders
    3. Suicidal
  n. Obstetrics/gynecology
    1. Vaginal bleeding
    2. Childbirth (normal and abnormal)
  o. Pediatric
    1. Respiratory distress
    2. Fever
    3. Seizures

UNIT TERMINAL OBJECTIVE

8–2   At the completion of this unit, the paramedic student will be able to integrate the principles of general incident management and multiple casualty incident (MCI) management techniques in order to function effectively at major incidents.

COGNITIVE OBJECTIVES

At the completion of this unit, the paramedic student will be able to:

8–2.1   Explain the need for the incident management system (IMS)/incident command system (ICS) in managing emergency medical services incidents. (C-1)

8–2.2   Define the term multiple casualty incident (MCI). (C-1)

8–2.3   Define the term disaster management. (C-1)

8–2.4   Describe essential elements of scene size-up when arriving at a potential MCI. (C-1)

8–2.5   Describe the role of the paramedics and EMS systems in planning for MCIs and disasters. (C-1)

8–2.6   Define the following types of incidents and how they affect medical management: (C-1)
   a. Open or uncontained incident
   b. Closed or contained incident

8–2.7   Describe the functional components of the incident management system in terms of the following: (C-1)
   a. Command
   b. Finance
   c. Logistics
   d. Operations
   e. Planning

8–2.8   Differentiate between singular and unified command and when each is most applicable. (C-3)

8–2.9   Describe the role of command. (C-1)

8–2.10   Describe the need for transfer of command and procedures for transferring it. (C-1)

8–2.11   Differentiate between command procedures used at small, medium and large scale medical incidents. (C-1)

8–2.12   Explain the local/regional threshold for establishing command and implementation of the incident management system including threshold MCI declaration. (C-1)

8–2.13   List and describe the functions of the following groups and leaders in ICS as it pertains to EMS incidents: (C-1)
   a. Safety
   b. Logistics
   c. Rehabilitation (rehab)
   d. Staging
   e. Treatment
   f. Triage
   g. Transportation
   h. Extrication/rescue
   i. Disposition of deceased (morgue)
   j. Communications

8–2.14   Describe the methods and rationale for identifying specific functions and leaders for these functions in ICS. (C-1)

8–2.15   Describe the role of both command posts and emergency operations centers in MCI and disaster management. (C-1)

8–2.16   Describe the role of the physician at multiple casualty incidents. (C-1)

8–2.17   Define triage and describe the principles of triage. (C-1)

8–2.18   Describe the START (simple triage and rapid treatment) method of initial triage. (C-1)

8–2.19   Given a list of 20 patients with various multiple injuries, determine the appropriate triage priority with 90% accuracy. (C-3)

8–2.20   Given color coded tags and numerical priorities, assign the following terms to each: (C-1)
   a. Immediate
   b. Delayed
   c. Hold
   d. Deceased

8–2.21   Define primary and secondary triage. (C-1)

8–2.22   Describe when primary and secondary triage techniques should be implemented. (C-1)

8–2.23   Describe the need for and techniques used in tracking patients during multiple casualty incidents. (C-1)

8–2.24   Describe techniques used to allocate patients to hospitals and track them. (C-1)

8–2.25   Describe modifications of telecommunications procedures during multiple casualty incidents. (C-1)

8–2.26   List and describe the essential equipment to provide logistical support to MCI operations to include: (C-1)
   a. Airway, respiratory, and hemorrhage control
   b. Burn management
   c. Patient packaging/immobilization

8–2.27   List the physical and psychological signs of critical incident stress. (C-1)

8–2.28   Describe the role of critical incident stress management sessions in MCIs. (C-1)

8–2.29   Describe the role of the following exercises in preparation for MCIs: (C-1)
   a. Tabletop exercises
   b. Small and large MCI drills

AFFECTIVE OBJECTIVES

At the completion of this unit, the paramedic student will be able to:

8–2.30   Understand the rationale for initiating incident command even at a small MCI event. (A-1)

8–2.31   Explain the rationale for having efficient and effective communications as part of an incident command/management system. (A-1)

8–2.32   Explain why common problems of an MCI can have an adverse effect on an entire incident. (A-1)

8–2.33   Explain the organizational benefits for having standard operating procedures (SOPs) for using the incident management system or incident command system. (A-1)

PSYCHOMOTOR OBJECTIVES

At the completion of this unit, the paramedic student will be able to:

8–2.34   Demonstrate the use of local/regional triage tagging system used for primary and secondary triage. (P-1)

8–2.35   Given a simulated tabletop multiple casualty incident, with 5–10 patients: (P-1)
   a. Establish unified or singular command

b. Conduct a scene assessment

c. Determine scene objectives

d. Formulate an incident plan

e. Request appropriate resources

f. Determine need for ICS expansion and groups

g. Coordinate communications and group leaders

h. Coordinate outside agencies

8–2.36 Demonstrate effective initial scene assessment and update (progress) reports. (P-1)

8–2.37 Given a classroom simulation of an MCI with 5–10 patients, fulfill the role of triage group leader. (P-3)

8–2.38 Given a classroom simulation of an MCI with 5–10 patients, fulfill the role of treatment group leader. (P-3)

8–2.39 Given a classroom simulation of an MCI with 5–10 patients, fulfill the role of transportation group leader. (P-3)

UNIT TERMINAL OBJECTIVE

8–3 At the completion of this unit, the paramedic student will be able to integrate the principles of rescue awareness and operations to safely rescue a patient from water, hazardous atmospheres, trenches, highways, and hazardous terrain.

COGNITIVE OBJECTIVES

At the completion of this unit, the paramedic student will be able to:

8–3.1 Define the term rescue. (C-1)

8–3.2 Explain the medical and mechanical aspects of rescue situations. (C-1)

8–3.3 Explain the role of the paramedic in delivering care at the site of the injury, continuing through the rescue process and to definitive care. (C-1)

8–3.4 Describe the phases of a rescue operation. (C-1)

8–3.5 List and describe the types of personal protective equipment needed to safely operate in the rescue environment to include: (C-1)

a. Head protection

b. Eye protection

c. Hand protection

d. Personal flotation devices

e. Thermal protection/layering systems

f. High visibility clothing

g. Specialized footwear

8–3.6 Explain the differences in risk between moving water and flat water rescue. (C-1)

8–3.7 Explain the effects of immersion hypothermia on the ability to survive sudden immersion and self rescue. (C-1)

8–3.8 Explain the phenomenon of the cold protective response in cold water drowning situations. (C-1)

8–3.9 Identify the risks associated with low head dams and the rescue complexities they pose. (C-1)

8–3.10 Given a picture of moving water, identify and explain the following features and hazards associated with: (C-2)

a. Hydraulics

b. Strainers

c. Dams/hydroelectric sites

8–3.11 Explain why water entry or go techniques are methods of last resort. (C-1)

8–3.12 Explain the rescue techniques associated with reach-throw-row-go. (C-1)

8–3.13 Given a list of rescue scenarios, identify the victim survivability profile and which are rescue versus body recovery situations. (C-1)

8–3.14 Explain the self rescue position if unexpectedly immersed in moving water. (C-1)

8–3.15 Given a series of pictures identify which would be considered "confined spaces" and potentially oxygen deficient. (C-3)

8–3.16 Identify the hazards associated with confined spaces and risks posed to potential rescuers to include: (C-1)

a. Oxygen deficiency

b. Chemical/toxic exposure/explosion

c. Engulfment

d. Machinery entrapment

e. Electricity

8–3.17 Identify components necessary to ensure site safety prior to confined space rescue attempts. (C-1)

8–3.18 Identify the poisonous gases commonly found in confined spaces to include: (C-1)

a. Hydrogen sulfide (H_2S)

b. Carbon dioxide (CO_2)

c. Carbon monoxide (CO)

d. Low/high oxygen concentrations (FiO_2)

e. Methane (CH_4)

f. Ammonia (NH_3)

g. Nitrogen dioxide (NO_2)

8–3.19 Explain the hazard of cave-in during trench rescue operations. (C-1)

8–3.20 Describe the effects of traffic flow on the highway rescue incident including limited access superhighway and regular access highways. (C-1)

8–3.21 List and describe the following techniques to reduce scene risk at highway incidents: (C-1)

a. Apparatus placement

b. Headlights and emergency vehicle lighting

c. Cones, flares

d. Reflective and high visibility clothing

8–3.22 List and describe the hazards associated with the following auto/truck components: (C-1)

a. Energy absorbing bumpers

b. Air bag/supplemental restraint systems

c. Catalytic converters and conventional fuel systems

d. Stored energy

e. Alternate fuel systems

8–3.23 Given a diagram of a passenger auto, identify the following structures: (C-1)

a. A, B, C, D posts

b. Fire wall

c. Unibody versus frame designs

8–3.24 Describe methods for emergency stabilization using rope, cribbing, jacks, spare tire, and come-a-longs for vehicles found on their: (C-1)

a. Wheels

b. Side

c. Roof

d. Inclines

8–3.25 Describe the electrical hazards commonly found at highway incidents (above and below ground). (C-1)

8–3.26 Explain the difference between tempered and safety glass, and identify its locations on a vehicle and how to break it safely. (C-3)

8–3.27 Explain typical door anatomy and methods to access through stuck doors. (C-1)

8–3.28 Explain SRS or "air bag" systems and methods to neutralize them. (C-1)

8–3.29 Define the following terms: (C-1)
a. Low angle
b. High angle
c. Belay
d. Rappel
e. Scrambling
f. Hasty rope slide

8–3.30 Describe the procedure for stokes litter packaging for low angle evacuations. (C-1)

8–3.31 Explain the procedures for low angle litter evacuation to include: (C-1)
a. Anchoring
b. Litter/rope attachment
c. Lowering and raising procedures

8–3.32 Explain techniques to be used in non-technical litter carries over rough terrain. (C-1)

8–3.33 Explain nontechnical high angle rescue procedures using aerial apparatus. (C-1)

8–3.34 Develop specific skill in emergency stabilization of vehicles and access procedures and an awareness of specific extrication strategies. (C-1)

8–3.35 Explain assessment procedures and modifications necessary when caring for entrapped patients. (C-1)

8–3.36 List the equipment necessary for an "off road" medical pack. (C-1)

8–3.37 Explain specific methods of improvisation for assessment, spinal immobilization, and extremity splinting. (C-1)

8–3.38 Explain the indications, contraindications, and methods of pain control for entrapped patients. (C-1)

8–3.39 Explain the need for and techniques of thermal control for entrapped patients. (C-1)

8–3.40 Explain the pathophysiology of "crush trauma" syndrome. (C-1)

8–3.41 Develop an understanding of the medical issues involved in providing care for a patient in a rescue environment. (C-1)

8–3.42 Develop proficiency in patient packaging and evacuation techniques that pertain to hazardous or rescue environments. (C-1)

8–3.43 Explain the different types of "stokes" or basket stretchers and the advantages and disadvantages associated with each. (C-1)

AFFECTIVE OBJECTIVES

None identified for this unit.

PSYCHOMOTOR OBJECTIVES

At the completion of this lesson, the paramedic student should be able to:

8–3.44 Using cribbing, ropes, lifting devices, spare tires, chains, and hand winches, demonstrate the following stabilization procedures: (P-1)
a. Stabilization on all four wheels
b. Stabilization on its side

c. Stabilization on its roof
d. Stabilization on an incline/embankment

8–3.45 Using basic hand tools demonstrate the following: (P-1)
a. Access through a stuck door
b. Access through safety and tempered glass
c. Access through the trunk
d. Access through the floor
e. Roof removal
f. Dash displacement/roll-up
g. Steering wheel/column displacement
h. Access through the roof

8–3.46 Demonstrate methods of "stokes" packaging for patients being: (P-1)
a. Vertically lifted (high angle)
b. Horizontally lifted (low angle)
c. Carried over rough terrain

8–3.47 Demonstrate methods of packaging for patients being vertically lifted without stokes litter stretcher packaging. (P-1)

8–3.48 Demonstrate the following litter carrying techniques: (P-1)
a. Stretcher lift straps
b. "Leap frogging"
c. Passing litters over and around obstructions

8–3.49 Demonstrate litter securing techniques for patients being evacuated by aerial apparatus. (P-1)

8–3.50 Demonstrate in-water spinal immobilization techniques. (P-1)

8–3.51 Demonstrate donning and properly adjusting a PFD. (P-1)

8–3.52 Demonstrate use of a throw bag. (P-1)

UNIT TERMINAL OBJECTIVE

8–4 At the completion of this unit, the paramedic student will be able to evaluate hazardous materials emergencies, call for appropriate resources, and work in the cold zone.

COGNITIVE OBJECTIVES

At the completion of this unit, the paramedic student will be able to:

8–4.1 Explain the role of the paramedic/EMS responder in terms of the following: (C-1)
a. Incident size-up
b. Assessment of toxicologic risk
c. Appropriate decontamination methods
d. Treatment of semi-decontaminated patients
e. Transportation of semi-decontaminated patients

8–4.2 Size-up a hazardous materials (haz-mat) incident and determine the following: (C-1)
a. Potential hazards to the rescuers, public, and environment
b. Potential risk of primary contamination to patients
c. Potential risk of secondary contamination to rescuers

8–4.3 Identify resources for substance identification, decontamination, and treatment information including the following: (C-1)
a. Poison control center
b. Medical control
c. Material safety data sheets (MSDS)
d. Reference textbooks
e. Computer databases (CAMEO)

    f. CHEMTREC
    g. Technical specialists
    h. Agency for toxic substances and disease registry

8–4.4 Explain the following terms/concepts: (C-1)
    a. Primary contamination risk
    b. Secondary contamination risk

8–4.5 List and describe the following routes of exposure: (C-1)
    a. Topical
    b. Respiratory
    c. Gastrointestinal
    d. Parenteral

8–4.6 Explain the following toxicologic principles: (C-1)
    a. Acute and delayed toxicity
    b. Route of exposure
    c. Local versus systemic effects
    d. Dose response
    e. Synergistic effects

8–4.7 Explain how the substance and route of contamination alter triage and decontamination methods. (C-1)

8–4.8 Explain the limitations of field decontamination procedures. (C-1)

8–4.9 Explain the use and limitations of personal protective equipment (PPE) in hazardous material situations. (C-1)

8–4.10 List and explain the common signs, symptoms, and treatment for the following substances: (C-1)
    a. Corrosives (acids/alkalis)
    b. Pulmonary irritants (ammonia/chlorine)
    c. Pesticides (carbamates/organophosphates)
    d. Chemical asphyxiants (cyanide/carbon monoxide)
    e. Hydrocarbon solvents (xylene, methylene chloride)

8–4.11 Explain the potential risk associated with invasive procedures performed on contaminated patients. (C-1)

8–4.12 Given a contaminated patient determine the level of decontamination necessary and: (C-1)
    a. Level of rescuer PPE
    b. Decontamination methods
    c. Treatment
    d. Transportation and patient isolation techniques

8–4.13 Identify local facilities and resources capable of treating patients exposed to hazardous materials. (C-1)

8–4.14 Determine the hazards present to the patient and paramedic given an incident involving hazardous materials. (C-2)

8–4.15 Define the following and explain their importance to the risk assessment process: (C-1)
    a. Boiling point
    b. Flammable/explosive limits
    c. Flash point
    d. Ignition temperature
    e. Specific gravity
    f. Vapor density
    g. Vapor pressure
    h. Water solubility
    i. Alpha radiation
    j. Beta radiation
    k. Gamma radiation

8–4.16 Define the toxicologic terms and their use in the risk assessment process: (C-1)
    a. Threshold limit value (TLV)
    b. Lethal concentration and doses (LD)

    c. Parts per million/billion (ppm/ppb)
    d. Immediately dangerous to life and health (IDLH)
    e. Permissible exposure limit (PEL)
    f. Short-term exposure limit (TLV–STEL)
    g. Ceiling level (TLV–C)

8–4.17 Given a specific hazardous material be able to do the following: (C-1)
    a. Research the appropriate information about its physical and chemical characteristics and hazards
    b. Suggest the appropriate medical response
    c. Determine risk of secondary contamination

8–4.18 Determine the factors which determine where and when to treat a patient to include: (C-1)
    a. Substance toxicity
    b. Patient condition
    c. Availability of decontamination

8–4.19 Determine the appropriate level of PPE to include: (C-1)
    a. Types, application, use, and limitations
    b. Use of chemical compatibility chart

8–4.20 Explain decontamination procedures when functioning in the following modes: (C-1)
    a. Critical patient rapid two step decontamination process
    b. Non-critical patient eight step decontamination process

8–4.21 Explain specific decontamination procedures. (C-1)

8–4.22 Explain the four most common decontamination solutions used to include: (C-1)
    a. Water
    b. Water and tincture of green soap
    c. Isopropyl alcohol
    d. Vegetable oil

8–4.23 Identify the areas of the body difficult to decontaminate to include: (C-1)
    a. Scalp/hair
    b. Ears/ear canals/nostrils
    c. Axilla
    d. Fingernails
    e. Navel
    f. Groin/buttocks/genitalia
    g. Behind knees
    h. Between toes, toe nails

8–4.24 Explain the medical monitoring procedures of hazardous material team members to be used both pre and post entry, to include: (C-1)
    a. Vital signs
    b. Body weight
    c. General health
    d. Neurologic status
    e. ECG

8–4.25 Explain the factors which influence the heat stress of hazardous material team personnel to include: (C-1)
    a. Hydration
    b. Physical fitness
    c. Ambient temperature
    d. Activity
    e. Level of PPE
    f. Duration of activity

8–4.26 Explain the documentation necessary for Haz-Mat medical monitoring and rehabilitation operations: (C-1)

a. The substance
b. The toxicity and danger of secondary contamination
c. Appropriate PPE and suit breakthrough time
d. Appropriate level of decontamination
e. Appropriate antidote and medical treatment
f. Transportation method

8–4.27 Given a simulated hazardous substance, use reference material to determine the appropriate actions. (C-3)

8–4.28 Integrate the principles and practices of hazardous materials response in an effective manner to prevent and limit contamination, morbidity, and mortality.

AFFECTIVE OBJECTIVES

None identified for this unit.

PSYCHOMOTOR OBJECTIVES

At the completion of this unit, the paramedic student will be able to:

8–4.29 Demonstrate the donning and doffing of appropriate PPE. (P-1)

8–4.30 Set up and demonstrate an emergency two step decontamination process. (P-1)

8–4.31 Set up and demonstrate an eight step decontamination process. (P-1)

UNIT TERMINAL OBJECTIVE

8–5 At the completion of this unit, the paramedic student will have an awareness of the human hazard of crime and violence and the safe operation at crime scenes and other emergencies.

COGNITIVE OBJECTIVES

At the completion of this unit, the paramedic student will be able to:

8–5.1 Explain how EMS providers are often mistaken for the police. (C-1)

8–5.2 Explain specific techniques for risk reduction when approaching the following types of routine EMS scenes: (C-1)
a. Highway encounters
b. Violent street incidents
c. Residences and "dark houses"

8–5.3 Describe warning signs of potentially violent situations. (C-1)

8–5.4 Explain emergency evasive techniques for potentially violent situations, including: (C-1)
a. Threats of physical violence
b. Firearms encounters
c. Edged weapon encounters

8–5.5 Explain EMS considerations for the following types of violent or potentially violent situations: (C-1)
a. Gangs and gang violence
b. Hostage/sniper situations
c. Clandestine drug labs
d. Domestic violence
e. Emotionally disturbed people
f. Hostage/sniper situations

8–5.6 Explain the following techniques: (C-1)
a. Field "contact and cover" procedures during assessment and care
b. Evasive tactics
c. Concealment techniques

8–5.7 Describe police evidence considerations and techniques to assist in evidence preservation. (C-1)

AFFECTIVE OBJECTIVES

None identified for this unit.

PSYCHOMOTOR OBJECTIVES

At the completion of this unit, the paramedic student will be able to:

8–5.8 Demonstrate the following techniques: (P-1)
a. Field "contact and cover" procedures during assessment and care
b. Evasive tactics
c. Concealment techniques

Index